Diagnostic Imaging: Radiology

Diagnostic Imaging: Radiology

Editor: Coby Hawkins

AMERICAN
MEDICAL PUBLISHERS
www.americanmedicalpublishers.com

AMERICAN
MEDICAL PUBLISHERS
www.americanmedicalpublishers.com

Cataloging-in-Publication Data

Diagnostic imaging : radiology / edited by Coby Hawkins.
p. cm.
Includes bibliographical references and index.
ISBN 979-8-88740-060-0
1. Medical radiology. 2. Diagnosis, Radioscopic. 3. Diagnostic imaging.
4. Radiotherapy. I. Hawkins, Coby.
R895 .D53 2023
616.075 7--dc23

American Medical Publishers,
41 Flatbush Avenue,
1st Floor, New York,
NY 11217, USA

ISBN 979-8-88740-060-0 (Hardback)

Contents

Preface

Every book is a source of knowledge and this one is no exception. The idea that led to the conceptualization of this book was the fact that the world is advancing rapidly; which makes it crucial to document the progress in every field. I am aware that a lot of data is already available, yet, there is a lot more to learn. Hence, I accepted the responsibility of editing this book and contributing my knowledge to the community.

Radiology is a medical discipline that uses imaging technology for diagnosing and treating diseases. It can be broadly divided into two categories, namely, diagnostic radiology and interventional radiology. Diagnostic radiology is used to view the structures or parts within the body. There are several types of imaging techniques including computed tomography (CT), fluoroscopy, magnetic resonance imaging (MRI), mammography, ultrasound, etc. Interventional radiology is a type of radiology that utilizes imaging techniques to help guide medical procedures. It uses minimally invasive procedures for treating different medical conditions. Angiography or angioplasty and stent placement, embolization to control bleeding, cancer treatments including tumor embolization using chemoembolization or Y-90 radioembolization, vertebroplasty, and kyphoplasty are a few important interventional radiology procedures. This book provides comprehensive insights into the field of radiology. A number of latest researches have been included to keep the readers up-to-date with the global concepts in this area of diagnostic imaging. This book will serve as an invaluable source for students and radiologists.

While editing this book, I had multiple visions for it. Then I finally narrowed down to make every chapter a sole standing text explaining a particular topic, so that they can be used independently. However, the umbrella subject sinews them into a common theme. This makes the book a unique platform of knowledge.

I would like to give the major credit of this book to the experts from every corner of the world, who took the time to share their expertise with us. Also, I owe the completion of this book to the never-ending support of my family, who supported me throughout the project.

Editor

1

The Agreement Rate between Radiographic Interpretation and Histopathologic Diagnosis of Jaw Lesions

Soulafa Almazrooa, Nada O. Binmadi, Hanadi M. Khalifa, Fatima M. Jadu, Ahmed M. Jan, and Dalia E. Meisha

Faculty of Dentistry, King Abdulaziz University, Jeddah, Saudi Arabia

Correspondence should be addressed to Fatima M. Jadu; fjadu@kau.edu.sa

Academic Editor: Paul Sijens

Background. To determine the agreement rate between histopathologic diagnosis and radiographic interpretation of jaw lesions. *Methods.* Cases with jaw pathologies that have diagnostically adequate histopathologic samples and radiographic examinations were reviewed retrospectively. Two board-certified oral and maxillofacial pathologists (OMFP) independently determined the histopathologic diagnosis, while two board-certified oral and maxillofacial radiologists (OMFR) determined the radiographic interpretations independently. Then the histopathologic diagnosis and the radiographic interpretation were compared for agreement. *Results.* A total of 104 cases (53% females) were included with a mean age of 31 years. The agreement rate between histopathologic diagnosis and radiographic interpretation was 49%. OMFP required OMFR consultations to reach a diagnosis in 16% of cases. The most commonly encountered lesions were by far odontogenic cysts of inflammatory origin and the agreement for this disease category was 49.1%. However, agreement rates were highest for the disease category of tumors (62.5%). *Conclusion.* The agreement rate between OMFP and OMFR was higher for tumors than cysts. Agreement rates between OMFP and OMFR improved with efficient consultation between the two disciplines.

1. Introduction

The oral and maxillofacial area is a complex region with many tissues and structures and is thus the site of much diverse pathology. Some of these pathologies affect the soft tissues, while others affect the osseous tissues and others affect both tissues. The clinical and radiographic findings play a significant role in diagnosis but histopathology is usually the major determinant of the diagnosis.

Biopsy is the gold standard for the diagnosis of many jaw pathologies [1]. The diagnosis assigned by a pathologist at the end of a biopsy report is often the basis on which many crucial decisions are based in regard to patient management and prognosis. Yet, the accuracy of a pathologists' ability to reach the correct diagnoses is an inadequately studied area. In the literature, the highest misdiagnosis rate was related to non-odontogenic tumors of the oral cavity, accounting for approximately 11.5%, followed by malignant tumors, accounting for approximately 9% [2].

The overall concordance between clinical findings and histopathologic diagnosis ranges between 50 and 99% [2–4]. However, there is no data on the concordance between radiographic interpretation and histopathologic diagnosis of jaw lesions. Therefore, in the current study, we investigated the agreement rate between radiographic interpretation and histopathologic diagnosis of jaw lesions.

2. Materials and Methods

In this retrospective review, the records of all patients referred to a university-based oral and maxillofacial pathology service over a three-year period were reviewed. Inclusion criteria included the availability of diagnostically adequate histopathologic samples and diagnostically adequate imaging with reports of jaw lesions based on the 2017 World Health Organization (WHO) classification of odontogenic and maxillofacial lesions [5]. This descriptive study took place

TABLE 1: Descriptive statistics for the cases included in the study (N=104).

Study Variable	*Descriptive Statistics* *Mean* ± *SD (range)*
Age (years)	30.7± 16.2 (4-76)
	% *(N)*
Gender (female)	53.8% (56)
Location (mandible)	53.8% (56)
Disease category:	
(i) Odontogenic cysts of inflammatory origin	52.9% (55)
(ii) Odontogenic developmental cysts and non-odontogenic cysts	28.8% (30)
(iii) Tumors (benign and malignant)	15.4% (16)
(iv) Fibro-osseous lesions	2.9% (3)
Advanced imaging	18.3% (19)

SD: standard deviation; advanced imaging: any three-dimensional imaging such as computed tomography, cone beam computed tomography, or magnetic resonance imaging.

at the Faculty of Dentistry of King Abdulaziz University, Jeddah, Saudi Arabia. Data collection commenced after ethical approval from the research ethics board (Number 009-15) was obtained. The guidelines of the Helsinki Declaration were followed diligently. Each patient was assigned a unique number that linked the clinical, radiographic, and histopathologic information. However, this information was available only to the principal investigator so that no connection can be made to the patient.

Two board-certified oral and maxillofacial pathologists (OMFP) reviewed the histopathology samples and their diagnosis was based on the 2017 World Health Organization (WHO) classification of odontogenic and maxillofacial bone lesions [5]. Two board-certified oral radiologists (OMFR) reviewed and interpreted the radiographic images. Brief clinical information was available to both disciplines as age, gender, location, and pertinent medical history, if any. The histopathology requisition form did not consistently include reference to the availability of imaging for each case.

All available images were reviewed including periapical and bitewing radiographs, panoramic radiographs, cone beam computed tomography (CT), multidetector CT, and magnetic resonance imaging (MRI) examinations. Disagreements among the disciplines were resolved by consensus.

Cases were allocated into disease categories consistent with the 2017 World Health Organization (WHO) classification of odontogenic and maxillofacial lesions [5]. Then, the histopathologic diagnosis was compared to the radiographic interpretation and each case was given one of three codes based on the agreement between the two disciplines: (0) no agreement, (1) agreement, and (2) if communication was needed between the two disciplines to reach a diagnosis. Statistics were done using the Statistical Package for Social Sciences (SPSS 22, Windows, SPSS Inc., Chicago, USA). Percent agreement was calculated.

3. Results

The initial sample included 311 cases. Of these, only 128 cases (41%) had a diagnostically adequate histopathologic sample. Furthermore, eighty-one percent of cases of the 128 cases had diagnostically adequate images. One hundred and four cases were included in this study.

Table 1 exhibits the descriptive statistics for the cases included in the study sample. The mean age was 31 years with a wide range of age from 4 years to 76 years. There was almost equal representation in terms of gender and location of the pathology (maxilla versus mandible). In terms of the disease categories, the most prevalent category was odontogenic cysts of inflammatory origin (55%), while fibroosseous lesions (FOL) were the least prevalent (2.9%). Only 18% of cases had some form of advanced imaging defined as any three-dimensional imaging such as computed tomography, cone beam computed tomography, or magnetic resonance imaging.

In sixteen percent of cases, OMFP required OMFR consultation to reach a diagnosis. Agreement between OMFP and OMFR was demonstrated in almost half of the cases (49%), whereas no agreement was reached in 35% of cases (Figure 1).

The need for communication between OMFP and OMFR varied according to the disease category. Communication was not needed for 93.8% of cases under the tumors category and 89.1% of cases under the odontogenic cysts of inflammatory origin category (Figure 2). The odds of needing communication between OMFP and OMFR were about 2.5 times higher for odontogenic cysts of developmental origin and non-odontogenic cysts compared to odontogenic cysts of inflammatory origin but did not reach statistical significance (odds ratio (OR): 2.5, 95% CI of OR: 0.7-8.2). While the odds of needing communication were half for tumor cases compared to cases with odontogenic cysts of inflammatory origin (OR: 0.5, 95% CI of OR: 0.06- 4.9). The need of communication between OMFP and OMFR was three times more with cases having advanced imaging compared to cases with conventional imaging only (OR: 3.2, 95% CI of OR: 1-10.4).

The percent agreement between OMFP and OMFR in this sample varied according to the disease category and was highest for the tumors category (62.5%). This was followed

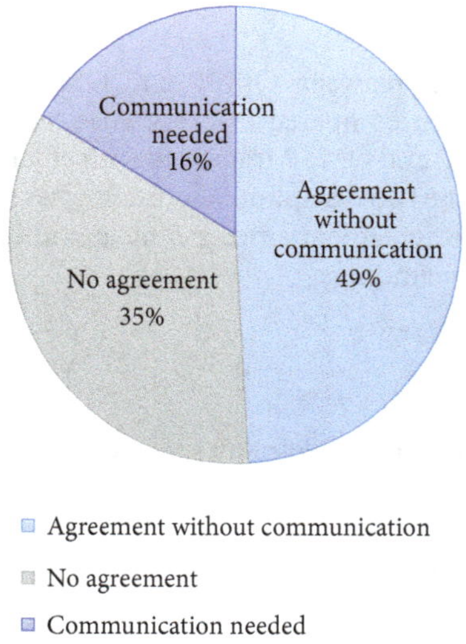

FIGURE 1: Agreement and need of communication to reach a diagnosis between oral and maxillofacial pathologist (OMFP) and oral and maxillofacial radiologist (OMFR).

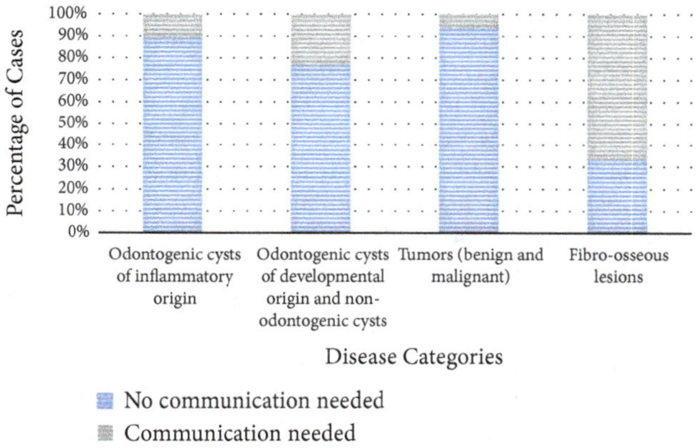

FIGURE 2: Comparison of percentage of cases that did and did not require communication between oral and maxillofacial pathologist (OMFP) and oral and maxillofacial radiologist (OMFR) in relation to disease categories.

by odontogenic cysts of inflammatory origin (49.1%) and odontogenic cysts of developmental origin as well as non-odontogenic cysts (46.7%). For the FOLs disease category, there was no agreement at all between OMFR and OMFR. These results are demonstrated in Figure 3. The odds of agreement between OMFP and OMFR were about twice times higher for tumors compared to odontogenic cysts of inflammatory origin but did not reach statistical significance (OR= 1.7, 95% CI of OR: 0.6- 5.4). While the odds of agreement were almost comparable for cysts of developmental origin compared to odontogenic cysts of inflammatory origin cases (OR= 0.9, 95% CI of OR: 0.4-2.2).

4. Discussion

Reaching an accurate diagnosis is a fundamental step in the process of patient management and treatment planning. The process of reaching a correct diagnosis is not an easy one

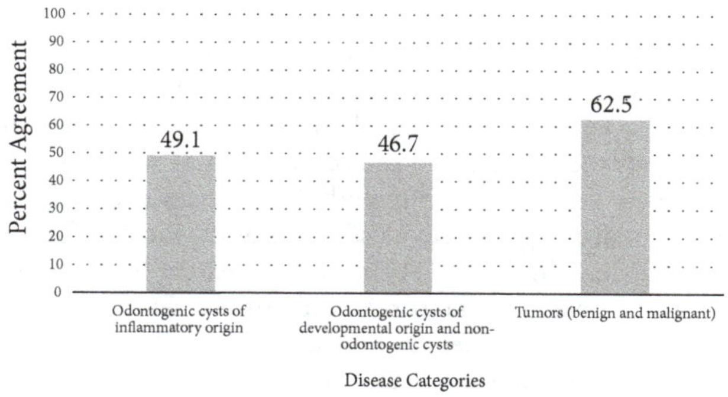

FIGURE 3: Percent agreement between histopathologic diagnosis and radiographic interpretation based on disease categories.

and proceeds through several stages that requires input from numerous outlets including clinical findings, imaging findings, and histopathology findings. Therefore, it is essential that these data be collected in a thorough manner to ensure completeness. It is also crucial that these data be correlated to ensure comprehensiveness.

Cohen's kappa is the most commonly used measure to assess inter-rater reliability [6]; however Kappa was incalculable in this study because the histopathologic diagnosis is the gold standard and therefore was constant. This is a recognized limitation of Kappa [7]. Percent agreement was calculated instead and was found to be 49% between radiographic interpretation and histopathologic diagnosis, which is lower than other published studies. A study by Sarabadani et al. in 2013 found the concordance between radiology and histopathology for central jaw lesions to be 71.4% [8], whereas the concordance between clinical impression and histopathology diagnosis was 80.4% [8]. Several studies have investigated the concordance between clinical and histopathology without any regard for imaging data. This may be due to the few number of cases with available imaging.

The most commonly encountered disease category was odontogenic cysts of inflammatory origin. This disease category accounted for 53% of cases included in this review; however, the agreement rate for this entity was only 49%. This is due to the fact that differentiating periapical granulomas from cysts is challenging from an imaging perspective. From a practical perspective, this differentiation may not be necessary since both conditions are usually treated similarly. Agreement rates were highest for tumors perhaps because the features of these lesions are undebatable or perhaps because the reviewers were not required to assign a specific disease label. This measure was taken because from an imaging perspective it is usually easy to recognize malignant features but it is difficult to pinpoint the exact type of malignancy.

The radiographic images that were examined in the current study were not limited to a specific type or number and included any images that were available for each case. These included conventional images as well as advanced imaging, such as cone beam computed tomography (CBCT), conventional computed tomography (CT), and magnetic resonance imaging (MRI). The accuracy of each type of imaging varies, which ultimately influences the accuracy of the interpretation. We predict that the agreement between radiographic interpretation and histopathology diagnosis may have been higher, had all the available images been of the advanced type. Advanced imaging is the standard of care in most cases with pathology because the three-dimensional imaging provides significantly more information regarding the features, behavior, and extent of the lesion, which improves the interpretation process. Future studies should examine the effect of imaging type on the agreement rate with histopathologic diagnosis.

Approximately 16% of the osseous lesions reviewed in this study required communication between OMFP and OMFR before a final histopathologic diagnosis was assigned. This was especially true for FOL as 67% required communication with the radiologist. FOL lesions such as fibrous dysplasia for example are known to be challenging in terms of histopathologic diagnosis, their features can be confused with those of other forms of fibro-osseous lesions and with osteomyelitis and even well differentiated osteogenic sarcoma [9–11]. Three vastly different conditions with extremely different management approaches. For these cases, imaging plays a significant role and communication between the OMFP and OMFR becomes of paramount importance.

Gephardt at al. reported that missing information such as the anatomic location of the lesion can result in revision or even changing of a histopathologic diagnostic decision [12]. Furthermore, other studies have demonstrated that amended histopathology reports after consultation with the clinician or radiologist lead to major changes in management in 3.8% of cases and minor changes in 2.9% of cases [13]. Therefore, it is essential for OMFP to communicate efficiently with all specialists involved in the patients' care, including clinicians, surgeons, and radiologists, to obtain all necessary information for an accurate diagnosis, especially if the necessary information is missing from the requisition form [12, 14, 15]. The simple act of communication has the potential to significantly reduce the chances of misdiagnosis and to ultimately improve patient outcome. Therefore, we strongly advocate all methods of communication, whether verbal or non-verbal, electronic or otherwise as long as they are eventually documented. In addition, we strongly advocate that each healthcare institution has specific policies on communication between specialists.

Limitations of this study include that the clinical differential diagnosis details included in the pathology requisition form were brief and inconsistent. This prevented the possibility of investigating the concordance between the clinical diagnosis and the radiographic impression with histopathology diagnosis. Although the role of clinical findings was not examined in this study, it should not be undermined or overlooked. Another limitation is having a relatively small proportion of cases identified as tumors (15.4%). This limited the possibility of assessing the differences in agreement between benign and malignant tumors, if any. In addition, the generalizability of the agreement rate for the FOL disease category was limited because only 3% of cases were diagnosed as FOL.

5. Conclusion

Agreement rates between OMFP and OMFR were higher for tumors when compared to cysts. Also, agreement rates between OMFP and OMFR improved with efficient consultation between the two disciplines. Future studies should aim to investigate the agreement among clinical, radiographic, and histopathologic findings.

Disclosure

The research did not receive any specific grant from funding agencies in the public, commercial, or not-for-profit sectors.

References

[1] R. J. Melrose, J. P. Handlers, S. Kerpel et al., "The use of biopsy in dental practice. The position of the American Academy of Oral and Maxillofacial Pathology," *Gen Dent*, vol. 55, no. 5, pp. 457–461, 2007.

[2] U. Tatli, O. Erdogan, A. Uguz, Y. Ustun, Y. Sertdemir, and I. Damlar, "Diagnostic concordance characteristics of oral cavity lesions," *The Scientific World Journal*, vol. 2013, Article ID 785929, 7 pages, 2013.

[3] K. J. Patel, H. L. De Silva, D. C. Tong, and R. M. Love, "Concordance between clinical and histopathologic diagnoses of oral mucosal lesions," *Journal of Oral and Maxillofacial Surgery: Official Journal of the American Association of Oral and Maxillofacial Surgeons*, vol. 69, no. 1, pp. 125–133, 2011.

[4] S. Fattahi, S. Vosoughhosseini, M. Moradzadeh Khiavi, S. Mostafazadeh, and A. Gheisar, "Consistency rates of clinical diagnosis and histopathological reports of oral lesions: a retrospective study," *Journal of Dental Research, Dental Clinics, Dental Prospects*, vol. 8, no. 2, pp. 111–113, 2014.

[5] A. K. El-Naggar, J. K. C. Chan, J. R. Grandis, T. Takata, and P. J. Slootweg, *WHO Classification of Head and Neck Tumours. WHO Classification of Tumours*, IARC Press, Lyon, France, 2017.

[6] J. Cohen, "A coefficient of agreement for nominal scales," *Educational and Psychological Measurement*, vol. 20, no. 1, pp. 37–46, 1960.

[7] Q. Xie, "Agree or disagree? A demonstration of an alternative statistic to cohens kappa for measuring the extent and reliability of agreement between observers," in *Proceedings of the Federal Committee on Statistical Methodology Research Conference*, The Council of Professional Associations on Federal Statistics, Washington, DC, USA, 2013.

[8] J. Sarabadani, A. Javadzadeh, M. Imanimoghaddam, N. Mohtasham, and M. Amirchaghmaghi, "Evaluating the accuracy rates of clinical and radiographic diagnoses compared with histopathologic diagnosis of oral exophytic lesions," *Journal of Dental Materials and Techniques*, vol. 2, no. 4, pp. 130–137, 2013.

[9] J. H. Bennett, G. Thomas, A. W. Evans, and P. M. Speight, "Osteosarcoma of the jaws: a 30-year retrospective review," *Oral Surgery, Oral Medicine, Oral Pathology, Oral Radiology, and Endodontology*, vol. 90, no. 3, pp. 323–333, 2000.

[10] F. Bertoni, P. Bacchini, N. Fabbri et al., "Osteosarcoma. Low-grade intraosseous-type osteosarcoma, histologically

resembling parosteal osteosarcoma, fibrous dysplasia, and desmoplastic fibroma," *Cancer*, vol. 71, no. 2, pp. 338–345, 1993.

[11] A.-M. Kurt, K. K. Unni, R. A. McLeod, and D. J. Pritchard, "Low-grade intraosseous osteosarcoma," *Cancer*, vol. 65, no. 6, pp. 1418–1428, 1990.

[12] R. E. Nakhleh, C. Gephardt, and R. J. Zarbo, "Necessity of clinical information in surgical pathology," *Archives of Pathology & Laboratory Medicine*, vol. 123, no. 7, pp. 615–619, 1999.

[13] H. M. McBroom and A. D. Ramsay, "The clinicopathological meeting: a means of auditing diagnostic performance," *The American Journal of Surgical Pathology*, vol. 17, no. 1, pp. 75–80, 1993.

[14] R. E. Nakhleh, "Quality in surgical pathology communication and reporting," *Archives of Pathology & Laboratory Medicine*, vol. 135, no. 11, pp. 1394–1397, 2011.

[15] D. Suleiman, "Pathologist-clinician collaboration: a marriage of necessity toward improving the quality of patient care," *Annals of Nigerian Medicine*, vol. 9, no. 1, pp. 1–3, 2015.

2

Prevalence and Risk Factors of Work-Related Lower Back Pain among Radiographers in the State of Kuwait

Hesham N. Alrowayeh,[1] **Musaed Z. Alnaser**,[2] **Talal A. Alshatti**,[1] **and Raed S. Saeed**[3]

[1]*Kuwait University, Faculty of Allied Health Sciences, Physical Therapy Department, Kuwait City, Kuwait*
[2]*Kuwait University, Faculty of Allied Health Sciences, Occupational Therapy Department, Kuwait City, Kuwait*
[3]*Kuwait University, Faculty of Allied Health Sciences, Radiological Science Department, Kuwait City, Kuwait*

Correspondence should be addressed to Hesham N. Alrowayeh; hrowayeh@hsc.edu.kw

Academic Editor: Alfonso Fausto

Background. Work-related lower back pain (WrLBP) is a global health issue and a rising concern in the State of Kuwait. The prevalence and the risk factors of WrLBP among radiographers are not well documented. *Objective.* The purpose of the study was to determine the one-year prevalence, characteristics, impact, and physical risk factors of WrLBP among radiographers in the State of Kuwait. *Methods.* A self-administered questionnaire was distributed to 200 radiographers. The questionnaire collected data on demographics, physical risk factors, and the occurrence of WrLBP in the previous 12 months. Descriptive statistics, frequency calculations, and chi-square analyses were performed. *Results.* One hundred forty-six radiographers completed and returned the questionnaires with a response rate of 73% (146/200). The one-year prevalence of WrLBP was 16%. The prevalence of WrLBP was not significantly associated with the participants' demographics. Although WrLBP was significantly associated with work demands, the overall impact of WrLBP on work duties was minimal. *Conclusions.* The occurrence of WrLBP among radiographers in Kuwait was low, particularly when compared to healthcare providers involved in more patient handling and direct contact. However, various physical risk factors were identified. Further research is needed to investigate the effect of a treatment and prevention program on the prevalence of WrLBP.

1. Introduction

Healthcare professionals are often at risk of sustaining work-related musculoskeletal disorders (WMSDs) during the performance of work duties. The National Institute for Occupational Safety and Health [1] has defined WMSD as "an injury of the muscles, tendons, ligaments, nerves, joints, cartilage, bones, or blood vessels in the arms, legs, head, neck, or back that is caused or aggravated by work tasks such as lifting, pushing, and pulling. Symptoms include pain, stiffness, swelling, numbness, and tingling." The lower back area is reported to be the most common location for WMSDs among healthcare professionals [2–4].

Several studies have investigated the prevalence of work-related lower back pain (WrLBP) among radiographers worldwide [5–8]. The 12-month WrLBP prevalence ranged from 59.6% to 83% [5–7]. Various physical and psychosocial work-related risk factors have been suggested [6–8]. Psychosocial risk factors for the development of lower back injuries among radiographers remain controversial, whereas physical risk factors have been well established [6–8].

Few studies have investigated the prevalence of WrLBP among healthcare professionals in the State of Kuwait [3, 9–11]. Of these, only one study specified the lifetime prevalence of WrLBP and possible risk factors among a small group of radiographers [9]. The lifetime prevalence was 25.7%, and transferring and lifting patients were identified as predisposing physical risk factors in the development of WrLBP.

Radiographers are mainly involved in the positioning of patients and equipment [12] in order to get the clearest and most accurate image possible. They are rarely involved in transferring and lifting patients. Thus, the study by Landry et al. [9] most probably overestimated the prevalence and misrepresented the physical risk factors (transferring or lifting patients) among radiographers in the State of Kuwait. Also, new advances in imaging technology should help to further reduce the physical workload and result in a lower prevalence of WrLPB. Furthermore, approximately 1,000 radiographers are currently working in the State of Kuwait [13]. Landry et al. [9], however, surveyed only a small proportion of them. In fact, the exact number of radiographers who participated in the study was not specified as radiographers were included in the "other healthcare professionals" category. This category also included physical therapists, laboratory technicians, pharmacists, and analgesic technicians. This may have biased the results and reduced generalizability. Thus, we aimed to examine WrLBP in a large group of radiographers working in the State of Kuwait and to report prevalence, characteristics, overall impact, and physical risk factors. The results of this study will contribute to the development of prevention and intervention strategies.

2. Methods

2.1. Participants. Radiographers of all nationalities who practiced in public or private hospitals in the State of Kuwait were randomly invited to participate in this study. Power analysis was performed, and 140 participants were deemed enough. All participants read and signed the informed consent form approved by the Ethical Review Board of Kuwait University.

2.2. Instrument. A three-part, self-administered questionnaire was used in this study. Part one collected information regarding the participants including age, gender, level of education, family history, exercise habits, and current work situation (i.e., duration of employment, work settings, and professional rank). Part two assessed the occurrence of WrLBP during the preceding 12 months using the Nordic questionnaire [14] and severity of the worst episode of WrLPB using the visual analogue scale (VAS). Part three assessed the physical risk factors associated with WrLBP and work demands. Participants rated how often they perform certain activities (sitting, standing, and so on) in their current job using 4-point scale varying from never to always. Excessive work demands were rated using yes/no scale.

2.3. Procedures. Two hundred questionnaires were distributed by a radiographer (fourth author) to prospective participants. The questionnaire was explained to each participant, and the radiographer provided a contact phone number in case further explanation should be required. Completed questionnaires were collected by the same radiographer after one week. The study protocol was approved by the Ethical Review Board of Kuwait University.

2.4. Data Analyses. Descriptive statistics were used to estimate the prevalence of WrLBP and analyze demographic variables. Frequencies, cross-tabulations, and chi-square tests were used to compare WrLBP prevalence by demographic variable (gender, age, and so on), work history (experience, setting, specialty, and so on), and physical risk factors. Statistical significance was set at $P < 0.05$.

3. Results

3.1. Participation Rate. One hundred forty-six radiographers completed the questionnaire; the response rate was 73% (146/200). No question was missing more than 5% of the responses. The time taken to complete the questionnaire was 5 to 10 minutes.

3.2. Participant Characteristics. Data regarding questionnaire responses are shown in Table 1. A higher proportion of male than female radiographers participated in this study. The mean age of participants was 37.8 ± 9.7 years (range, 23–66 years). Approximately two-thirds of radiographers were middle-aged (between 20 and 40 years). The majority of respondents (79%) were not of Kuwaiti nationality. Over 60% of participants (64%) had more than 10 years of clinical experience (mean of 15.0 ± 9.5 years). Almost all of the radiographers worked in public hospitals (95%), and most worked at least 40 hours per week (87%); the mean number of working hours was 45.7 ± 13.2 hours. Almost 39% of participants were ranked as radiographer practitioners (RS), and 52% of the participants held entry-level degrees or higher (i.e., BSc, MSc, or PhD).

3.3. Prevalence and Characteristics of WrLBP. The one-year prevalence of WrLBP among radiographers in this study was 16% (24/146). Almost half of the affected radiographers experienced only one episode of WrLBP (47%), and most cases lasted one to seven days (57%; Table 2). Stiffness and pain, which developed gradually, were the most common symptoms. The mean severity of the worst episode of WrLBP experienced over the past 12 months was 5.13 out of 10 using the VAS. Radiographers were mostly seen by a general practitioner, and the majority received treatment with aspirin or ibuprofen.

The prevalence of work-related lower back complaints was significantly associated with work demands ($p = 0.002$; Table 3). It was however not significantly associated with gender, age, area of specialty, professional experience, workings hours, exercise, or co-worker or supervisor support (Table 3).

3.4. Work Activity and the Prevalence of WrLBP. WrLBP was significantly associated with the following work activities: standing, sitting, walking for prolonged periods, working with one's hands above shoulder height, reaching, lifting less than 5 kg, pushing and pulling loads, bending and/or twisting the upper body ($p < 0.05$), and squatting ($p < 0.005$) (Table 4). WrLBP was, however, not significantly associated

Table 1: Study participant demographics.

Gender	No.	%
Male	87	60
Female	59	40
Age		
20–30 years	33	23
31–40 years	70	49
41–50 years	24	17
51+ years	17	12
Nationality		
Kuwaiti	30	20
Egyptian	25	17
Filipino	30	20
Indian	44	30
Other	17	12
Education		
Diploma	68	48
BSc	72	50
MSc	2	1
PhD	1	1
Professional rank		
Junior RS	27	19
RS	54	39
Senior RS	36	26
RS specialist	10	7
Senior RS specialist	9	7
Superintendent RS	3	2
Professional experience		
0–10 years	49	36
11–20 years	57	42
21+ years	30	22
Working hours		
<10–19 hours	10	7
20–39 hours	9	6
40+ hours	123	87
Work settings		
General hospital	134	95
Private hospital/clinic	7	5
Areas of specialty		
General	31	22
Special	89	62
Both	24	17

Column values do not always add up to the total number of questionnaire respondents due to missing data. Others nationalities include Iranian, Jordanian, Polish, Sudanese, Syrian, and Yemeni. For areas of specialty, special includes CT, MRI, fluoroscopy, and mammography.

with working posture ($p = 0.15$) or with slipping or falling during the transport of loads ($p = 0.16$) (Table 4).

3.5. Impact of LBP on Work. Figure 1 shows the impact of LBP on work. Absence from work due to WrLBP ranged from one to seven days. The majority of radiographers (63.6%, 14/22) who complained of WrLBP did not take any sick leave. Two-thirds of radiographers (65.2%, 15/23) were aware that WrLBP can interfere with daily work activities. Thus, most radiographers (60.8%, 14/23) made changes in their work habits such as changing their area of practice or amount of patient contact.

Table 2: Characteristics of LBP among radiographers working in Kuwait.

	LBP	
Number of spells	No.	%
1	9	47
2 to 5	7	37
6+	3	16
Longest spell		
1 to 7 days	13	57
2 to 3 weeks	5	22
3to 4 weeks	2	9
3+ months	3	13
Nature of complaints		
Stiffness	10	50
Nagging feeling	0	0
Numbness	2	10
Tingling	0	0
Loss of strength	1	5
Cramp and spasm	2	10
Pain	5	25
Onset of complaints		
Sudden	10	44
Gradual	13	57
Expert seen		
No visit	6	40
Physical therapist	3	20
General practitioner	4	27
A specialist	2	13
Treatment received		
PT	3	21
Drugs	6	43
No treatment	5	36

Column values do not always add up to the total number of questionnaire respondents due to missing data.

4. Discussion

We report three key findings in our study. First, WrLBP was not common among radiographers working in the State of Kuwait. Second, WrLBP was significantly associated with work demands but not with demographics, work settings, exercise habits, or co-worker or supervisor support. Third, work duties were not affected by WrLBP.

4.1. Prevalence Rate and Characteristics of LBP. The one-year prevalence rate of WrLBP reported by radiographers in our study (16%) was lower than most rates reported worldwide. Studies from Italy, the United States of America (USA), the Netherlands, and Canada have reported prevalence rates of almost 60% [7], 72% to 77% [5], 76% [8], and 83% [6], respectively. The disparity between our results and these results might be due to the widespread availability of radiographer assistants in Kuwait. A lower prevalence of WrLBP has previously been reported among physical therapists in Kuwait compared to those around the world as a result of the abundant help available to them [3]. Work-related physical load is significantly associated with the occurrence of musculoskeletal injuries [2], and the availability of assistants helps to reduce the physical load that radiographers must bear.

TABLE 3: Prevalence and association of LBP among radiographers working in Kuwait with demographics, work settings, exercise habits, and physical risk factors.

Gender	LBP	
	P	X^2 value
Male Female	0.470	0.522
Age 20–30 31–40 41–50 51+	0.745	1.233
Area of specialty General Special Both	0.074	5.217
Professional experience 1–10 11–20 21+	0.822	0.393
Working hours <10 10–19 20–29 30–39 40+	0.985	0.149
Exercise Yes No	0.267	1.233
Work demands Yes No	0.002*	9.473
Co-worker support Yes No	0.6	0.275
Supervisor support Yes No	0.15	1.739

For area of specialty, special includes CT, MRI, fluoroscopy, and mammography. * indicates statistically significant difference at $P = 0.05$.

TABLE 4: Prevalence of LBP among radiographers working in Kuwait and association with physical risk factors (work activity).

Work activity	LBP	
	P	X^2 value
Standing	0.012*	6.255
Sitting	0.024*	5.128
Walking	0.022*	5.232
Squatting	0.006*	7.657
Overhead activity	0.025*	5.011
Reaching	0.011*	6.487
Lifting less than 5 kg	0.020*	5.400
Pushing/pulling	0.020*	5.400
Slipping/falling	0.169	1.889
Bending/twisting	0.048*	3.980
Improper body mechanism	0.150	2.069

* indicates statistically significant association at $P = 0.05$.

The one-year prevalence rate of WrLBP among radiographers in the State of Kuwait was lower than that reported among local physical and occupational therapists [3, 10, 11, 15]. It was also lower than that reported among physical therapists [16–21], occupational therapists [20, 21], and nurses [22–24] around the world. The high prevalence of WrLBP among these health professionals could be associated with patient handling such as transferring and lifting. As the work duties of radiographers require minimal patient handling, the prevalence of WrLBP was very low in this professional group. This finding clearly supports the notion that an increase in patient handling is associated with a growing risk of injury. The prevalence of WrLBP among radiographers in the State of Kuwait was lower also than the prevalence rate among dentists [2, 25, 26]. The lack of patient handling, however, cannot explain this difference as dental practice does not involve lifting or transferring patients. One possible explanation for the difference might be the length of time spent in static postures during work activities [26]. Ratzon et al. [26] found a significant association between length of time spent sustaining an activity and WrLBP.

4.2. Demographics, Exercise Habits, Co-Worker or Supervisor Support, Work Demands, and Work Settings. Age is a potential risk factor for the development of WrLBP among physical therapists and nurses [3, 24]. Age, however, as a risk factor for the development of WrLBP among radiographers is controversial [5, 7]. We found no significant association between age and the prevalence of WrLBP. This finding is in agreement with the results reported by Wright and Witt [5] but differs from those reported by Lorusso et al. [7].

In this study, there was no significant association between the prevalence of WrLBP and gender. This finding is in agreement with the results reported by Lorusso et al. [7] among radiographers. However, they contradict the findings reported among other healthcare professionals [3, 24]. These studies have shown that female healthcare professionals are more at risk of sustaining musculoskeletal injuries than males [3, 24] as a result of anatomical and physiological differences [3].

In accordance with the finding reported by Landry et al. [9], we found no significant association between exercise and the prevalence of WrLBP among radiographers in this study. This was unexpected as physical activity promotes and maintains health and fitness and should therefore reduce the risk of injury. This suggests that physical activity is not sufficient to prevent WrLBP where static and awkward postures are involved in the performance of work duties.

WrLBP among radiographers in this study was not significantly associated with co-worker or supervisor support. This was similar to the results of Bos et al. [8]. However, since the perception of one's work or meaning of work is subjective and can differ greatly from one individual to another, the association between psychosocial factors such as support and WrLBP might be inconsistently reported.

Previous studies [7, 27] have reported a positive association between length of employment and WrLBP. However, the results of this study were not in agreement. The specialty area is a potential risk factor in the development of work-

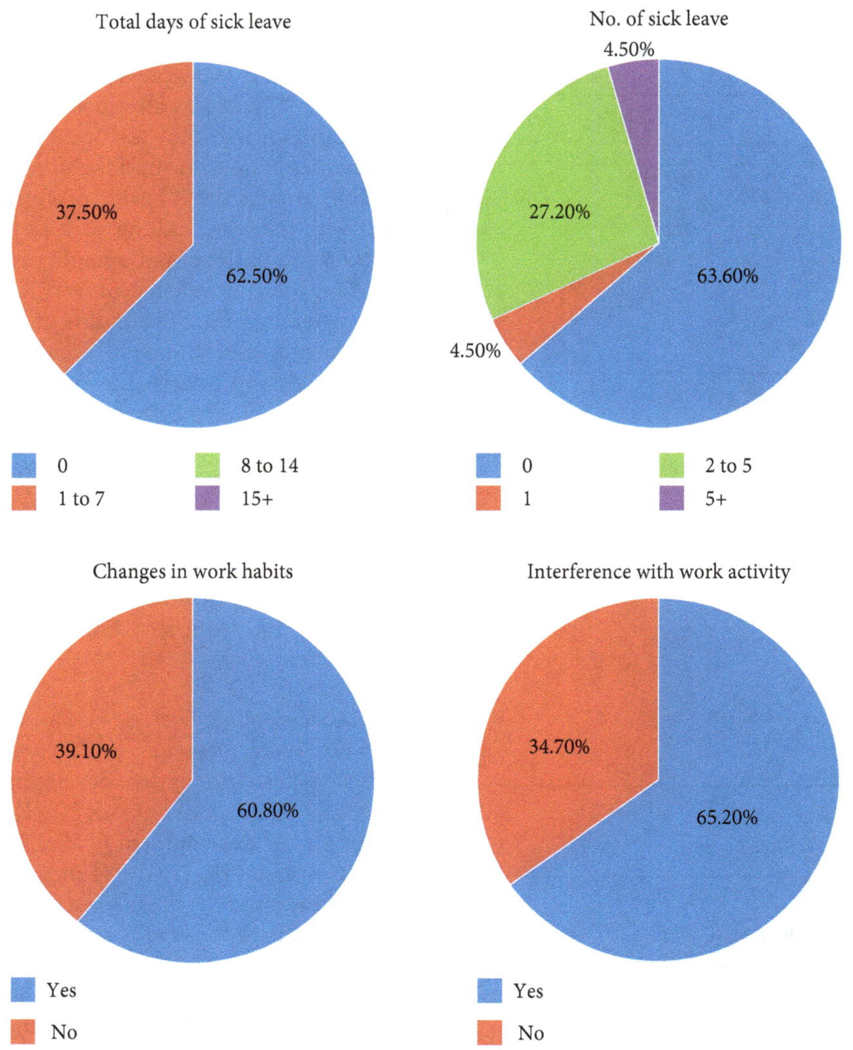

FIGURE 1: Impact of LBP on radiographers working in Kuwait. Percentage/number values do not always add up to the total percentage/number of questionnaire respondents due to missing data.

related musculoskeletal pain. However, the nonsignificant association between area of specialty and prevalence of WrLBP reported in this study contradicts the findings previously reported among nurses [24], physical therapists [19], and dental office personnel [28]. A possible explanation is that areas of practice in radiography do not vary significantly in work activities and tasks, and in turn no change in the rate of prevalence of WrLBP is observed. Finally, as far as we are aware, there is a lack of studies regarding the association between working hours and prevalence of WrLBP among radiographers; we report a nonsignificant association.

4.3. Work Activity and the Occurrences of WrLBP. Like most studies conducted among healthcare professionals, we found that work-related physical activities were significantly associated with the occurrence of WrLBP. In this study, standing, sitting, or walking for prolonged periods of time increased the prevalence of WrLBP, indicating that cumulative physical burdens increase the prevalence of WrLBP among radiographers.

Common activities in radiological units include helping to wheel and position patients, moving X-ray machines, carrying cassettes, pushing mobile units, and moving buck trays. These duties involve squatting, static posture, working with one's hands above shoulder height, reaching far, pushing, and bending and/or twisting. These activities increase the physical load on the lower back area and intensify muscular contractions. They were significantly associated with the prevalence of WrLBP among radiographers in the present study. Therefore, using ergonomic procedures to position patients and handle equipment during clinical practice may reduce the prevalence of WrLBP. This possibility is the subject of ongoing research.

4.4. LBP Effect on Work. The overall effect of LBP on work was minimal. The majority of radiographers in this study did not take any sick leave from work as a result of their WrLBP. The total number of days of work lost due to LBP was 56. This is very low compared to the number of lost workdays reported by nurses [24] and physical therapists [3]. Studies have reported a loss of 202 days by nurses and 75 to 219 days by physical therapists as a result of WrLBP. These professionals frequently engage in handling, lifting, and transferring patients. They spend more time in direct contact with patients than radiographers as a result of their work duties. This might explain the difference in the impact of WrLBP.

No change in the way radiographers practiced was reported despite the fact that the majority were aware that WrLBP might interfere with their daily work activities. Furthermore, the majority of respondents did not take any sick leave to rest and recover from their WrLBP but rather continued their normal working routine. The mean VAS was 5.12 for the worst pain suffered by these radiographers during an attack of WrLBP over the past 12 months. This VAS score indicates mild to moderate pain. Absence from work might increase when LBP becomes severe [29]. In addition, the majority of radiographers received analgesic drugs during attacks of WrLBP. This rendered the mild to moderate pain tolerable enough for the radiographers to work comfortably.

4.5. Limitations. The main limitation of this study was recall bias. The study relied on self-reported data, and participants may not have remembered all incidents of WrLBP. Furthermore, participants may have underestimated their work-related back injuries to avoid being stereotyped by their superiors or viewed negatively based on their injury history.

5. Conclusion and Recommendation

The prevalence of WrLBP among radiographers in the State of Kuwait was low. However, various work-related physical risk factors were identified. Further research to evaluate the effect of a treatment and prevention program on the prevalence of WrLBP is needed. Similarly, further research is needed to document the prevalence of WMSDs in all anatomical areas of the body among radiographers in the State of Kuwait.

References

[1] National Institute for Occupational Safety and Health, *NIOSH Hazard Review: Occupational Hazards in Home Healthcare*, National Institute for Occupational Safety and Health, Cincinnati, OH, USA, 2010.

[2] E. C. Alexopoulos, I.-C. Stathi, and F. Charizani, "Prevalence of musculoskeletal disorders in dentists," *BMC Musculoskeletal Disorders*, vol. 5, no. 1, p. 16, 2004.

[3] H. N. Alrowayeh, T. A. Alshatti, S. H. Aljadi, M. Fares, M. M. Alshamire, and S. S. Alwazan, "Prevalence, characteristics, and impacts of work-related musculoskeletal disorders: a survey among physical therapists in the state of Kuwait," *BMC Musculoskeletal Disorders*, vol. 11, no. 1, p. 116, 2010.

[4] M. Z. Alnaser, "Occupational musculoskeletal injuries in the health care environment and its impact on occupational therapy practitioners: a systemic review," *Work*, vol. 29, no. 2, pp. 89–100, 2007.

[5] D. L. Wright and P. L. Witt, "Initial study of back pain among radiographers," *Radiologic Technology*, vol. 64, pp. 283–289, 1993.

[6] S. Kumar, L. Moro, and Y. Narayan, "Perceived physical stress at work and musculoskeletal discomfort in X-ray technologists," *Ergonomics*, vol. 47, no. 2, pp. 189–201, 2004.

[7] A. Lorusso, S. Bruno, and N. L'ABBATE, "Musculoskeletal complaints among Italian X-ray technologists," *Industrial Health*, vol. 45, no. 5, pp. 705–708, 2007.

[8] E. Bos, B. Krol, L. van der Star, and J. Groothoff, "Risk factors and musculoskeletal complaints in non-specialized nurses, IC nurses, operation room nurses, and X-ray technologists," *International Archives of Occupational and Environmental Health*, vol. 80, no. 3, pp. 198–206, 2007.

[9] M. D. Landry, S. R. Raman, C. Sulway, Y. M. Golightly, and E. Hamdan, "Prevalence and risk factors associated with low back pain among health care providers in a Kuwait hospital," *Spine*, vol. 33, no. 5, pp. 539–545, 2008.

[10] M. Z. Alnaser and S. H. Aljadi, "Physical therapists with work-related musculoskeletal disorders in the State of Kuwait: a comparison across countries and health care professions," *Work*, vol. 63, no. 2, pp. 261–268, 2019.

[11] D. Shehab, K. Al-Jarallah, M. A. A. Moussa, and N. Adham, "Prevalence of low back pain among physical therapists in Kuwait," *Medical Principles and Practice*, vol. 12, no. 4, pp. 224–230, 2003.

[12] American Society for Radiology Technologists. Careers in radiologic technology. Retrieved from https://www.asrt.org/main/career-center/careers-in-radiologic-technology (accessed October 2019).

[13] Ministry of Health, *Ministry Statistics: Annual Health Report 2018*, Ministry of Health, Kuwait, 2019, https://www.moh.gov.kw/en/Ministry-Statistics.

[14] I. Kuorinka, B. Jonsson, A. Kilbom et al., "Standardised Nordic questionnaires for the analysis of musculoskeletal symptoms," *Applied Ergonomics*, vol. 18, no. 3, pp. 233–237, 1987.

[15] M. Z. Alnaser, "Occupational therapy practitioners with occupational musculoskeletal injuries: prevalence and risk factors," *Journal of Occupational Rehabilitation*, vol. 25, no. 4, pp. 763–769, 2015.

[16] J. E. Cromie, V. J. Robertson, and M. O. Best, "Work-related musculoskeletal disorders in physical therapists: prevalence, severity, risks, and responses," *Physical Therapy*, vol. 80, no. 4, pp. 336–351, 2000.

[17] W. Glover, A. McGregor, C. Sullivan, and J. Hague, "Work-related musculoskeletal disorders affecting members of the Chartered Society of Physiotherapy," *Physiotherapy*, vol. 91, no. 3, pp. 138–147, 2005.

[18] B. O. Adegoke, A. K. Akodu, and A. L. Oyeyemi, "Work-related musculoskeletal disorders among Nigerian Physiotherapists," *BMC Musculoskeletal Disorders*, vol. 9, no. 1, pp. 112–120, 2008.

[19] B. E. Bork, T. M. Cook, J. C. Rosecrance et al., "Work-related musculoskeletal disorders among physical therapists," *Physical Therapy*, vol. 76, no. 8, pp. 827–835, 1996.

[20] M. S. Islam, M. M. Habib, M. A. Hafez, N. Nahar, D. Lindstrom-Hazel, and M. K. Rahman, "Musculoskeletal complaints among physiotherapy and occupational therapy rehabilitation professionals in Bangladesh," *Work*, vol. 50, no. 3, pp. 379–386, 2015.

[21] A. R. Darragh, W. Huddleston, and P. King, "Work-related musculoskeletal injuries and disorders Occupational and physical therapists," *American Journal of Occupational Therapy*, vol. 63, no. 3, pp. 351–362, 2009.

[22] Y. B. Yip, "A study of work stress, patient handling activities and the risk of low back pain among nurses," *Journal of Advanced Nursing*, vol. 36, no. 6, pp. 794–804, 2001.

[23] C. Sopajareeya, C. Viwatwongkasem, and P. Lapvongwatana, "Prevalence and risk factors of low Back pain among nurses in a Thai public hospital," *Medical Journal of the Medical Association of Thailand*, vol. 92, no. 7, pp. S93–S99, 2009.

[24] L. Sikiru and S. Hanifa, "Prevalence and risk factors of low back pain among nurses in a typical Nigerian hospital," *African Health Sciences*, vol. 10, no. 1, pp. 26–30, 2010.

[25] L. Finsen, H. Christensen, and M. Bakke, "Musculoskeletal disorders among dentists and variation In dental work," *Applied Ergonomics*, vol. 29, no. 2, pp. 119–125, 1998.

[26] N. Z. Ratzon, T. Yaros, and A. Mizlik, "Musculoskeletal symptoms among dentists in relation to work posture," *Work*, vol. 15, no. 3, pp. 153–158, 2000.

[27] S. D. Miller and J. E. O'brien, "Prevalence of back pain among radiation therapists," *Radiologic Technology*, vol. 62, no. 6, pp. 460–466, 1991.

[28] J. A. Lalumandier, S. D. McPhee, C. B. Parrott, and M Vendemia, "Musculoskeletal pain: prevalence, prevention, and differences among dental office personnel," *General Dentistry*, vol. 49, pp. 160–166, 2001.

[29] K. M. Dunn and P. R. Croft, "Classification of low back pain in primary care: using "bothersomeness" to identify the most severe cases," *Spine*, vol. 30, no. 16, pp. 1887–1892, 2005.

3

Exposure Levels of Adult Patients during Radiographic Examinations: Sinuses and Coastal Grill Cases at the Ngaoundere Regional Hospital, Cameroon

Guiswe Gnowe,[1,2] **Fouda H. P. Ekobena,**[3] **Amvene J. Mbo,**[4] **and Guena M. Neossi**[1,5]

[1] *Department of Biomedical Sciences, Faculty of Sciences, University of Ngaoundere, Cameroon*
[2] *Higher Institute of Sciences, Health Technics and Management of Garoua, Cameroon*
[3] *University Institute of Technology, University of Ngaoundere, Cameroon*
[4] *Faculty of Medicine and Biomedical Sciences of Garoua, Cameroon*
[5] *Department of Radiology and Medical Imaging, Regional Hospital of Ngaoundere, Cameroon*

Correspondence should be addressed to Guiswe Gnowe; gnoweguiswe@gmail.com

Academic Editor: Paul Sijens

Background. The purpose of this study was to estimate the doses delivered to adult patients during explorations of the sinuses and coastal grill whose attention in dosimetric terms is neglected because of the low demand for diagnosis. But yet dosimetric values are very high. *Materials and Methods.* The present study was transversely descriptive and was conducted between April and July 2016. The data were collected on 50 adult patients of mass of 70±10kg at the Regional Hospital of Ngaoundere (HRN). The dose at the entrance of the patients' skin was evaluated through the theoretical methods derived from the Davies model according to the 75th percentile calculations. *Results and Discussion.* The entrance skin doses obtained in mGy were, respectively, of 7.2±0.2 for sinuses and 5.27±0.1 for coastal grill. The present study found many variations in doses during radiological investigations. These variations allowed us to understand that the notions of quality of the radiographic image, insurance, and quality control of the radiological equipment are tributary, abstract, and often theoretical because doses delivered are not sufficiently optimized. *Conclusion.* The dosimetric analysis remains very worrying because the various procedures show that an improvement of the practices especially with respect to the technical parameters and the protocols must be considered. Therefore a strengthening of radiological protection skills of radiological manipulators (continuing education and retraining) would contribute to a better protection of patients.

1. Introduction

In radiology, patient dosimetry is a good match between image quality and the low dose process. Continuous evaluation by means of periodic inspections and the fight to reduce the doses delivered should be at the center of the activities (after the structure in charge through effective monitoring in the field and in all structures equipped with X-ray tubes). In fact, the doses delivered to patients during medical imaging examinations are not sufficiently controlled and the working protocols for a given examination differ from one hospital service to another. These variations indicate that good imaging technique is needed to reduce the dose to patients at the lowest practicable level to respond to the clinic and make the diagnosis [1]. These large variations in the doses delivered to patients for the same examination also show a crucial importance for the study of dose variations [2], for quality assurance and standardization of protocols [3], in order to guarantee the optimization of doses to patients. We must give ourselves the means to measure and to evaluate this energy and to verify that patients are not overexposed during standard radiography.

Patient dosimetry is a functional operation parameter such as high voltage or kilovolt (kV), current intensity or milliamperage (mAs), morphotype, posteroanterior (PA), anteroposterior (AP), focus-skin distance (FSD), and field and filtration [4]. It should be noted that the diagnosis is dependent on the quality of the radiological image and therefore of the dose at the entrance surface of the skin. In radiology, the dosimetric quantities selected for the Diagnostic Reference Levels (DRLs) determinations are the input dose (ESD in mGy) and the Dose-Area Product (DAP in Gy.cm^2) [5].

The entrance skin dose (ESD) in conventional radiography can be obtained by calculation from mathematical methods or measured by a thermoluminescent dosimeter (TLD) [6]. These methods have relatively small differences. The calculation or mathematical method appears reliable and is an effective alternative for measuring the entrance skin dose [7]. The determination of patient doses is an essential part of the optimization process, such as the adequacy of the image and radiation in radiological examination. The optimization of doses delivered during the radiological examinations, by the determination of the DRLs, the control of the quality of the installations, and radiological procedure, makes it possible to minimize the risk related to these irradiations by reducing the dose received by the patient. The concept of DRL is specific to medical exposures and should not be confused with that of "individual dose limit" which is applied in these areas of radiation protection of workers and the public. Reference levels are tools for improving practices and optimizing doses. These levels exist only for routine explorations in radiological examination. Respect for the reference levels is not, by itself, a criterion of good practice. The primary goal, inseparable from dosimetry, is the diagnostic quality of low dose images [5].

Our objectives were the following:

(i) Determine the sociodemographic profiles of the patients received for these particular examinations.

(ii) Determine the dose levels delivered to adult patients based on radiological exploration by theoretical models of dose calculation.

(iii) Compare the results obtained with those obtained elsewhere according to our realities.

2. Materials and Methods

The study was monocentric, descriptive, and transversal. It took place between April and July 2016 (four months), in the Radiology and Medical Imaging Department of the Ngaoundéré Regional Hospital. This department is equipped with a GENERAL ELECTRIC X-ray tube, model 5192454, whose maximum voltage was around 150 kV.

2.1. Target. Included in this study were all adult subjects irrespective of sex and age who had undergone a blondeau radiographic examination and coastal grill during the period. The data collected include age, sex, and anthropometric data of patients with weights between 60 and 80 kg.

2.2. Collection and Statistical Analysis. The information was collected using a sheet adapted according to the model of the Institute of Radiation Protection and Nuclear Safety (IRNS) dosimetric evaluation. The irradiation parameters used (kV, mAs), the geometric parameters (FFD, FSD), and the anthropometric data (age, sex, and weight) were processed and analyzed with the strictest anonymity. The calculations, the output of the tube, and the entrance skin dose (ESD) patients were donned by Sphinx Plus^2 V.5.1.0.6 and Excel 2010.

2.3. Calculation of the Dose. The irradiation and geometric parameters involved in the calculation of the dose at the entrance of the skin were calculated (by means of 75th percentiles, standard deviations). The calculation of the dose at the entrance of the skin began by calculating the output (output) of the X-ray tube according to the model of [8]:

$$\frac{O}{P}(mR) = A \times 6,53 \times 10^{-4} \left(\frac{mR}{mAs}\right) \left(kV^2\right)^{-1} \times kV^2 \times mAs \quad (1)$$

where A is a constant equal to 0.5; 0.8 and 1 are for single-phase, three-phase, and high frequency tubes generators. As part of our study, the X-ray tube was three phases. The yields obtained in (mR) were converted to mGy, mAs^{-1} by multiplication at a factor of 0.00877/mAs [9].

Then, the calculation of the dose at the entrance of the skin proper for each patient was according to the Davies model [10]. This is thanks to the values of irradiation parameters and geometric and output values. We chose this model because it integrates all the elements directly, involved in the realization of radiographic examinations and the definition of the dose at the entrance of the skin [11]. The logic of the arrangement of radiographic parameters in this formula obeys well to that realized during the obtaining of the radiographic images.

$$ESD\,(mGy) = \left(\frac{O}{P}\right) \times \left(\frac{kV}{80}\right)^2 \times mAs \times \left(\frac{100}{FSD}\right)^2 \times BSF \quad (2)$$

Only images of good qualities accepted for interpretation were considered. The study was authorized by the ethics committee of the hospital structure.

3. Results

The results obtained only were presented in Table 4.

3.1. Sociodemographic Data. For 50 subjects, men were more represented than women (66%), with a sex ratio (H/F=1.94).

Regarding the male sex: the mean age was 40.33 and the standard deviation was 8.54 years; the range of age was 26-48 years for sinuses.

The mean age was 27.2 and the standard deviation was 6.64 years; the range of age was 20-38 years for coastal grill.

With regard to the female sex: the mean age of the women was 27.2 and the standard deviation was 6.64 years; the range of age was between 20 and 38 years for sinuses. The mean age was 33.16 and the standard deviation was 6.22 years; the range of age was between 32 and 41 years for coastal grill.

3.2. Yield of X-Ray Tube. The different values of the output are essential for the process of optimizing the dose delivered and the quality of the images. They are directly a function of the high voltage (kV) and the load (mAs). For sinuses, in mGy. $(mAs)^{-1}$, the output ranged from 0.19 to 0.29 in PA. For coastal grill, in mGy $(mAs)^{-1}$, output ranged from 0.19 to 0.25 in AP.

3.3. Overall Knowledge of the Irradiation Parameters Used during Exams. The parameters presented in this study are those that made it possible to obtain good quality according to the different morphotypes of the patients. These parameters are very important in the process of optimizing the dose delivered and improving the quality of the images. After calculation (mGy), the third quartile was 7.02 and standard deviation was 0.2 for sinuses. The minimum and maximum entrance skin dose ranged from 5.8 to 12.2 in PA. The third quartile was 5.27 and standard deviation was 0.1 for coastal grill. The minimum and maximum entrance skin dose skin ranged from 4.98 to 7.67 in AP.

3.4. Study of Comparative Values. The values obtained (mGy) were compared with those obtained elsewhere by the same approaches. The entrance skin dose was 7.02±0.2 for sinuses in PA. The entrance skin dose was 5.27±0.1 for coastal grill in AP.

4. Discussion

The population of our study consisted of patients admitted to the Radiology Department of the Regional Hospital of Ngaoundere. The study included 50 adult patients of more than 20 years, both sexes, with a weight between 60 and 80 kg. X-ray examinations were performed by manipulators of different rank and seniority. The parameters used for the same examination were variable according to the habits of each manipulator. Many manipulators do not have the same rules of good practice. These different parameters were observable on the quality of the snapshots and the disparity of the input doses delivered to the patients. The results obtained were calculated using the 75th percentile method. The good practicing in radiographic involves a permanent adaptation of the technical procedure related to the equipment, the choice of parameters (irradiation and geometry), and possible accessories, which constantly influence the dose received by the patient. The resumption of radiographic examinations is an important preventable or at least reducible factor of overexposure of patients. Effective remediation and reduction measures such as periodic assessment and dosimetric testing must be considered.

4.1. Perception of Sociodemographic Data. Table 1 presents the sociodemographic data of the patients. Ages, sex, and weight of the patient are the most important parameters in considering the interpretation of radiological images. The technical choices of performing an examination are also a function of the morphotype of the patient. Therefore, some clinicians would ignore the importance of these parameters for imaging, coupled with the fact that some patients in our environment are not always able to accurately age [12]. Much more according to [13], the level of awareness of clinicians in Cameroon is very low and superficial, which affects the quality of their imaging demands. Despite the compliance of certain test reports, it should be noted that contact with the patient during imaging examinations should allow us to complete the missing parameters.

TABLE 1: Sociodemographic characteristics.

Radiography	Sex	Amount	Age (years)	Weight (kg)
Sinuses	M	14	26-48 40.33±8.54	65-78 71.33±5.77
	F	11	26-54 33.57±9.04	61-78 69.42±5.02
Coastal grill	M	19	20-38 27.2±6.64	63-78 68.5±3.62
	F	6	32-41 33.16±6.22	65-76 70.33±4.52

M: male, F: female.

TABLE 2: Output of X-ray tube in mR and mGy. $(mAs)^{-1}$.

Radiography	Projection	Output (mR)		Output mGy. $(mAs)^{-1}$	
		Min	Max	Min	Max
Sinuses	PA	22.07	33.43	0.19	0.29
Coastal grill	AP	22.07	29.38	0.19	0.25

PA: posteroanterior, AP: anteroposterior, Min: minimum, max: maximum.

4.2. Importance of X-Ray Tube Performance. Table 2 presents the estimation of the X-ray tube yielding from the theoretical model proposed by [8]. It is important to consider tube efficiencies for each specific run to control tube power and to take corrective action if deviations from normal are noted. Obtaining a quality image is the primary function of the efficiency of the X-ray tube. The power of the tube becomes an optimization factor in the evaluation of the "dead" performance of the X-ray tube. The devices are calibrated beforehand by the manufacturers and the parameters applied on the console for any examination are not the same at the exit of the tube.

4.3. State of Exposure and Context. Table 3 presents the following:

(i) The result of the exploration of the sinuses was in the order of 7.02-0.2 mGy. This result was greater than 3.2 mGy estimated by [14], but similar to 5.06 mGy, estimated by [15]. Mali and Cameroon share some common points of delay in the radiation protection of patients.

(ii) At the end of the exploration of the coastal grill, we obtained 5.27±0.1mGy. This result appears very high to our knowledge because the thoracic framework is a bone structure. It can be explored from low settings. According to [16], the reduction in voltage and charge (mAs) has been shown to be effective in reducing the dose delivered by 40% without impairing the diagnostic quality of images, especially for bone structures.

TABLE 3: Technical parameters used.

Radiography	Projection	m	mAs	DFF	FSD	ESD Min	ESD Max	3rd quartile	SD
Sinuses	PA	65-80 66.1±1.5	32-50 41.9±2.4	1.3-1.5 1.2±0.04	1.0-1.3 1.1±0.04	5.8	12.2	7.02	0.2
Coastal grill	AP	65-75 66.7±2.0	40-55 43.2±2.1	1.5-1.8 1.6±0.07	1.2-1.5 1.3±0.06	4.98	7.67	5.27	0.1

kV: kilovolt, mAs: milliampere second, FFD: focus-film distance, FSD: focus-skin distance, ESD: entrance skin dose, SD: standard deviation.

TABLE 4: Comparison between our values and some of them.

Radiography	Projection	Our study	DRL Europe	Mali [15]	Saudi Arabia [14]
Sinuses	PA	7.02±0.2	-	5.06	3.2
Coastal grill	AP	5.27±0,1	-	-	-

4.4. Knowledge of Radiation Protection during Standard Radiological Examinations. Table 4 presents a comparative statement between our results and others elsewhere. This table indicates that the values are obtained by [14, 15]. These differences were specifically associated with exceeding nominal values as proposed by the manufacturer despite the absence of protocols. This study is devoted to examinations that are weakly "realized" and whose evaluation in dosimetric terms is often not considered. Yet, they are strongly radiating. We note that these results cannot be extrapolated to all radiology departments in Cameroon because the study was based on the principle of voluntary. Nevertheless, these values are indicatives from the dosimetric point of view. Despite the existence of a law governing radiation protection and an agency in charge of radiation protection, the absence of technical protocols in the examination room makes it difficult to control the doses delivered to patients. As observed elsewhere, the absence of texts in favor of radioprotection and or extracts in this radiology department proves the embryonic state of radiation protection of patients in this department. In practice, it is possible to avoid unnecessary radiation despite attendance routine trainees and make good quality pictures. But this observation is still very alarming, when X-rays are carried out daily by some caregivers who have no background profile of the field but rather converted into radiology manipulators. The latter then have no idea or then a rough knowledge of the texts in favor of radiation protection. All these observations point to [17]; unlike developed countries, in the sub-Saharan African countries, particularly in Cameroon, legislative and regulatory frameworks are either nonexistent or are implemented in an approximate manner and the practices of radiation protection of patients are poorly documented in a context of expanding medical imaging. If the report is real, it is necessary to note the embryonic and precarious state of the standards and devices in favor of the radioprotection of the patients. Moreover, the lack of qualified personnel in radiation protection and the lack of resources and continuing training in radiological protection should only lead to approximate visions of radiation protection if the manipulators were recycled; endowing more than the manipulation console offers a platform for adjustment irradiation parameters and therefore dosimetric controls. As imaging spreads to the most remote areas of the country, there is an urgent need to optimize work protocols. This optimization of the protocols could be achieved by continuous training; the display in the examination rooms of the working protocols and a permanent comparison of the values to the references and permanent correction measures could partly reduce the observed radiology differences.

5. Conclusion

The risk of irradiation is potentiated by the nonobservance of the basic principles of patient protection. Far from trivializing the exposure of patients to the ionizing radiation, we must instead be vigilant and educate staff about it and we are proposing the measures to reduce the skin entrance doses. However, the dosimetric analysis remains very worrying. The analysis of the different procedures shows that an improvement of the practices especially with respect to the technical parameters and the protocols, combined with a reinforcement of the radioprotection competences of the radiology manipulators (continuous training and recycling), will contribute to a better radioprotection of the patients. The creation of a regulatory framework allowing not only the radiation protection of the patients but also the personnel must be effective on the ground, by means of the periodic controls and the evaluations of the professional practices. This work is also an essential call to work in the mastery of technical and standardization of examination protocols to control and optimize the doses delivered to patients for a better match of the image quality and the low dose over the area.

References

[1] D. Z. Joseph, O. Chinedu, N. Favious, G. Luntsi, L. Shem, and Y. Dlama, "Rationale for implementing dose reference level as a quality assurance tool in medical radiography in Nigeria," *IOSR Journal of Dental and Medical Sciences*, vol. 13, no. 12, pp. 41–45, 2014.

[2] J. Gray, "Reference values-what are they?" *American Association of Physicist in Medicine*, vol. 24, pp. 9-10, 1999.

[3] O. E. Kwasi, D. N. Scutt, W. Matt, H. V. Kwaku, and D. T. Klenam, "Evaluation of patient radiation dose from skull X-ray examinations in Ghana," *Journal of Medical and Biomedical Science*, vol. 12, 2012.

[4] A. Nasr, N. Khidir, Y. Mohamed et al., "A review study on patients radiation dose from diagnostic radiography," *International Journal of Science and Research*, vol. 2, pp. 372–378, 2013.

[5] Y. S. Cordoliani, P. Grenier, H. Beauvais, J. E. Grellet, D. E. Marshall, and M. Bourguignon, "Le point sur les procédures en radiologie conventionnelle et en tomodensitométrie," *Médecine Nucléaire Imagerie Fonctionnelle et Métabolique*, vol. 26, no. 5, pp. 241–246, 2002.

[6] C. J. Olowookere, I. A. Babalola, N. N. Jibiri, R. I. Obed, L. L. Bamidele, and E. O. A. Jetumobi, "A preliminary radiation dose audit in some nigerian hospitals : need for determination of national diagnostic reference levels (NDRLs)," *The Pacific Journal of Science and Technology*, vol. 13, no. 1, pp. 487–495, 2012.

[7] V. Tsapaki, I. A. Tsalafoutas, I. Chinofoti et al., "Radiation doses to patients undergoing standard radiographic examinations: a comparison between two methods," *British Journal of Radiology*, vol. 80, no. 950, pp. 107–112, 2007.

[8] K. Suchart and T. Montree, "An estimation of X-radiation output using mathematic model american," *Journal of Applied Sciences*, vol. 8, no. 9, pp. 923–926, 2011.

[9] K. Faulkner, D. A. Broadhead, and R. M. Harrison, "Patient dosimetry measurement methods," *Applied Radiation and Isotopes*, vol. 50, pp. 113–123, 1999.

[10] M. Davies, H. Mc Callum, G. White, J. Brown, and M. Hlem, "Patient dose audit in diagnostic radiography using custom designed software," *Radiography*, vol. 3, pp. 17–25, 1997.

[11] C. J. Olowookere, I. A. Babalola, M. O. Olayiwola, G. Odina, R. I. Obed, and T. O. Bello, "Comparison of five models for assessing patient dose from radiological examinations," *African Journal Medical Physik, Biomed Eng & Sc*, vol. 1, pp. 21–29, 2009.

[12] B. Moifo, M. Kamgnie, N. Ndeh Fointama, J. Tambe, H. Tebere, and F. J. Gonsu, "Évaluation de la conformité des demandes d'examens d'imagerie médicale : une expérience en Afrique subsaharienne," *Médecine et Santé Tropicales*, vol. 24, pp. 392–396, 2014.

[13] B. Moifo, U. Tene, J. R. Moulion Tapouh et al., "Knowledge on irradiation, medical imaging prescriptions, and clinical imaging referral guidelines among physicians in sub-saharan African country (Cameroon)," *Radiology Research and Pratice*, pp. 1–7, 2017.

[14] J. George, J. P. Eatough, P. J. Mountford, C. J. Koller, J. Oxtoby, and G. Frain, "Patient dose optimization in plain radiography based on standard exposure factors," *British Journal of Radiology*, vol. 77, no. 922, pp. 858–863, 2004.

[15] T. Sounkalo, *Étude Comparative de la Dose Patient À la Dose de Référence Dans le Service de Radiologie et d'Imagerie Médicale de L'Hôpital Gabriel Touré (HGT) À Propos de 70 Cas [Thèse de Médecine]*, Université de Bamako, Faculté de Médecine, de Pharmacie et d'Odontostomatologie (FMPOS), 2006.

[16] S. Singh, M. K. Kalra, and M. A. Moore, "Dose reduction and compliance with pediatric CT protocols adapted to patient size, clinical indication, and number of prior studies," *Radiology*, vol. 252, pp. 200–208, 2009.

[17] Z. P. Ongolo, B. S. Nguehouo, J. Yomi, and S. et Nkoo Amvene, "Connaissances en matière de radioprotection: enquête auprès des personnels des services hospitaliers de radiodiagnostic, radiothérapie et médecine nucléaire à Yaoundé," *Communication orale Journées Françaises de Radiologie*, pp. 21–25, 2011.

4

Audit of Radiology Request Form for Completion and Usefulness of Clinical History: Teaching Hospital Experience, Ghana

Bashiru Babatunde Jimah

Department of Medical Imaging, College of Health Sciences, University of Cape Coast, Cape Coast, Ghana

Correspondence should be addressed to Bashiru Babatunde Jimah; jimah@uccsms.edu.gh

Academic Editor: Daniele La Forgia

Background. The role of the "traditional" radiologist has shifted from imaging centered to patient focus, which underscores the utmost importance of the clinical radiologist in the multidisciplinary team in patient management. For the clinical radiologist to effectively play this key role, the referring clinician must provide adequate and useful patient information to assist the radiologist in making a diagnosis or provide differential diagnosis. The objectives were to assess the level of completion of the radiology request form and to determine whether the clinical history provided aided in the final impression/diagnosis. *Materials and Method.* We conducted a prospective review of 500 radiology request forms at the Cape Coast Teaching Hospital (CCTH) between September and October 2018. The forms were consecutively sampled and reviewed for each field/area such as patient's name, age, and clinical history. Data were analyzed descriptively for the level of completeness and usefulness of clinical history entered by the clinician. *Results.* No request form was completed in full. All the request forms did not have X-ray serial number and previous examination details documented. The proportions of forms with various fields completed were as follows: more than 90% of the forms had patient's name, investigation required, date of the request, doctor's name, and clinical history fields filled. The patient's age, patient's ward/address, and doctor's address were filled in 88%, 75%, and 18.4%, respectively. Twenty percent of the request forms were not useful to the radiologist in the final diagnosis. *Conclusion.* A significant proportion of radiology request forms are incompletely filled and therefore denies the radiologist, the critical information needed to make a diagnosis, or narrow differential diagnosis.

1. Introduction

The concept of "Lean Thinking in Healthcare" is an adoption from the auto and manufacturing industry which seeks to improve workflow, efficiency, and customer satisfaction [1]. This concept has been used in the United States and United Kingdom to improve the efficiency of pathology and emergency departments [1]. The concept, if implemented, can improve patient satisfaction by removing waste in the radiology department, from request form writing to delivery of reports to patients. The entire principle of the concept of "Lean Thinking" in the radiology department is beyond the scope of the current write up and will be discussed extensively in the upcoming paper "*The concept of Lean Thinking in Radiology, what must change in Ghana.*" This paper focuses on the completion of the various aspects of the request form and ways to improve the form.

The management of patient requires a multidisciplinary approach involving the radiologist and the clinician. Utmost importance of the clinical radiologist is the reflection of the evolving role of the "traditional" radiologist from an imaging centered to patient focus [2]. The radiologist role is to aid other colleagues in reaching their diagnosis and, since the advent of interventional radiology, provide treatment for various conditions. For the clinical radiologist to function effectively, it is imperative that the referring clinician provides adequately filled requisition forms.

The radiology request forms are clinical and legal documents, completed by a referring clinician or his/her surrogate, and serve to communicate the procedure required and the reasons for the procedure [3]. The guidelines of the Royal College of Radiologist (RCR) suggest that this request form should be completed adequately and legibly to avoid any misinterpretation [4]. A comparison of the American College of Radiology and the Royal College of Radiology shows that a radiology request form should contain the following information [5, 6]: the clinical background; the question to be answered; the patient's name, age, address, and telephone number; the ward; the name and signature of the requesting doctor; the name of the consultant responsible for the patient's well-being; and the date.

The forms provide the clinical question to be answered by the radiologist. Some diseases have similar radiographic patterns, and their elucidation requires adequate patient information. An incompletely filled form will make it difficult for the radiologist to narrow the differential diagnosis for certain imaging patterns. It may also lead to unnecessary investigations, increased hospital stay, repeated exposure to radiation, and delayed management of the patient with increased cost to the patient and the hospital.

The aim of this study is to assess the level of completion of the radiology request form and whether the clinical information provided aided in the final impression by the radiologist. This study did not assess the appropriateness of the request form.

2. Materials and Methods

A prospective review of the radiology request was conducted at the Cape Coast Teaching Hospital (CCTH) between September and October 2018. The Cape Coast Teaching Hospital is located within the Cape Coast Metropolis in the central region of Ghana. It is a 234-bed facility and serves as a tertiary referral center for the central and western regions. It serves as a teaching hospital for the University of Cape Coast School of Medical Sciences and Allied Health Science faculty. It is a residency training center for the Ghana College of Physicians and Surgeons.

Prior to the study, ethical approval was sought from the Ethical Review Committee of the Cape Coast Teaching Hospital.

The CCTH Department of Radiology receives paper request forms for various imaging modalities. The request forms are presented by the patients on the day of their investigation. A total of 500 readily available request forms were analyzed within one-month period of the study from inpatient and outpatient clinics of the CCTH, private hospitals, and public hospitals within central and western regions. The modalities included plain radiographs for radiologist's report (35), computed tomography scan (77), general ultrasonography: abdomen, pelvis, and small parts (300), vascular ultrasound scan (35), hysterosalpingography (21), mammography (24), and special studies (8) (barium enema, barium swallow, barium meal, MCUG, RUG, and distal loopogram).

We assessed each request form for the filling of all the fields on the form (demographics of patients/patient identifiers (age, name, and address), history/clinical information, investigation requested, demographics of the referring physician (name and address), X-ray serial number, previous serial number/previous exam details, and date of the request. The audit did not assess the appropriateness of the investigation requested.

Data were analyzed descriptively using percentages. The clinical history was considered "useful" if it contributed to the final impression/diagnosis and "not useful" if it did not contribute to the final impression/diagnosis.

3. Results

A total of 500 request forms were analyzed in the study. None of the forms were completely filled. Details of form completion are as shown in Figure 1. Almost all the request forms had the patients name filled (99.6%) except two (0.4%). The investigation requested was filled in 99.4%, and only three were not filled. The date and doctor's name were filled in 98.4% and 94%, respectively. The other fields such as the clinical history, age, patient's ward/address, and doctor's address/station were completed, respectively, in 92.2%, 88%, 75%, and 18.4%. X-ray serial number and previous serial number/previous exam details were not filled in any of the forms.

Figure 2 shows the level of usefulness of clinical information of request forms. Twenty percent (100/500) of the request forms (includes request forms with no clinical history and request forms with unhelpful clinical information) were not useful, which implies that they did not contribute to the final diagnosis or impression.

A total of 35 vascular ultrasound scan were requested which included peripheral venous and arterial studies. 31 (88.5%) of the requests were nonspecific (venous or arterial or both), and only 4 were specific for venous Doppler (Figure 3).

Fifty percent (250/500) of the request forms had abbreviations that did not suit the internationally recognized, particularly in areas such as the age, patient's ward/address, clinical history, and investigation (Table 1).

4. Discussion

Management of the patient requires a multidisciplinary approach that is based on adequate communication between the various team members, in order to provide the patient with the best possible service [2–4]. The radiology request form is an important communication tool between the managing clinician and the radiologist [3, 4, 6]. At CCTH, multidisciplinary board meetings and interdepartmental clinical meetings are organized routinely to review clinical activities within a period. The radiology requisition form has been an item often discussed to increase awareness of the importance of the information provided on the request form and to sensitize referring clinicians to adequately fill the form to aid the radiologist to narrow the differential diagnosis for certain imaging patterns.

Most studies show that there is a global deficiency in the completion of the radiology requisition form [2, 3, 6–9]. The study findings showed that none of the request form was completely filled. This is consistent with the findings by

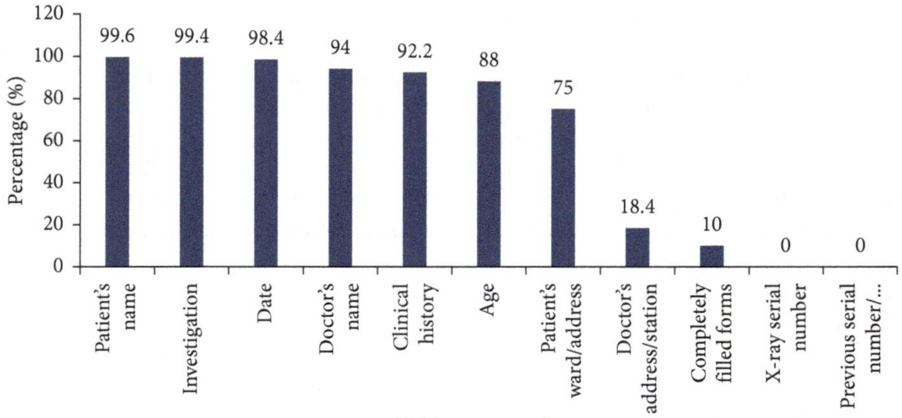

FIGURE 1: Proportion of forms with fields completely field.

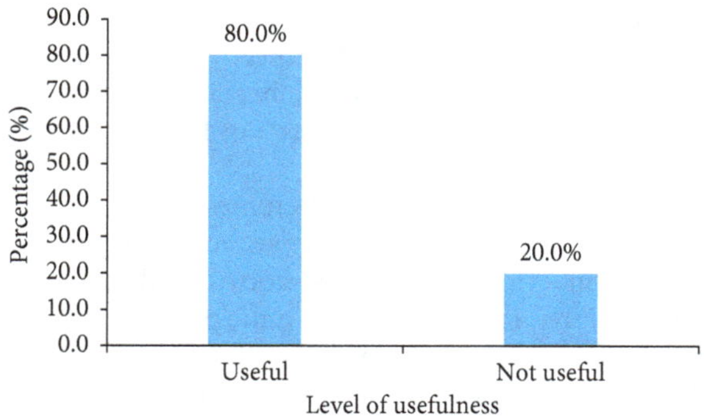

FIGURE 2: Usefulness of clinical information provided.

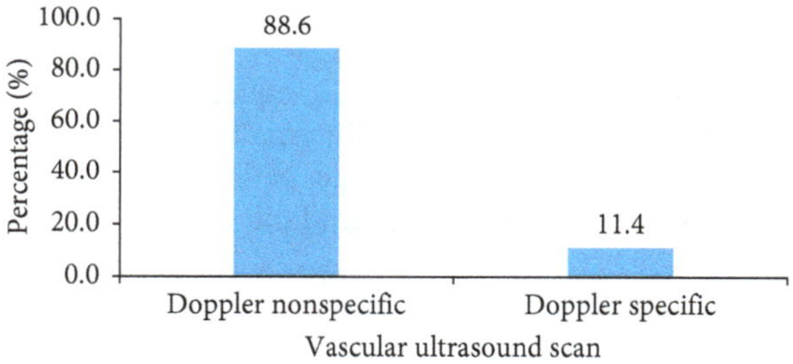

FIGURE 3: Category of request for vascular ultrasound.

Akinola et al. [6], and Depasquale and Crockford [2] found 4% of request forms fully filled. Seventy-five percent ($n = 375$) had patient's ward/address fully filled in this study, similar to the findings by Depasquale and Crockford [2] who found 77% of request form had addresses in their study, contrary to Akinola et al. [6] who found only 2.1% of request form with addresses. For most inpatients, the addresses will help the imaging department submit the report to reduce waiting time.

The findings showed that 99.6% of the forms had the names of the patients adequately filled. Similar observation was made by Agi et al. [8] who reported that all the forms reviewed had the names of the patients properly filled. Patient identifiers such as name are of utmost importance and must be included at all times.

It was surprising to see that 3 (0.6%) of the request form did not have any stated investigation to be performed, contrary to Agi et al. [8] who had 100% of the investigated stated. The radiologist had to take a clinical history from the patient and decide on the appropriate procedure. Such omissions may increase the waiting time, increase cost of transportation, and ultimately patient dissatisfaction.

The doctor's name and doctor's ward/address were found in 94% and 18.4%, respectively. In the study done by Akintomide et al. [7], 86% of the forms had medical officer's name provided and 24.4% of the medical officers provided their names in Akinola et al.'s [6] study. We observed that the doctors who provided their ward/address (18.4%) were predominantly on National Health Insurance request forms which makes it mandatory in others for claims to be paid. Occasionally, radiologists seek clarification on the information provided. The absence of doctor's information may deny the radiologist the needed patient information. This may potentially increase the reporting time or provide a wide range of differential diagnosis which may not help in the management of the patient.

Arterial or venous disease often has specific presenting complaint and must be stated. Most health facilities do not accept the National Health Insurance for Doppler investigations, and most patients do not have private insurance. Clients therefore have to pay out-of-pocket for these investigations. Cost of performing both arterial and venous studies as stated in Figure 4 is likely in the range of 1000–1400 Ghana Cedis. For only venous studies, the cost is likely 400–600 Ghana Cedis or 600–800 Ghana Cedis for arterial studies. It is therefore important to refer clinician's state clearly what is required to avoid unnecessary cost to the patient.

The result shows that 13.2% of the clinical information provided was not useful in arriving at the final impression, and 6.8% of the request forms analyzed did not provide any clinical information at all. This means that 20% of the request forms were not useful to the radiologist. Akinola et al. [6] found that request forms that provided adequate clinical history received radiologist reports that were more helpful in the management of the patients. This study shows that 80%

Table 1: Abbreviations on request forms that are not internationally recognized, CCTH.

Abbreviation	Referring clinician meaning	Internationally accepted meaning
A	Adult	Adenine, adenosine, alanine, ampere/amp, artery, vitamin A
MMW	Male medical ward	Medium molecular weight
FMW	Female medical ward	Formulated molecular weight
FSW	Female surgical ward	No medical meaning
CLD	Chronic liver disease	Chronic lung disease, cholestatic liver disease
HPT	Hypertension	Home pregnancy test
LAP	Lower abdominal pain	Left atrial pressures, laparoscopy/laparoscopic

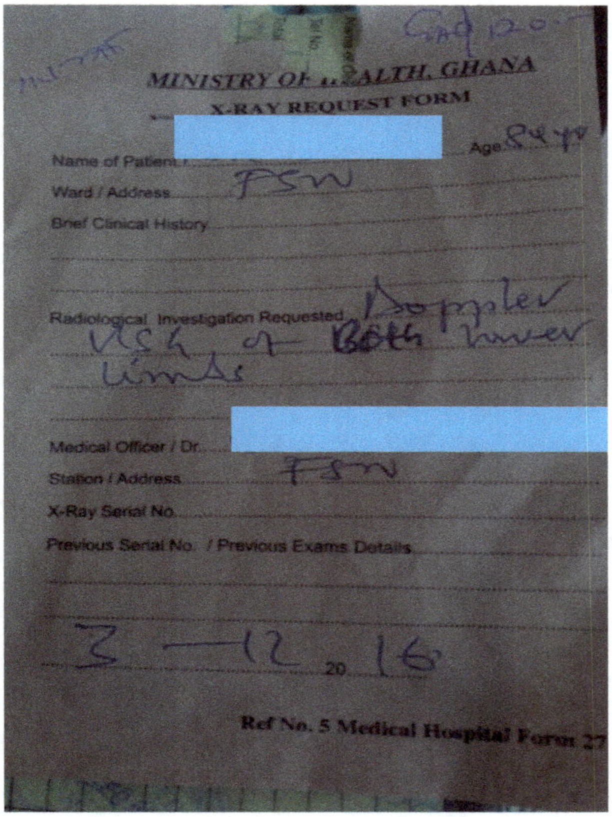
MINISTRY OF ..ALTH, GHANA
X-RAY REQUEST FORM
Name of Patient ... Age 84 yrs
Ward / Address ... FSW
Brief Clinical History ...
Radiological Investigation Requested ... Doppler USG of Both lower limbs
Medical Officer / Dr. ...
Station / Address ... FSW
X-Ray Serial No. ...
Previous Serial No. / Previous Exams Details ...
3—12 20 16
Ref No. 5 Medical Hospital Form 27

Figure 4: A sample of a request form. No clinical history is provided. The investigation requested is not specific as it has cost implications to the patient. The X-ray serial number and previous examination details were not provided. Unknown medical abbreviation is noted at ward/address.

of the request forms received had useful clinical information. This could be due to the prior in-service training to the various departments about the need to adequately fill the request forms. This finding is compared to the 100% clinical history found by Akinola et al. [6] and 71% by Akintomide et al. [7].

The radiology request form does not include the clinical question to be answered by the radiologist, and therefore, the radiologist must deduce the question from the clinical information provided by the clinician. The clinical question to be answered and the clinical information provided are important for the radiologist to decide whether the investigation requested will answer the question asked, to avoid exposing the patient to unnecessary radiation, decide on the protocol for the study, and aid in the final diagnosis or differential diagnoses [2, 6, 10]. Periodic education of referring clinicians is imperative to ram home this message.

Our review further showed that more than 50% of the request forms had abbreviations that are not internationally recognized. Fields with such abbreviations included the age, ward's/patient's address, clinical history, and investigation. Typical example is FMW, in our institution, which refers to female surgical ward but internationally represents formulated molecular weight [11]. Other internationally recognized abbreviations are OPD (outpatient department), AKI (acute kidney injury), HCC (hepatocellular carcinoma), CKD (chronic kidney disease), TIA (transient ischemic attack), CVA (cerebrovascular accident), RIF (right iliac fossa), LT (left), RT (right), ? (query/question), # (fracture), CXR (chest radiograph), USG (ultrasonography), CT (computed tomography), mammo (mammography), HSG (hysterosalpingography), ICSOL (intracranial space occupying lesion), Paeds (paediatrics), and RUG (retrograde urethrogram) [11].

Our review showed that all the referring doctors failed to include their contacts to allow the radiologist to probe for further information. This observation in practice is contrary to the guidelines proposed by the Royal College of radiology calling on referring clinician to provide the contact details [4, 5]. In our experience at our institution, referring clinicians are contacted through the hospital or regional platforms. Despite the perceived challenges, effective communication is necessary between radiologist and referring clinicians, and it must be a concern for a multidisciplinary management team.

5. Conclusion

A significant proportion of radiology request forms are incompletely filled and therefore denies the radiologist, the critical information needed to make a diagnosis or narrow differential diagnosis. Attitudinal change among referring clinicians in filling radiology request form will be essential in effective diagnosis and management of patients.

5.1. Recommendation. In line with the study findings and discussions on the possible actions or changes that could be implemented in order to reach this goal, we recommend the following:

(i) The Ministry of Health/Ghana Health Service should review the current radiology request form to suit international best practice and ensure its adoption by all health facilities (both public and private)

(ii) The X-ray serial number and previous serial number/previous exam details must be removed from the current request form and replaced with findings of previous exams if any

(iii) The transition from the paper-based to the paperless system in most hospitals, including Cape Coast Teaching Hospital, should ensure that electronic request forms meet the international best practice

(iv) All electronic request forms should ensure that all aspects of the forms are filled before it can be transmitted to the imaging department

(v) Frontline staff at the imaging department should be trained to return any inadequately completed forms to referring clinician who still uses the paper-based forms

(vi) Completion of the request form should be part of the orientation for new doctors and periodic in-service training for all clinicians and physician assistants

Acknowledgments

The author acknowledges the contributions of Dr. Augustina Badu-Peprah and Prof. Rahman Ganiyu.

References

[1] T. P. Young, S. I. McClean, Young, and S. I. McClean, "A critical look at Lean Thinking in healthcare," *Quality and Safety in Health Care*, vol. 17, no. 5, pp. 382–386, 2008.

[2] R. Depasquale and M. Crockford, "Are radiology request forms adequately filled in? An audit assessing local practice," *Malta Medical Journal*, vol. 17, no. 4, pp. 36–38, 2005.

[3] M. D. Cohen, S. Curtin, and R. Lee, "Evaluation of the quality of radiology requisitions for intensive care unit patients," *Academic Radiology*, vol. 13, no. 2, pp. 236–240, 2006.

[4] D. Remedios and P. McCoubrie, "Making the best use of clinical radiology services: a new approach to referral guidelines," *Clinical Radiology*, vol. 62, no. 10, pp. 919-920, 2007.

[5] Royal College of Radiologists, *Making the Best Use of a Department of Clinical Radiology: Guidelines for Doctors*, Royal College of Radiologists (RCR), London, UK, 5th edition, 2003.

[6] R. Akinola, M. Akinkunmi, K. Wright, and O. Orogbemi, "Radiology request forms: are they adequately filled by clinicians?" *The Internet Journal of Radiology*, vol. 12, no. 1, 2012.

[7] A. Akintomide, A. Ikpeme, A. Ngaji, N. Ani, and A. Udofia, "An audit of the completion of radiology request forms and the request practice," *Journal of Family Medicine and Primary Care*, vol. 4, no. 3, p. 328, 2015.

[8] C. Agi, P. J. Alagoa, and B. G. Fente, "A simple audit of radiological request forms at the university of port harcourt teaching hospital," *IPageifil*, vol. 15, no. 4, pp. 2–5, 2015.

[9] J. Prasad, D. K. A. Meena, D. k. Meena, and D. Meena, "Imaging of intracranial space occupying lesions: a prospective study in a tertiary care centre in northern westran Rajasthan," *The International Journal of Current Advanced Research*, vol. 6, no. 4, pp. 3254–3256, 2017.

[10] Glick, Yair J. B. D. Medical Abbreviations and Acronyms (I) Radiology Reference Article Radiopaedia, 2020.

[11] All Acronyms Abbreviations for Medical:Medical Related Acronyms and Abbreviations, 2020.

5

Occurrence of the Elongated Styloid Process on Digital Panoramic Radiographs in the Riyadh Population

Lingam Amara Swapna[1] **Nada Tarek AlMegbil**[1] **Alhanouf Othman Almutlaq**[1] **and Pradeep Koppolu**[2]

[1]*Department of Surgical and Diagnostic Sciences, College of Dentistry, Dar Al Uloom University, Riyadh 13314, Saudi Arabia*
[2]*Department of Preventive Dental Sciences, College of Dentistry, Dar Al Uloom University, Riyadh 13314, Saudi Arabia*

Correspondence should be addressed to Lingam Amara Swapna; laswapna123@gmail.com

Academic Editor: Maryam Tofangchiha

Background. Patients with an elongated styloid process might present with dysphagia and pain in the cervicofacial region. These patients could be misdiagnosed as other orofacial pathologies. *Aim.* The present study attempted to assess the prevalence of the elongated styloid process on digital panoramic radiographs in the Riyadh population. *Materials and Methods.* The present prospective randomized study was conducted on the panoramic digital radiographs of 300 randomly selected patients visiting a private dental hospital to identify any elongation of the styloid process. Only the radiographs without any magnification errors were considered. The styloid process length was measured using the Sidexis measuring tool and entered in an Excel spreadsheet with other demographic data. A length beyond 30 mm was considered styloid process elongation. The data were subjected to statistical analysis. *Results.* The symptoms of styloid process elongation were higher among females (78.6%), and this difference was statistically significant ($\chi^2 = 7.182$; $P = 0.007$). No statistically significant association was observed between styloid process elongation and symptoms between different age groups. Females exhibited a significant longer mean length of the styloid process than males. The present study exhibited a 27.3% prevalence for the elongation and calcification of the styloid process. *Conclusion.* Given the significant prevalence of the elongated styloid process in our study, we recommend it to be considered as one of the differential diagnosis for pain or discomfort in the orofacial region.

1. Introduction

The styloid process is a slender bony process starting from the lower portion of the temporal bone anteromedial to the stylomastoid foramen [1]. The term styloid has originated from the Greek word "stylos," which means "pillar" [2]. The process is attached to the lesser cornu of the hyoid bone through the styloid ligament and is flanked on both sides by the external and internal carotid arteries [3]. The normal length of the styloid process is from 15 mm to 30 mm. A length of >30 mm is regarded as elongated [4]. The prevalence of an elongated styloid process in the general population ranges 2%–52% in various studies [5, 6].

The symptomatic elongation of the styloid process is termed as Eagle syndrome. This pathology was first reported in 1937 by the otorhinolaryngologist, Eagle, who termed it stylalgia [7]. Patients with Eagle syndrome present with dysphagia, pain in the cervicofacial region and neck, and pain at the mandibular angle, which aggravate with neck rotation or tongue protrusion. These features may be due to the pressure that the elongated styloid process exerts on the adjacent neurovascular structures [8]. However, the presentation of this pathology may be confusing in a clinical setting and may be misinterpreted as unerupted or impacted tooth, cranial nerve neuralgias, temporal arthritis, temporomandibular joint disorders, migraine, pharyngotonsillitis, and benign and malignant tumors [9, 10]. This may lead to unnecessary invasive diagnostic and therapeutic procedures. Additionally, an elongated styloid process may also cause stroke due to the compression of carotid arteries [11].

Thus, an elongated styloid process must be diagnosed accurately and considered as a differential diagnosis in orofacial pain. Therefore, the present study attempts to evaluate the prevalence of styloid process elongation and its association with demographic factors in the population in Riyadh.

2. Materials and Methods

The present cross-sectional observational study was conducted in 300 patients above 14 years of age in Dar Al Uloom University Hospital, Riyadh, Saudi Arabia, from August 2020 to April 2021, after institutional ethics clearance. The study was conducted according to the guidelines of the Declaration of Helsinki and approved by the Institutional Review Board of College of Dentistry, Dar Al Uloom University, Riyadh, KSA (COD/IRB/2020/5). Both verbal and written consent was obtained from all patients. The patients visiting the dental clinics were randomly selected. Radiographs clearly exhibiting bilateral styloid processes with minimal or no magnification were included in the study. Radiographs exhibiting magnification errors were excluded from the study.

The digital panoramic radiographs of all 300 patients were obtained, and data regarding the same were obtained from the university hospital systems (Sidexis). These panoramic radiographs were taken with a digital panoramic orthophos XG system (Sirona Company) using exposure factors as per manufacturer' instruction. The length of the styloid process was measured from the junction of the process and the tympanic plate to the tip of the process. In case of a segmented styloid process, the measurement was performed in the same manner. The ossification of the stylohyoid or stylomandibular ligaments, if present, was considered a part of the elongated styloid process, and measurements were performed accordingly. A styloid process greater than 30 mm long was considered as elongated.

The patients were interviewed in either Arabic or English depending on their comfort. Extraoral examination was then carried out. The neck region of the patients was palpated for any signs of styloid process elongation. Additional patient information was obtained from the hospital electronic file system (Open Dental). A Sidexis ruler was used to calculate the length of the styloid process in the radiographs (Figure 1).

The data were collected and entered in MS Excel. The results were analyzed using SPSS version 22.0. The association between the different parameters was analyzed using the chi-square test, and $P < 0.05$ was considered statistically significant.

3. Results

The characteristics of the study population are given in Table 1. In the present study, majority of the samples were males ($n = 166$; 55.3%). The majority of patients were in the age group of 20–29 years (34%), followed by 30–39 years (23.3%), 40–49 years (19.3%), above 50 years (12.7%), and less than 20 years (10.7%). The prevalence of elongation and calcification patterns of the styloid process was 27.3% ($n = 82$). Among the patients with positive symptoms ($n = 28$; 9.3%), 4.7% ($n = 14$) exhibited symptoms on the right side and 6% ($n = 18$) exhibited symptoms on the left side. Of these, 4 patients had bilateral symptoms.

Chi-square analysis displayed no statistically significant association among styloid process elongation ($\chi^2 = 4.909$; $P = 0.297$), symptoms ($\chi^2 = 3.357$; $P = 0.5$), and sides of the symptoms ($\chi^2 = 3.78$; $P = 0.706$) with different age groups. Chi-square analysis displayed significantly higher symptoms of styloid process elongation in females (78.6%) compared with males (21.4%) ($\chi^2 = 7.182$; $P = 0.007$). No significant difference was observed in the occurrence of styloid process elongation and symptoms on left and right between males and females ($P > 0.05$).

Table 2 provides the association of styloid process elongation, symptoms, and sides of the symptoms between different age groups. No statistically significant association was observed between styloid process elongation ($\chi^2 = 4.909$; $P = 0.297$), symptoms ($\chi^2 = 3.357$; $P = 0.5$), and sides of the symptoms ($\chi^2 = 3.78$; $P = 0.706$) between different age groups.

Table 3 provides the association of styloid process elongation, symptoms, and sides of the symptoms between males and females. No statistically significant difference was observed between styloid process elongation between males and females ($P > 0.05$). However, the symptoms of styloid process elongation were higher among females (78.6%), and this difference was statistically significant ($\chi^2 = 7.182$; $P = 0.007$).

4. Discussion

Eagle syndrome may cause symptoms such as orofacial pain, which might be confusing to clinicians [8]. All clinicians must be aware of the clinical and radiological signs and symptoms of styloid process elongation to accurately diagnose and treat symptoms in the cervicofacial region. The present study thus attempts to evaluate the prevalence of styloid process elongation in the Riyadh population and its association with demographic factors.

The present study was conducted on digital panoramic radiographs. Numerous imaging modalities can be used for the diagnosis of styloid process elongation. These include modalities such as lateral skull radiograph, Towne's view, anterioposterior skull radiograph, and computed tomography (CT) scan [12]. However, digital panoramic radiographs can be easily performed and interpreted. Additionally, they expose the patients to a lower radiation dose and cost much lesser than CT. Thus, this procedure can be easily used for epidemiological evaluations [13]. Furthermore, digital panoramic radiographs are commonly prescribed for orofacial pain, and a styloid process elongation is usually an accidental finding on these radiographs. So, we opted for this diagnostic modality in the present study.

The present study exhibited a prevalence of 27.3% for the elongation and calcification of the styloid process. This finding was concurrent with those of Bozkir et al., Keur et al.,

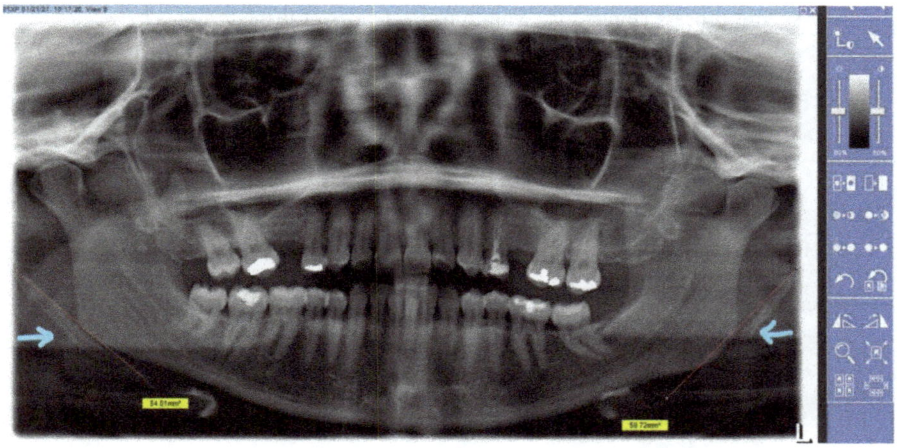

FIGURE 1: Measuring the elongated styloid process on both sides.

TABLE 1: Characteristics of the study population.

Age and sex distribution in the population				
			Frequency	%
Age groups	Less than 20 years		32	10.7
	20–29		102	34
	30–39		70	23.3
	40–49		58	19.3
	Above 50 years		38	12.7
Sex	Female		134	44.7
	Male		166	55.3
Mean age among sexes				
		N	Mean age	SD
Sex	Female	134	31.49	11.70
	Male	166	35.47	13.67
Total		300	33.69	12.94
Distribution of elongation of the styloid process				
			Frequency	%
Elongated	No		218	72.7
	Yes		82	27.3
Distribution of symptoms between sides				
			Frequency	%
Symptoms	No		172	90.7
	Yes		28	9.3
Symptoms right	No		286	95.3
	Yes		14	4.7
Symptoms left	No		282	94
	Yes		18	6

N, number of samples; SD, standard deviation.

and Scaf et al., who exhibit prevalence rates less than 30% [14]. However, this finding was in contrast with the findings of AlZarea and Bagga et al. [2, 6]. Bagga et al. reported a prevalence of 52.1% for the elongated styloid process. This difference in prevalence may be explained by the differing geographic area as the study was conducted in Mathura. The authors explained this high prevalence by the fact that majority of the population perform strenuous works such as carrying heavy weights on their heads and chew hard foods such as gutka and areca nut, which may promote the ossification of the ligaments attached to the styloid process [6]. However, the study on AlZ area, exhibiting a prevalence of 43.93% for the elongated styloid process, was conducted in Saudi Arabia itself. However, the population studied was >60 years of age. As the present study included patients as young as 14 years, the age difference in the study population may account for the difference in prevalence.

The difference in the length of the styloid process between different age groups in this study was statistically nonsignificant. This finding was in contrast to the findings of More and Asrani, Bruno et al., and Jamal et al., who reported a progressive increase in the length of the styloid process with aging [12–15]. Additionally, the present study presented a longer mean length of the styloid process in females (right side: 16.04 ± 16.88 mm; left side: 16.44 ± 17.31 mm) compared with males (right side: 12.51 ± 16.38 mm; left side: 13.86 ± 16.89 mm). This finding is in contrast with those of More and Asrani and Jamal et al., who reported longer styloid processes in males as compared with females [12, 15]. However, these findings were concurrent with the findings of Magat and Ozcan, who reported no significant difference in the length of the styloid process between males and females, and Ferrario et al., who reported a longer styloid process length in females [16, 17].

Out of the 34 females with elongated styloid processes in the present study, 22 (78.60%) exhibited symptoms, whereas only 6 (21.40%) of the 48 males with elongated processes exhibited symptoms. This difference was statistically significant ($P = 0.007$). This may be due to the lower pain threshold in females [18].

The present study has certain limitations. Langlais et al. classified the radiographic images of the elongated styloid process into three types based on morphology of elongation, namely, type I: elongated, type II: pseudoarticulated, and type III: segmented [19]. The present study did not take this classification under consideration. The relatively small sample size and the single-centre design of the study prevent the generalization of the findings. Additionally, digital panoramic radiography is prone to magnification errors, which may confound findings. Future multicentre studies with a larger sample size will further strengthen the findings of this study.

TABLE 2: Association of styloid process elongation, symptoms, and sides of the symptoms between different age groups.

Mean length among age groups (in mm)			
Age groups		Right	Left
	N	32	32
Less than 20 years	Mean	13.40	12.73
	SD	17.03	15.03
	N	102	102
20–29	Mean	12.85	11.43
	SD	17.01	16.93
	N	70	70
30–39	Mean	16.22	19.81
	SD	17.56	18.07
	N	58	58
40–49	Mean	13.77	16.69
	SD	15.89	17.14
	N	38	38
Above 50 years	Mean	14.54	15.15
	SD	16.06	16.23
	N	300	300
Total	Mean	14.09	15.01
	SD	16.64	17.07

Association of styloid process elongation among different age groups										
			Age groups					χ^2 value	P value
			Less than 20 years	20–29	30–39	40–49	Above 50 years		
Elongated	No	N	28	70	44	46	30	4.909	0.297
	Yes	N	4	32	26	12	8		
Symptoms	No	N	30	88	64	52	38	3.357	0.5
	Yes	N	2	14	6	6	0		

*Statistical significance set at 0.05; N, number of samples; χ^2 value, chi-square value.

TABLE 3: Association of styloid process elongation, symptoms, and sides of the symptoms between males and females.

Mean length among males and females (in mm)			
Sex		Right	Left
	N	134	134
Female	Mean	16.04	16.44
	SD	16.88	17.31
	N	166	166
Male	Mean	12.51	13.86
	SD	16.38	16.89
	N	300	300
Total	Mean	14.09	15.01
	SD	16.64	17.07

Association of styloid process elongation among males and females						
			Sex		χ^2 value	P value
			Female	Male		
Elongated	No	N	100	118	0.234	0.628
	Yes	N	34	48		
Symptoms	No	N	112	160	7.182	0.007*
	Yes	N	22	6		

*Statistical significance set at 0.05; N, number of samples; χ^2 value, chi-square value.

5. Conclusion

As styloid process elongation may be an accidental finding during radiographic examination, practitioners must remember to look for the same when patients visit with pain in the cervicofacial region. The present study exhibited a prevalence of 27.3% for the elongation and calcification of the styloid process. Thus, it must be considered as a differential diagnosis for pain or discomfort in the orofacial region.

Consent

Informed consent was obtained from all subjects involved in the study.

Authors' Contributions

A.L conceptualized, collected resources, visualized, reviewed, and edited the study. A.L, A.A, P.K, and N.A developed methodology. N.A, A.A, and A.L developed software, validated and investigated the study, and wrote the original draft. N.A and A.A performed formal analysis. A.L and P.K involved in data curation and supervised the study. All authors have read and agreed to the published version of the manuscript.

Acknowledgments

The authors extend their appreciation to the Deanship of Postgraduate and Scientific Research at Dar Al Uloom University, Riyadh, KSA, for supporting this work.

References

[1] S. Standring, *Gray's Anatomy the Anatomical Basis of Clinical Practice*, Elsevier, Amsterdam, Netherlands, 39th edition, p. 470, 2005, Skull and Mandible.

[2] B. K. AlZarea, "Prevalence and pattern of the elongated styloid process among geriatric patients in Saudi Arabia," *Clinical Interventions in Aging*, vol. 12, no. 30, pp. 611-617, 2017.

[3] Iannucci, M. Joen, and L. Jansen Howerton, *Dental Radiography: Principles and Techniques*, Elsevier, St. Louis, Missouri, 2017.

[4] J. Alkhabuli, H. Zakaria, and A. Muayad, "Prevalence of stylohyoid complex elongation among patients attending RAK College of dental sciences clinic," *Acta Stomatologica Croatica*, vol. 54, no. 1, pp. 60–68, 2020.

[5] E. M. Vieira, O. A. Guedes, S. D. Morais, C. R. Musis, P. A. Albuquerque, and Á. H. Borges, "Prevalence of elongated styloid process in a central Brazilian population," *Journal of Clinical and Diagnostic Research: JCDR*, vol. 9, pp. ZC90–ZC92, 2015.

[6] M. B. Bagga, C. A. Kumar, and G. Yeluri, "Clinicoradiologic evaluation of styloid process calcification," *Imaging Science in Dentistry*, vol. 42, no. 3, pp. 155-161, 2012.

[7] W. W. Eagle, "Elongated styloid processes: report of two cases," *Archives of Otolaryngology-Head and Neck Surgery*, vol. 25, no. 5, pp. 584–587, 1937.

[8] D. Raina, R. Gothi, and S. Rajan, "Eagle syndrome," *Indian Journal of Radiology and Imaging*, vol. 19, no. 02, pp. 107-108, 2009.

[9] M. A. Baseer and M. S. Alenazy, "Eagle's syndrome: a rare case of young female," *Dental Research Journal*, vol. 10, pp. 568–570, 2013.

[10] G. Krennmair and E. Piehslinger, "Variations of ossification in the stylohyoid chain," *Cranio*, vol. 21, no. 1, pp. 31–37, 2003.

[11] F. Asutay, N. F. Erdem, Y. Atalay, A. H. Acar, and H. Asutay, "Prevalence of elongated styloid process and eagle syndrome in east eagean population," *Bezmialem Science*, vol. 7, no. 1, pp. 28–32, 2019.

[12] C. B. More and M. K. Asrani, "Evaluation of the styloid process on digital panoramic radiographs," *The Indian Journal of Radiology & Imaging*, vol. 20, no. 4, pp. 261–265, 2010.

[13] G. Bruno, A. De Stefani, P. Balasso, S. Mazzoleni, and A. Gracco, "Elongated styloid process: an epidemiological study on digital panoramic radiographs," *Journal of Clinical and Experimental Dentistry*, vol. 9, no. 12, pp. e1446–52, 2017.

[14] G. Scaf, D. Q. d. Freitas, and L. d. C. M. Loffredo, "Diagnostic reproducibility of the elongated styloid process," *Journal of Applied Oral Science*, vol. 11, no. 2, pp. 120–124, 2003.

[15] B. T. Jamal, K. K. Ravikumar, S. H. Alyawar et al., "Prevalence of elongated styloid process and elongation pattern on digital panoramic radiographs in Saudi Population, Jeddah," *International Journal of Psychosocial Rehabilitation*, vol. 3, pp. 37–39, 2018.

[16] G. Magat and S. Ozcan, "Evaluation of styloid process morphology and calcification types in both genders with different ages and dental status," *Journal of Istanbul University Faculty of Dentistry*, vol. 51, no. 2, pp. 29–36, 2017.

[17] V. F. Ferrario, D. Sigurta, A. Daddona et al., "Calcification of the stylohyoid ligament: incidence and morphoquantative evaluation," *Oral Surgery, Oral Medicine, Oral Pathology*, vol. 69, no. 4, pp. 524–529, 1990.

[18] W. G. Lombana, S. E. G. Vidal, and G. Vida, "Pain and gender differences: a clinical approach," *Colombian Journal of Anesthesiology*, vol. 40, no. 3, pp. 207-212, 2012.

[19] R. P. Langlais, D. A. Miles, and M. L. Van Dis, "Elongated and mineralized stylohyoid ligament complex: a proposed classification and report of a case of Eagle's syndrome," *Oral Surgery, Oral Medicine, Oral Pathology*, vol. 61, no. 5, pp. 527–532, 1986.

6

Maxillary Incisive Canal Characteristics: A Radiographic Study Using Cone Beam Computerized Tomography

Penala Soumya[1], **Pradeep Koppolu**[2], **Krishnajaneya Reddy Pathakota**[3] **and Vani Chappidi**[4]

[1]*Department of Dentistry, Mahavir Institute of Medical Sciences, Vikarabad, Telangana, India*
[2]*Department of Preventive Dental Sciences, College of Dentistry, Dar Al Uloom University, Riyadh, Saudi Arabia*
[3]*Department of Peroiodontics, Sri Sai College of Dental Surgery, Vikarabad, India*
[4]*Department of Oral Medicine and Radiology, Sri Sai College of Dental Surgery, Vikarabad, Telangana, India*

Correspondence should be addressed to Penala Soumya; penalasoumya@gmail.com

Academic Editor: Paul Sijens

Background. The incisive canal located at the midline, posterior to the central incisor, is an important anatomic structure of this area to be considered while planning for immediate implant placement in maxillary central incisor region. The purpose of the present study is to assess incisive canal characteristics using CBCT sections. *Materials and Methods*. CBCT scans of 79 systemically healthy patients, with intact maxillary incisors, were evaluated by two calibrated and independent examiners. Assessments included (1) mesiodistal diameter, (2) labiopalatal diameter, (3) length of the incisive canal, (4) shape of incisive canal, and (5) width of the bone anterior to the incisive foramen. *Results*. The mean width of the foramen labiopalatally and mesiodistally was 3.12 ± 0.94 mm and 3.23 ± 0.98 mm, respectively. Mean canal length was 18.63 ± 2.35 mm and males have significantly longer incisive canal than females. The mean width of bone anterior to the incisive canal was 6.32 ± 1.43 mm. As age of the subjects increased, incisive foramen diameter and incisive canal length were found to be increased. Cylindrical shaped incisive canals were seen in most of the individuals followed by funnel shaped and hour-glass shaped canals, and banana-like canal is least prevalent type. *Conclusion*. The findings from the present study suggest that the diameter and length of incisive canal vary among different individuals and presence of very thin bone anterior to the canal would suggest that a pretreatment CBCT scan is a valuable tool to evaluate anatomic variations, morphology, and dimensions of incisive foramen before immediate implant placement in maxillary central incisor region.

1. Introduction

Immediate implant placement is gaining much of clinical importance in recent years and requires a thorough knowledge of important anatomic structures in concerned area. Implant placement in maxillary central incisor region is often challenging due to anatomical variations in dimensions of incisive canal and foramen. Incisive canal has two openings: incisive foramen and nasopalatine foramen [1]. The nasopalatine nerves and vessels traverse through this canal. Placement of implant into incisive canal results in nervous tissue injury, sensory dysfunction, and nonosseointegration of implant.

Several morphological alterations in the incisive canal shape have been described; Mardinger et al. [2] classified incisive canal shape as cylindrical, funnel like, banana like, and hour-glass like. Size, shape, position, and number of foramina vary in different individuals. Presence of wider foramina and thin alveolar bone anterior to the canal may make an implant placement almost impossible in this area.

Careful evaluation and planning are necessary before an immediate implant placement in anterior maxilla. Clinically sound and sophisticated radiograph techniques such as dental CTs can assist in diagnosing deficiencies. Preoperative CBCT of maxillary incisor region helps in diagnosing any anatomical difficulties before proceeding with an implant placement. CBCT is noninvasive, has high resolution, low dose of radiation, and financial advantage, and allows full 3D characterization of alveolar bone.

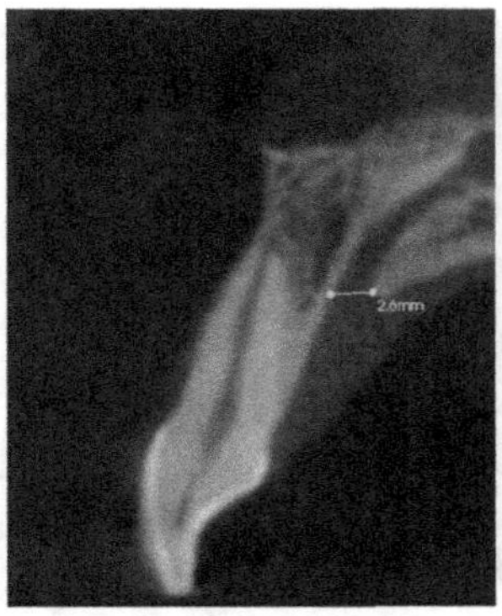

(a) Sagittal section showing measurement of labiopalatal width of incisive foramen

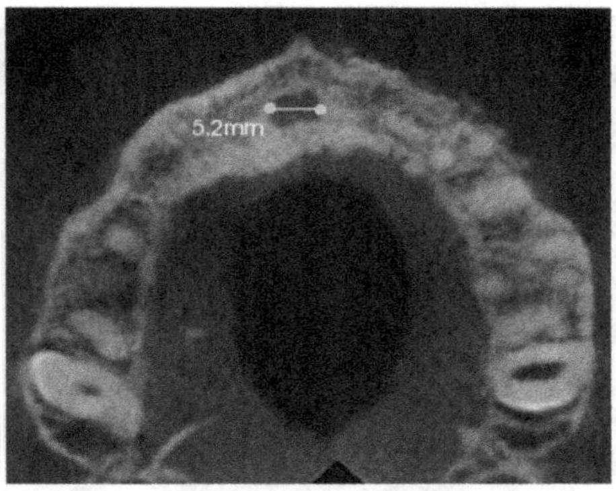

(b) Axial section showing measurement of mesiodistal width of incisive foramen

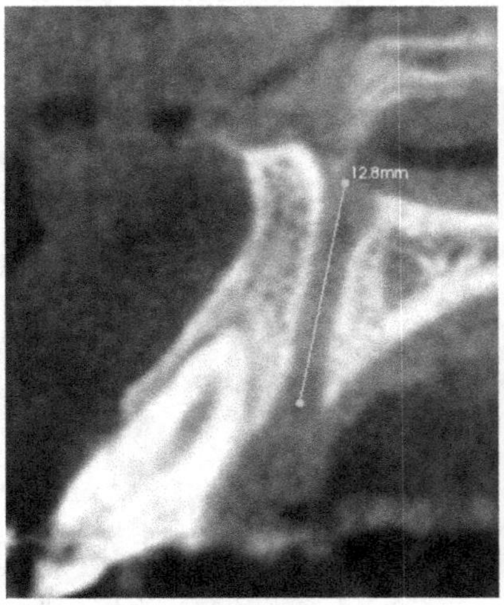

(c) Sagittal section showing measurement of length of incisive canal

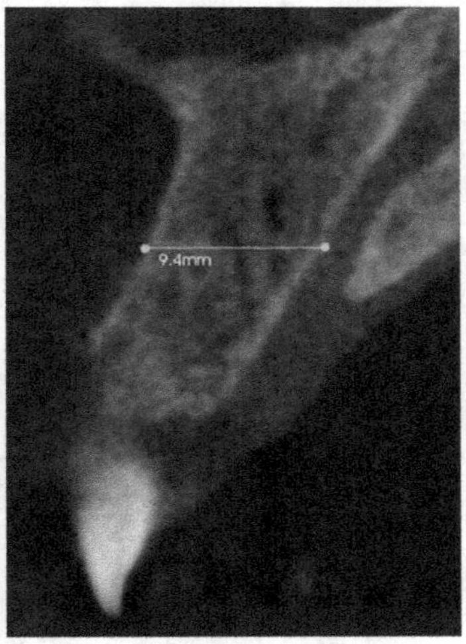

(d) Sagittal section showing measurement of width of labial bone anterior to the incisive canal

FIGURE 1

The aim of this study was to determine maxillary incisive canal characteristics in relation to the maxillary central incisors using CBCT images.

2. Materials and Methods

Hundred systemically healthy dentulous and/or partially edentulous patients (53 males and 47 females) aged between 17 and 72 years (with a mean age of 42.7 years) scheduled for implant insertion in different dental clinics in Hyderabad were included in the study. Written informed consent was obtained from all the patients and the Ethical Committee of Sri Sai College of Dental Surgery approved this study. Subjects with missing maxillary incisors, with evident nasopalatine pathology, and images with poor quality are excluded.

All CBCT scans were obtained with 1 mm slice thickness and the tomographic scanner CS 9000C 3D CBCT scanner with exposure settings of 120 kV, 15 mA, and 12-inch field of view was used to obtain CBCT scan. A software program, Care stream 3D Imaging software, was used to reconstruct the images and perform the measurements.

2.1. Interexaminer Calibration. Two observers were calibrated using 10 randomly selected scans. An assessment of the reproducibility of measurement between observers measuring the same quantity to one-tenth of a millimeter was calculated at a correlation of 0.95 for the 10 scans. Each of the two observers measured 79 scans independently at the exact same slice and magnification.

2.2. Parameters Evaluated. The following characteristics of incisive were evaluated:

(1) Width of the nasopalatine canal labiopalatally and mesiodistally (Figures 1(a) and 1(b))

(2) Length of the canal (Figure 1(c))

(3) Width of the bone anterior to the canal (Figure 1(d))

(4) Shape of the canal (Figures 2(a)–2(d))

Comparison of characteristics between males and females and correlation with age is done.

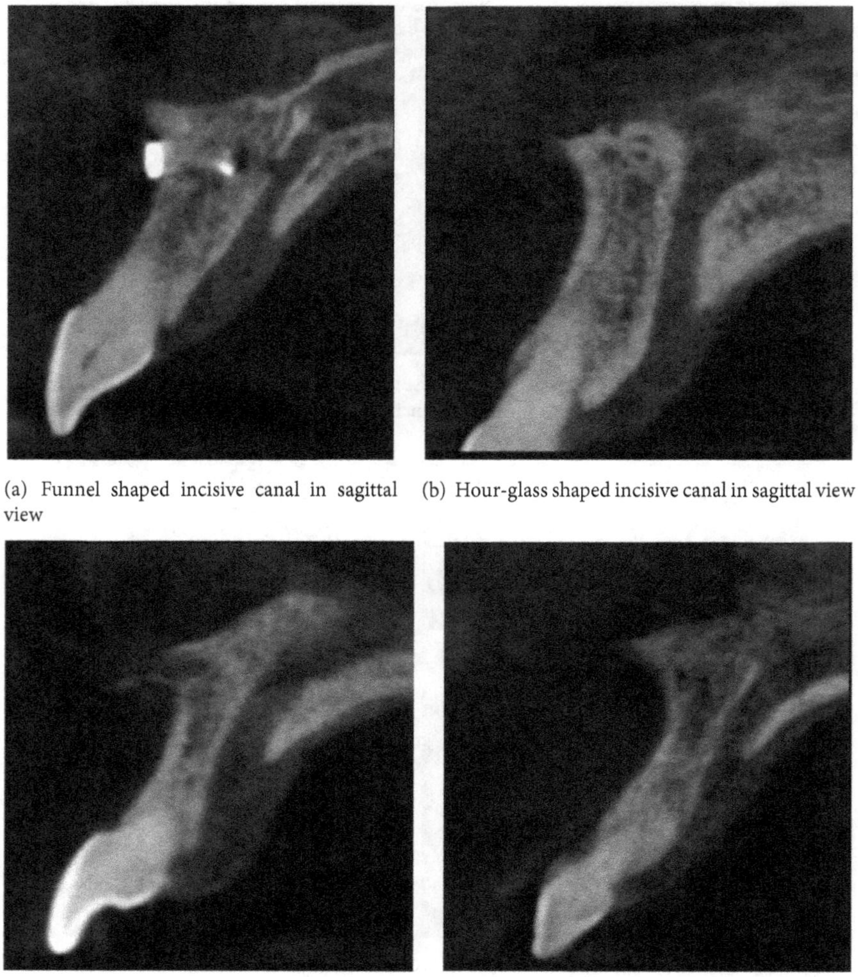

(a) Funnel shaped incisive canal in sagittal view (b) Hour-glass shaped incisive canal in sagittal view

(c) Cylindrical shaped incisive canal in sagittal view (d) Banana-like incisive canal in sagittal view

FIGURE 2

3. Statistical Analysis

Mean and standard deviations (SD) were calculated for all the variables. All statistical analysis was performed using SPSS version 18.0. Independent sample t test was used to compare the incisive canal characteristics between male and female subjects. Analysis of variance (ANOVA) was used to evaluate the influence of age on the incisive canal characteristics. A p value <0.05 was considered to be statistically significant and a p value <0.001 is considered to be highly statistically significant.

4. Results

Initially CT scans of 100 patients were assessed, of which 21 were excluded. A total of 79 scans were evaluated for the determined parameters. Mean length of canal was 18.63 ± 2.35 mm. Mean diameter of the nasopalatine canal mesiodistally was 3.23 ± 0.98 mm, and labiopalatally it was 3.12 ± 0.94 mm. Mean width of the bone anterior to the foramen was found to be 6.32 ± 1.43 mm (Table 1).

TABLE 1: Demographic variables and descriptive statistics of 79 individuals.

Descriptive statistics	Mean ± SD
Age	42.36 ± 16.44 years
Canal length	18.63 ± 2.35 mm
Mesiodistal width	3.23 ± 0.98 mm
Labiopalatal width	3.12 ± 0.94 mm
Width of the bone anterior to the canal	6.32 ± 1.43 mm

When the influence of age on the canal length was assessed, it was observed to be increasing with age. Younger individuals are found to have significantly smaller length of incisive canal when compared to older individuals and this was found to be statistically significant (Table 2). When males and females were compared, i.e., when the effect of gender was evaluated, there was no significant difference between male and female subjects (Table 2).

When the effect of age on the diameter of incisive canal was evaluated, there was a statistically significant (p<0.05)

TABLE 2: Comparison of incisive canal characteristics according to age using ANOVA.

Parameter	<30 years (n=23)	31-50 (n=23)	>50 (n=33)	p value
Canal length	14.7 ± 1.41	16.93 ± 1.25	19.13 ± 1.61	<0.0001*
Mesiodistal width	3 ± 0.75	2.92 ± 0.89	3.71 ± 1.07	0.003*
Labiopalatal width	2.81 ± 0.98	2.86 ± 0.87	3.6 ± 0.83	0.001*
Width of the bone anterior to the canal	6.73 ± 1.67	6.3 ± 1.33	6.02 ± 1.34	0.2

Values are presented as mean ± standard deviation.
*Statistically significant difference between the age groups.

TABLE 3: Comparison of incisive canal characteristics between male and female subjects.

Parameter	Male (n=43)	Female (n=36)	p value
Canal length	19.07 ± 1.09	18.38 ± 2.87	0.72
Mesiodistal width	3.25 ± 1.05	3.21 ± 0.92	0.42
Labiopalatal width	3.23 ± 0.89	2.99 ± 1.0	0.13
Width of the bone anterior to the canal	6.50 ± 1.52	6.10 ± 1.32	0.11

Values are presented as mean ± standard deviation.

increase in diameter of incisive foramen both labiopalatally and mesiodistally (Table 2) and when effect of gender was evaluated, there was no significant difference between males and females (Table 3).

Bone width anterior to the canal was in the range of 4 to 10.4 mm with a mean width of 6.32 ± 1.43 mm; when different age groups were compared, with increasing age there seems to be a decrease in mean width of bone anterior to the incisive canal, although it was not statistically significant (p=0.2) (Table 2).

Male subjects had a mean bone width of 6.50 ± 1.52 mm and female subjects had a width of 6.10 ± 1.32 mm anterior to the incisive canal. Females had a thin bone plate anterior to the incisive canal when compared to males, which was not statistically significant (Table 1).

Of the 79 scans evaluated most prevalent shape of the canal was found to be cylindrical followed by funnel shaped canal, hour-glass like canal, and banana-like canals (Figures 2(a)–2(d)).

5. Discussion

Close proximity of incisive canal to maxillary central incisor region and a thin anterior labial bone may sometimes hamper the immediate implant placement or one may end up in encroachment of the canal leading to sensory dysfunction and nonosseointegration. Careful planning and evaluation using CBCT help in diagnosing such anatomical deficiencies.

Several studies mentioned the anatomic features of this area. In the present study incisive canal characteristics were measured using CBCT sections. To the best of the authors' knowledge this was the first study evaluating the incisive canal characteristics using CBCT sections in Indian subjects.

Mean canal length was found to be 18.63 ± 2.35 mm, which is longer when compared to other studies. Tozum et al. [3] in their multicentered trial found a mean canal length of 10.86 ± 2.67. Liang et al. [4] examined 120 spiral CTs and found a length of 9.9 ± 2.6 mm. Song et al. [1] have demonstrated that mean length of canal in dentate maxillae is 12 mm (8.4 mm to 15.6 mm). Mraiwa et al. [5] reported a mean length of 8.1 ± 3.4 mm. The longer incisive canal length seen in the present study compared to other studies can be attributed to variations in the anatomical characteristics in Indian population.

Mean canal diameter measured 3.23 ± 0.98 mm and 3.12 ± 0.94 mm, mesiodistally and labiopalatally, respectively. In a similar study Tozum et al. [3] measured mean foramen diameter at two different points, i.e., superior and inferior orifice, and it was found to be 2.76 ± 1.40 mm and 2.93 ± 1.01 mm. In the present study foramen width was measured in two different CBCT sections (axial and sagittal sections) and the measurements were comparatively larger than Tozum et al. [3] study; this can be attributed to variations in the anatomical characteristics in Indian population.

Immediate implant placement is advantageous as it decreases the time elapse between tooth loss and restoration and reduces the number of surgical procedures. Initial stability of an implant placed in maxillary incisor area is primarily dependent on the width of the bone anterior to the canal and length of the bone apical to the roots. Although augmentation procedures can be done to modify the width of bone anterior to the canal, it is a determinant of dimensions of implant in that area. In the present study width of bone anterior to the canal was found to be 6.32 ± 1.43 mm. This value is in accordance with Tozum et al. [3] study, where they have found a mean width of 7.38 ± 1.42 mm.

In the present study no significant correlation was detected between gender and incisive canal characteristics. Many studies have reported gender influence on incisive canal characteristics (Mraiwa et al. [5], Mardinger et al. [2], Liang et al. [4], Song et al. [2], Bornstein et al. [6], Kovisto et al. [7], and Tozum et al. [3]). Mraiwala et al. [5] found no significance relation between gender and incisive canal characteristics, which is in accordance with the present study. Bornstein et al. [6] found higher canal length in males when compared to females. Liang et al. [4] reported greater canal length and width in males when compared to female subjects. Guncu et al. [8] examined CTs of 417 male and 516 female patients and concluded that there are statistically significant gender related differences in anatomical features of incisive canal like canal length, diameter, and bone thickness anterior to the incisive canal.

Age of the patient had a significant influence on the length of the incisive canal and diameter of incisive foramen; with increasing age there was an increase in incisive canal length and diameter of incisive foramen. Similarly, Bornstein et al. [6] reported that age of the subjects had a significant influence on the length of the incisive canal. However, Tozum et al. [3] and Mriawa et al. [5] could not find any relation between age and incisive canal characteristics.

Incisive canal morphology was classified in various ways. Mardinger et al. [2] classified the shape of the incisive canals based on how they look in cross sectional view of CBCT scans into cylindrical, funnel shaped, hour-glass shaped, and banana-like canals. In the present study the most predominant shape of the canal was cylindrical shaped followed by funnel shaped, hour-glass shaped, and banana-like. These results are in accordance with Guncu et al. study [8] in which the predominant canal shape was cylindrical; they further analyzed percentage of different shapes of incisive canal in males and females. Similarly Kajan et al. [9] reported predominance of cylindrical shaped incisive canal. In contrast to these studies Etoz et al. [10] examined 500 CBCT scans of dentate patients and found predominance of hour-glass shaped incisive canals.

In edentulous patients with severe atrophic maxilla, invasive procedures like removal of neurovascular bundle from the incisive canal and subsequent grafting of the incisive canal, followed by placement of dental implants, have been presented [11, 12]. A recent clinical study proposed removal of neurovascular bundle from the incisive canal and subsequent placement of implant in seven patients, with only few patients experiencing minor complications [13].

This signifies the importance of assessing incisive foramen characteristics before planning for implant placement; a clinician requires a thorough knowledge of incisive canal anatomical variations. CBCT is an advanced diagnostic aid which helps in diagnosing anatomical difficulties before planning for implant placement in maxillary incisor area.

6. Conclusion

Within the limitations of the study, the present study suggests that the diameter and length of incisive canal vary among different individuals and presence of very thin bone anterior to the canal would suggest that a pretreatment CBCT scan is a valuable tool to evaluate anatomic variations, morphology, and dimensions of incisive foramen before immediate implant placement in maxillary central incisor region. Findings from this study suggest that age has a significant influence over incisive canal characteristics.

Disclosure

This study is self-funded.

References

[1] W.-C. Song, D.-I. Jo, J.-Y. Lee et al., "Microanatomy of the incisive canal using three-dimensional reconstruction of microCT images: an ex vivo study," *Oral Surgery, Oral Medicine, Oral Pathology, Oral Radiology, and Endodontology*, vol. 108, no. 4, pp. 583–590, 2009.

[2] O. Mardinger, N. Namani-Sadan, G. Chaushu, and D. Schwartz-Arad, "Morphologic changes of the nasopalatine canal related to dental implantation: a radiologic study in different degrees of absorbed maxillae," *Journal of Periodontology*, vol. 79, no. 9, pp. 1659–1662, 2008.

[3] T. F. Tözüm, G. N. Güncü, Y. D. Yildirim et al., "Evaluation of maxillary incisive canal characteristics related to dental implant treatment with computerized tomography: a clinical multicenter study," *Journal of Periodontology*, vol. 83, no. 3, pp. 337–343, 2012.

[4] X. Liang, R. Jacobs, W. Martens et al., "Macro- and micro-anatomical, histological and computed tomography scan characterization of the nasopalatine canal," *Journal of Clinical Periodontology*, vol. 36, no. 7, pp. 598–603, 2009.

[5] N. Mraiwa, R. Jacobs, J. Van Cleynenbreugel et al., "The nasopalatine canal revisited using 2D and 3D CT imaging," *Dentomaxillofacial Radiology*, vol. 33, no. 6, pp. 396–402, 2004.

[6] M. M. Bornstein, R. Balsiger, P. Sendi, and T. Von Arx, "Morphology of the nasopalatine canal and dental implant surgery: a radiographic analysis of 100 consecutive patients using limited cone-beam computed tomography," *Clinical Oral Implants Research*, vol. 22, no. 3, pp. 295–301, 2011.

[7] T. Kovisto, M. Ahmad, and W. R. Bowles, "Proximity of the mandibular canal to the tooth apex," *Journal of Endodontics*, vol. 37, no. 3, pp. 311–315, 2011.

[8] G. N. Güncü, Y. D. Yildirim, H. G. Yilmaz et al., "Is there a gender difference in anatomic features of incisive canal and maxillary environmental bone?" *Clinical Oral Implants Research*, vol. 24, no. 9, pp. 1023–1026, 2013.

[9] Z. D. Kajan, J. Kia, S. Motevasseli, and S. R. Rezaian, "Evaluation of the nasopalatine canal with cone-beam computed tomography in an Iranian population," *Dental Research Journal*, vol. 12, no. 1, pp. 14–19, 2015.

[10] M. Etoz and Y. Sisman, "Evaluation of the nasopalatine canal and variations with cone-beam computed tomography," *Surgical and Radiologic Anatomy*, vol. 36, no. 8, pp. 805–812, 2014.

[11] J. B. Rosenquist and E. Nyström, "Occlusion of the incisal canal with bone chips. A procedure to facilitate insertion of implants in the anterior maxilla," *International Journal of Oral and Maxillofacial Surgery*, vol. 21, no. 4, pp. 210-211, 1992.

[12] Z. Artzi, C. E. Nemcovsky, I. Bitlitum, and P. Segal, "Displacement of the incisive foramen in conjunction with implant placement in the anterior maxilla without jeopardizing vitality of nasopalatine nerve and vessels: a novel surgical approach," *Clinical Oral Implants Research*, vol. 11, no. 5, pp. 505–510, 2000.

[13] M. Peñarrocha, C. Carrillo, R. Uribe, and B. García, "The nasopalatine canal as an anatomic buttress for implant placement in the severely atrophic maxilla: a pilot study," *The International Journal of Oral & Maxillofacial Implants*, vol. 24, no. 5, pp. 936–942, 2009.

7

A Concise Review and Required Precautions for COVID-19 Outbreak in Diagnostic and Interventional Radiology

Ali Kord,[1,2] **Behnam Rabiee**,[1] **Siwen Wang**,[3] **Sara Rostami**,[1] **Ron C. Gaba**,[1,2] **and Karen L. Xie**[1]

[1]*Department of Radiology, University of Illinois at Chicago, Chicago, IL, USA*
[2]*Division of Interventional Radiology, University of Illinois at Chicago, Chicago, IL, USA*
[3]*Biomedical Visualization Graduate Program, University of Illinois at Chicago, Chicago, IL, USA*

Correspondence should be addressed to Ali Kord; alikord@uic.edu

Academic Editor: Henrique M. Lederman

A global outbreak of a novel coronavirus (COVID-19) pneumonia began in December 2019 in Wuhan, China. The World Health Organization (WHO) announced a pandemic on March 11, 2020. The rapid rise in the case numbers and mortality led to the saturation of hospitals in many countries. COVID-19 patients usually present with fever, fatigue, dry cough, and dyspnea. Given the shortage of diagnostic kits in many countries and very high sensitivity of computed tomography (CT) for diagnosis of COVID-19 in clinically suspicious patients, the chest CT has been implemented among the primary initial methods of diagnosis before the confirmatory laboratory tests. This puts radiologists and radiology staff on the front line of this alarming pandemic. This report summarizes chest CT findings of COVID-19 patients to facilitate diagnosis and reviews a list of necessary precautions and safety measures for diagnostic and interventional radiology personnel. These precautionary plans are extremely important to avoid contamination of the health-care providers, as well as cross-contamination between patients.

1. Introduction

Beginning on December 31, 2019, the World Health Organization (WHO) was informed of a cluster of cases of pneumonia with unknown causes reported in Wuhan, Hubei province, China [1]. The patients presented with progressive pneumonia symptoms including fever, dry cough, fatigue, and respiratory distress.

A novel coronavirus, severe acute respiratory syndrome coronavirus 2 (SARS-CoV-2, previously known as 2019-nCoV), was isolated from the respiratory tract secretions of the patients by January 7, 2020 [2–4], and the disease was named as coronavirus disease 2019 (COVID-19) soon thereafter.

2. What Is Known About COVID-19

Being a member of the Coronaviridae family, the novel coronavirus (2019-nCoV) is a nonsegmented, enveloped, positive-sense, single-strand ribonucleic acid virus [5, 6]. This virus has a significant capability to infect humans through an interaction between the viral S protein and the angiotensin-converting enzyme 2 receptors on human respiratory endothelial cells [3]. It spread rapidly inside China and transmitted to other countries [4, 7]. As early as 45 days after the first notice, more than 60,000 cases were reported worldwide, with 1,525 mortalities, providing the preliminary estimation of a 2% mortality rate [4, 8–11]. By March 11, 2020, WHO officially announced COVID-19 as a pandemic, declaring a worldwide health emergency state [12]. As of this report on May 14, 2020, the number of cases worldwide has reached 4,258,666 in more than 216 countries with 294,190 deaths, which estimates the mortality rate of 6.9% [11]. These numbers highlight the significant virulence of the novel coronavirus.

Two previous outbreaks of coronavirus, severe acute respiratory syndrome (SARS) and Middle East respiratory syndrome (MERS) coronavirus, which had high mortality of

11% and 30%, respectively, have alarmed the medical community to the potential of these respiratory infections [5, 13]. Despite their high mortality, comparing the number of cases and countries affected by the epidemics demonstrates that the transmission rate of those viruses was significantly lower than that of the novel coronavirus (2019-nCoV); MERS affected a total of 2,500 cases in 27 countries, and SARS infected 8,422 cases in 29 countries [5, 14]. This highlights the increased risks of disease exposure and transmission to front-line health-care professionals in treating the patients and the importance of taking necessary precautions and safety measures to protect the health-care personnel during the current pandemic [15, 16].

3. Radiology Personnel Are among the Front-Line Caregivers for COVID-19

The diagnostic gold standard for viral infections is usually a real-time polymerase chain reaction (RT-PCR) of the respiratory tract specimens. In general, nasopharyngeal or throat swabs are used for viral diagnostics. Sputum and feces specimens can certainly add to the diagnostic yield if nasopharyngeal or throat swabs are negative for COVID-19. Furthermore, although bronchoalveolar lavage is a very relevant specimen, it may not be always possible in severely ill patients. In COVID-19 cases, the routine RT-PCR from nasopharyngeal swaps has a significantly limited sensitivity of 60–70%, especially in the early days of infection [17, 18], which may be due to sample error and the choice of specimen. On the other hand, chest computed tomography (CT) has been investigated as a tool to primarily diagnose the patients with COVID-19 pneumonia, which showed a high sensitivity of 97% in selected patients, even before the PCR test read positive [18]. Therefore, in many countries, a chest CT has been implemented among the primary methods of diagnosis, although sufficient data are lacking. This puts radiologists and radiology staff on the front line of this alarming pandemic. Hence, taking the necessary precautions is deemed to be essential to protect the radiology personnel, while maintaining their efficiency to provide service to the patients.

Radiologic findings of COVID-19 patients can be nonspecific and overlap with pneumonia caused by other viruses. The chest radiograph may be not sensitive enough to detect early disease changes (Figure 1). Typical CT features are described as bilateral multiple lobular and subsegmental areas of consolidation in patients admitted in the intensive care unit (ICU) and bilateral ground-glass opacity and subsegmental areas of consolidation in non-ICU patients (Figure 1) [14]. The abnormalities are typically in peripheral and lower-lobe distributions (Figure 2). Another study indicated that the findings could be unilateral in up to 25% of the cases [19]. In resolving cases with less severe disease, later, chest CT images showed bilateral ground-glass opacities, whereas the consolidation had resolved [13]. In more severe cases leading to death, serial chest CT showed progressively worsening bilateral consolidation during a course of 7 days [5]. Overall, the radiologic findings are similar to those of MERS and SARS [13] and can also overlap with atypical pneumonia, cytomegalovirus pulmonary involvement, as well as H1N1 influenza. Specifically, in the high risk groups with prior pulmonary diseases, CT findings may be less specific. Therefore, gathering a relevant history and physical examination could help raise the alarm for COVID-19 in such patients with the aforementioned chest CT findings.

4. How to Stay Safe while Providing Critical Patient Care

The novel coronavirus (2019-nCoV) is highly contagious, and the main route of transmission is believed to be respiratory droplets. The virus can stay active for several hours to days on multiple surfaces under artificial conditions, and touching the face or the mucosal surfaces of the body with contaminated hands could probably lead to infection. While the highest risk of transmission via droplets is within 3 feet (91.44 cm) of the source, they can contaminate up to 6 feet (183 cm) [5, 20].

According to the latest WHO and Center for Disease Control and Prevention (CDC) guidelines and considering the ongoing research on the subject, the necessary precautionary recommendations fall under three main categories: patient-centered precautions, provider-centered precautions, and equipment-centered precautions (Figure 3). We added an additional category for Interventional Radiology- (IR-) specific precautions. Some of the patient-centered and provider-centered precautions may also be useful and overlap with the operation room precautions.

4.1. Patient-Centered Precautions. All patients should be screened for relevant symptoms. Patients who meet the criteria for a person under investigation (PUI) require isolation and additional precautions to provide triage and care.

To minimize the risk of cross-infection, patients with different infection risks should be separated by space where possible or by time otherwise [21]. Additionally, procedures on PUI should be separated by place and time from other patients [21].

The transfer of PUIs should be kept at a minimum. Utilizing portable radiology equipment in this setting proved to be a very effective safety measure in the SARS epidemic [5, 13, 22, 23]. For complicated cases in which patient transfer is inevitable, assigning dedicated procedural rooms and predetermined transport routes and performing a cleaning protocol according to infectious disease control protocol afterward will greatly minimize the risk of cross-contamination. It is important that the COVID-19 patients wear a surgical mask during the transfer and, if possible, during the procedures which require direct provider contact.

4.2. Provider-Centered Precautions. Based on the experience of the SARS epidemic, it is clear that the risk of virus transmission to the providers is significantly reduced by using droplet and contact precautions [13, 23–25]. The current evidence suggests asymptomatic transmission even through the incubation period [26]. This highlights the

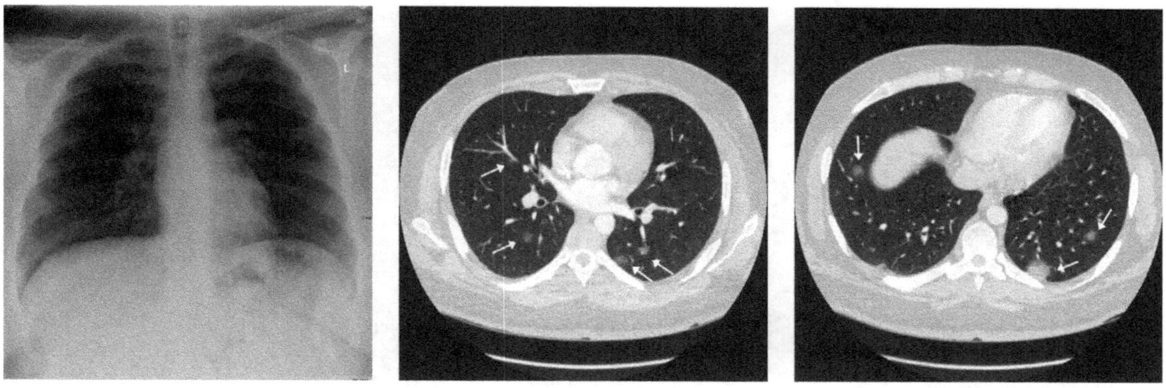

(a) (b) (c)

Figure 1: A 26-year-old male with a recent diagnosis of diabetes presented with several days of progressive myalgia, cough, chills, and dyspnea and intermittent generalized crampy mild abdominal pain. (a) The chest radiograph was negative for consolidation. (b, c) The CT pulmonary arteriogram was performed for the same patient to rule out pulmonary embolism and showed multiple patchy, lower-lobe-prominent, nodular ground-glass opacities (arrows). The patient was tested positive for COVID-19.

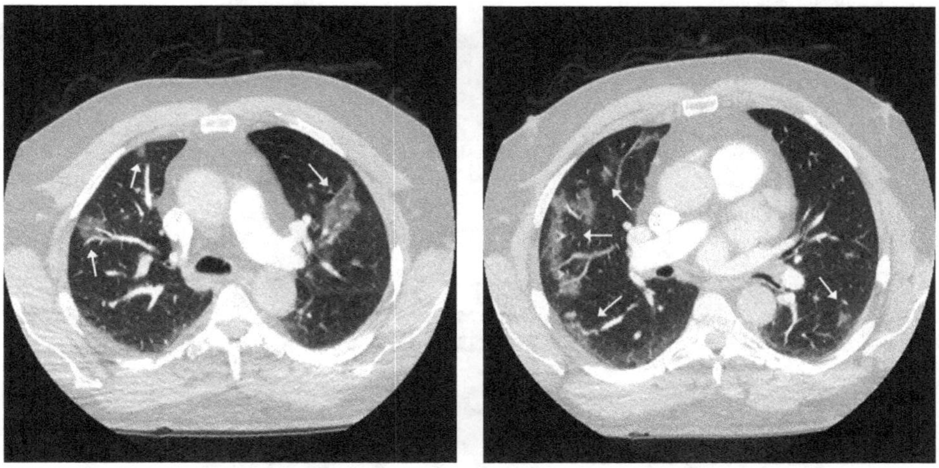

(a) (b)

Figure 2: A 67-year-old male with a past medical history of sudden cardiac arrest with the placement of a defibrillator and a recent travel history to Europe presented with nonproductive cough, myalgia, and fever. (a, b) The CT pulmonary arteriogram was performed to rule out pulmonary embolism and demonstrated multiple patchy, peripheral, more organized ground-glass opacities (arrows) compared to the patient in Figure 1. The patient was tested positive for COVID-19.

importance of the use of minimum personal protective equipment (PPE) for all staff during all procedures, preferably everywhere or, at least, at the involved centers.

The latest recommendations of WHO include respiratory protection with a standard face mask for the health-care providers while interacting with all patients, unless aerosol-generating procedures are performed [5, 27, 28]. Additionally, CDC recommends strict airborne precaution using an N95 mask or higher when in close contact with a confirmed COVID-19 case, or a PUI [5]. Furthermore, necessary PPE includes a disposable (if resources are limited, autoclavable) fluid-resistant isolation gown, disposable gloves with the emphasis of coverage over gown cuffs, protective goggles, and, if available, a face shield [29]. Recent studies also reported the possibility of transmission via ocular surface mucosa, which highlights the importance of ocular protection wear such as glasses or face shields as well [30, 31].

Rapid spread of COVID-19 pandemic highlights the importance of the awareness and effective measures to prevent transmission of microorganisms, particularly highly resistant microorganisms. Therefore, it is important to be mindful of general infection prevention protocols, such as hand hygiene for everyone including patients and health-care providers. In addition, lessons learned from the present outbreak management of COVID-19 call for a continuing quality improvement program in place for the infection prevention and control to prepare for potential outbreaks in the future.

4.3. Equipment-Centered Precautions. The use of portable imaging devices is highly recommended specifically for the confirmed COVID-19 patients, as well as the PUI. These devices should be carefully disinfected before and after the procedures. All the routinely used equipment including CT

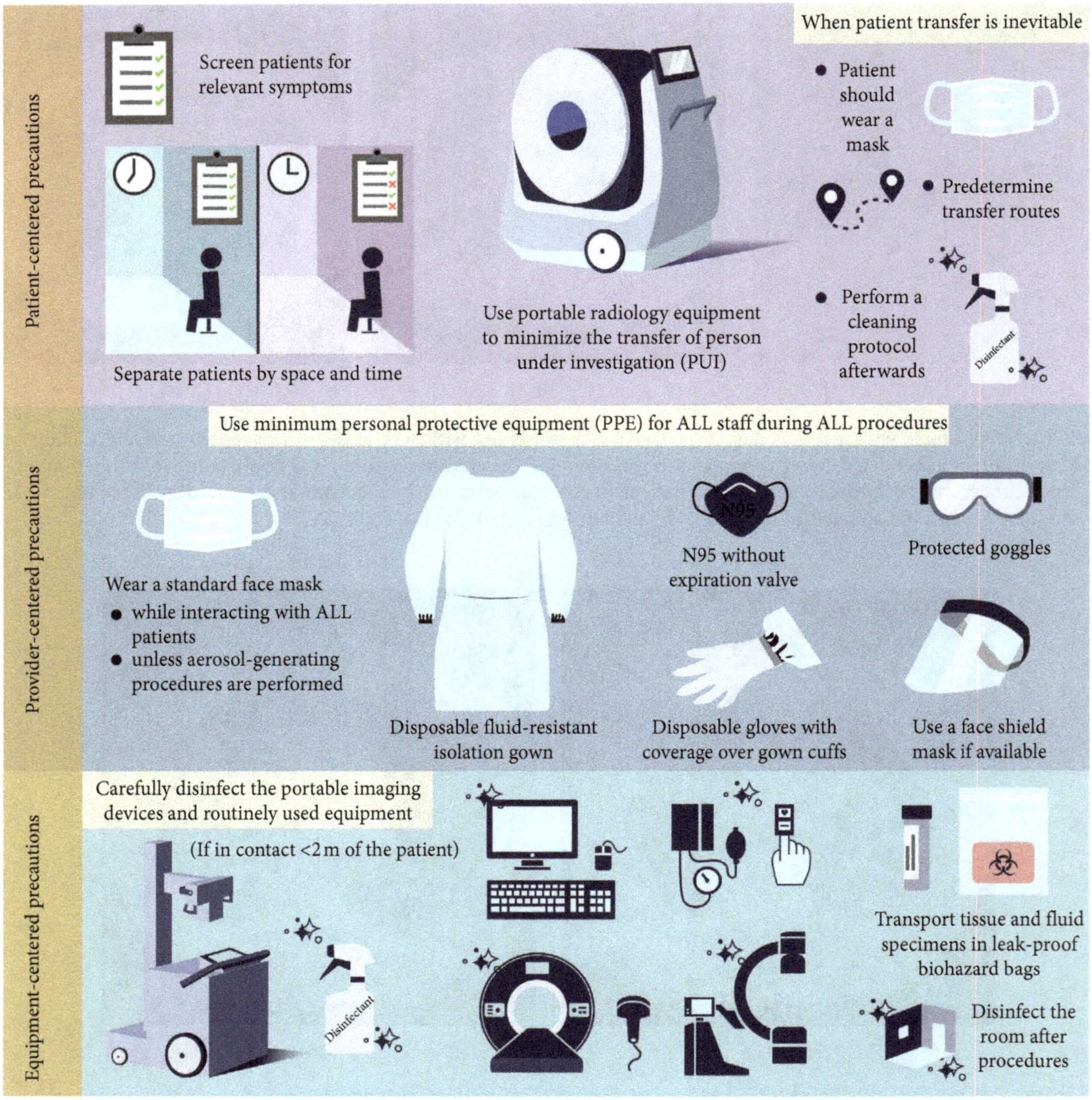

FIGURE 3: Proposed precautions for diagnostic radiology for COVID-19 outbreak based on the WHO and CDC recommendations.

and magnetic resonance imaging (MRI) machines, ultrasound transducers, blood pressure monitoring cuffs, pulse oximeters, and reading room mice, keyboard, monitors, and surfaces, as well as interventional radiology suite equipment, should be disinfected following every COVID-19 suspect encounter, if in contact <2 m of the patient, which should be avoided whenever possible [5].

CDC recommendations include washing with soap and water on the possible surfaces and equipment or alternatively use of at least intermediate-level disinfectants such as ethyl alcohol, isopropyl alcohol, and iodophor germicidal detergent solution [5]. It is important to note that ethanol solutions should contain at least 70% ethanol for surfaces and at least 60% ethanol for hand sanitizers, according to CDC guidelines [32]. Education of the staff on the decontamination protocols plays an important role to prevent cross-contaminations in these settings [33].

Tissue and fluid specimens are considered infectious and must be transported in leak-proof biohazard bags by trained personnel to ensure safe handling practices and spill decontamination procedures [21]. Disinfection of the room and medical equipment must be performed after procedures on these patients as well [21].

4.4. Interventional Radiology-Specific Precautions. Specific precautions should be taken for interventional radiology suites to lower the risk of disease spread [34]. While the interventional radiology team may continue with urgent (e.g., oncologic and dialysis management procedures) and emergent (e.g., abscess drainage) procedures, elective cases should be deferred in the interest of resource conservation and exposure risk mitigation. To this end, it may be useful to generate a stratification system for procedure urgency to guide scheduling; a proposed protocol may be to assign

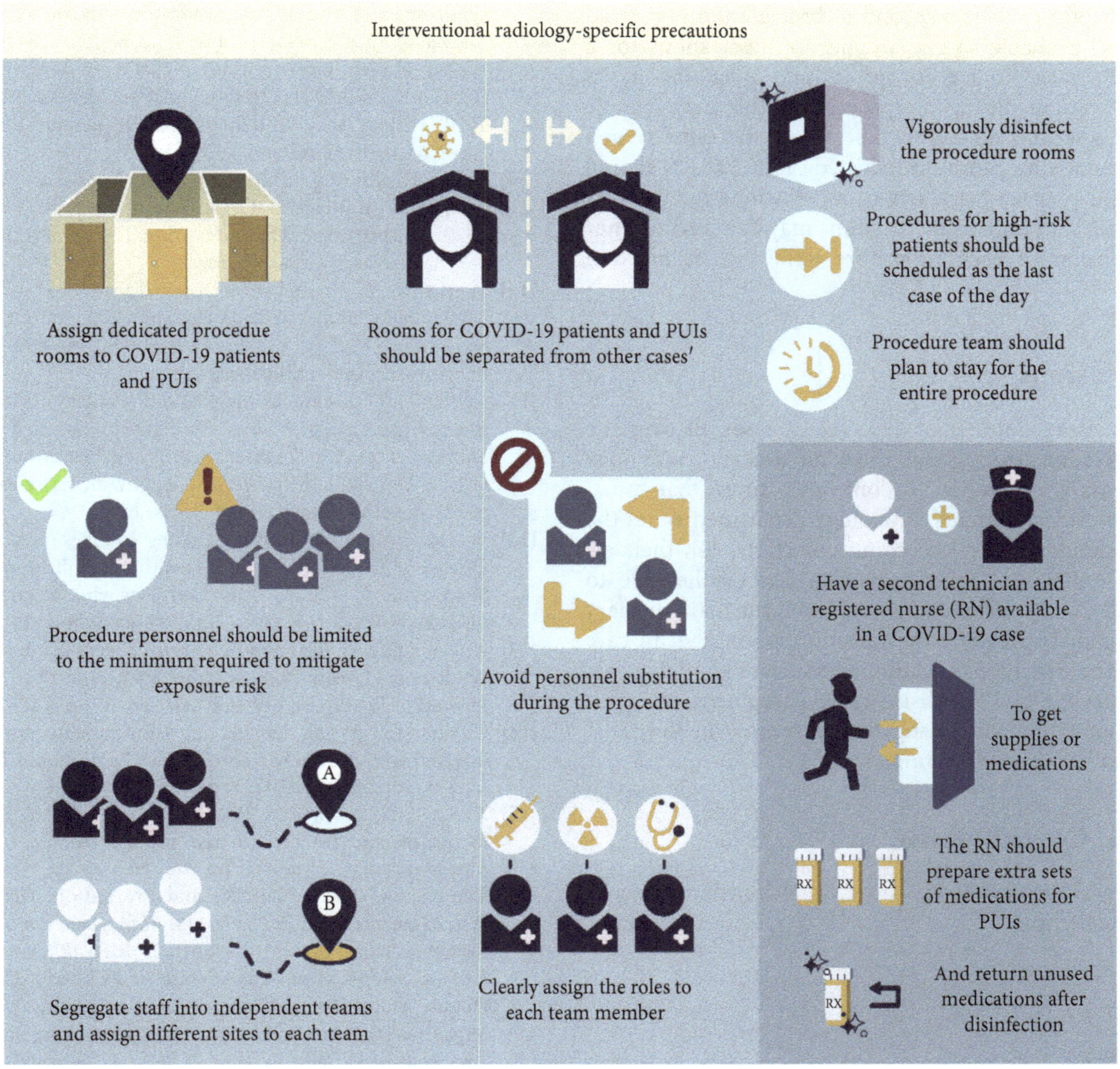

FIGURE 4: Proposed precautions for interventional radiology for COVID-19 outbreak based on the WHO and CDC recommendations and ongoing studies.

procedures color codes to indicate urgency (red = schedule within 2 weeks, orange = schedule within 2–4 weeks, yellow = schedule within 4–8 weeks, and green = schedule after 8 weeks). Regardless of the system used, scheduling alterations require more targeted patient triage and communication of measures taken to protect patients [21]. A proposed protocol for the COVID-19 outbreak, adapted from our institutional protocol, has been summarized in the following paragraphs and Figure 4. Regarding outpatient clinic visits, these can be performed as telehealth visits using video or phone conferencing.

While portable procedure performance is preferred, specific and dedicated procedure rooms should be dedicated to the PUIs or confirmed COVID-19 patients, and these rooms should be separated from other procedure rooms [23]. The procedure rooms should be vigorously disinfected following each procedure on a suspected patient. If possible, performing the procedure on COVID-19 patients or PUIs should be scheduled as the last case of the day to minimize the risk of cross-contamination.

Procedure personnel should be limited to the minimum required for safe and effective performance, in order to minimize exposure risk to the personnel. The procedure team should plan to stay for the entire procedure from start to finish (i.e., no breaks or substitute personnel). Medical doctor coverage should be limited to a single person in order to keep the risk of infection and losing manpower to a minimum unless case complexity requires multiple doctors. No nonessential personnel (e.g., medical students) should scrub into cases during the COVID-19 outbreak. For medical teams covering multiple hospitals, assigning different sites to each subteam will minimize the cross-contamination risk [21, 23]. In the case of intrahospital transmission, segregation of staff into independent teams will be needed to prevent a shutdown of the entire service should there be a need for quarantine [21, 23]. The assigned role of each member of the provider team should be clear to minimize confusion during the probable overflow hours, which will require more detailed protocols than usual.

It is helpful to have a second technician and registered nurse (RN) available to get supplies or medications for a COVID-19 case to prevent procedural personnel from leaving the room during the procedure. This may include assigning a second on-call technician for the same reason and particularly for more complicated cases. The RN should predict and prepare extra sets of medications for the suspicious case, and unused medications may be returned after the conclusion of each procedure following disinfection protocol.

5. Conclusions

With the rising number of COVID-19 cases all over the world, including throughout the United States, radiology departments are expected to confront a more than usual volume of critical patients. Radiology departments and the IR team should be in close communication with their affiliated hospital units and providers. Strict adherence to WHO and CDC policies and guidelines is the main primary defense against spreading the infection among health-care workers. These include measurements such as hand hygiene, appropriate use of PPE, disinfecting equipment and procedure rooms, and educating the personnel on the most current policies and recommendations.

Authors' Contributions

Ali Kord and Behnam Rabiee have equal contributions and listed alphabetically.

References

[1] World Health Organization, *Coronavirus–China*, World Health Organization, Geneva, Switzerland, 2020, https://www.who.int/csr/don/12-january-2020-novel-coronavirus-china/en/.

[2] World Health Organization, *Coronavirus Disease (COVID-19) Outbreak*, World Health Organization, Geneva, Switzerland, 2019, https://www.who.int/emergencies/diseases/novel-coronavirus-2019.

[3] X. Xu, P. Chen, J. Wang et al., "Evolution of the novel coronavirus from the ongoing Wuhan outbreak and modeling of its spike protein for risk of human transmission," *Science China Life Sciences*, vol. 63, no. 3, pp. 457–460, 2015.

[4] H. Shi, X. Han, N. Jiang et al., "Radiological findings from 81 patients with COVID-19 pneumonia in Wuhan, China: a descriptive study," *The Lancet Infectious Diseases*, vol. 20, no. 4, pp. 425–434, 2020.

[5] S. Kooraki, M. Hosseiny, L. Myers, and A. Gholamrezanezhad, "Coronavirus outbreak: what the department of radiology should know," *Journal of the American College of Radiology*, vol. 17, no. 4, pp. 447–451, 2020.

[6] S. R. Weiss and J. L. Leibowitz, "Coronavirus pathogenesis," in *Advances in Virus Research*, vol. 81, pp. 85–164, Academic Press, Cambridge, MA, USA, 2019.

[7] M. Hosseiny, S. Kooraki, A. Gholamrezanezhad, S. Reddy, and L. Myers, "Radiology perspective of coronavirus disease 2019 (COVID-19): lessons from severe acute respiratory syndrome and Middle East respiratory syndrome," *American Journal of Roentgenology*, vol. 214, no. 5, pp. 1078–1082, 2020.

[8] World Health Organization, *Novel Coronavirus–Thailand (Ex-China)*, World Health Organization, Geneva, Switzerland, 2020, https://www.who.int/csr/don/14-january-2020-novel-coronavirus-thailand/en/.

[9] World Health Organization, *Novel Coronavirus—Japan (Ex-China)*, World Health Organization, Geneva, Switzerland, 2020, https://www.who.int/csr/don/17-january-2020-novel-coronavirus-japan-ex-china/en/.

[10] World Health Organization, *Novel Coronavirus—Republic of Korea (ex-China)*, World Health Organization, Geneva, Switzerland, 2020, https://www.who.int/csr/don/21anuary-noveloronavirus-epublicforeaxhina/en/.

[11] Centers for Disease Control and Prevention, *First Travel-Related Case of 2019 Novel Coronavirus Detected in United States*, Centers for Disease Control and Prevention, Atlanta, GA, USA, 2020, https://www.cdc.gov/media/releases/2020/p0121-novel-coronavirus-travel-case.html.

[12] World Health Organization, *Rolling Updates on Coronavirus Disease (COVID-19)*, World Health Organization, Geneva, Switzerland, 2019, https://www.who.int/emergencies/diseases/novel-coronavirus-2019/events-as-they-happen.

[13] A. Gogna, K. H. Tay, and B. S. Tan, "Severe acute respiratory syndrome: 11 years later—a radiology perspective," *American Journal of Roentgenology*, vol. 203, no. 4, pp. 746–748, 2014.

[14] C. Huang, Y. Wang, X. Li et al., "Clinical features of patients infected with 2019 novel coronavirus in Wuhan, China," *The Lancet*, vol. 395, no. 10223, pp. 497–506, 2020.

[15] K. Ng, B. H. Poon, T. H. Puar et al., "COVID-19 and the risk to health care workers: a case report," *Annals of Internal Medicine*, vol. 172, no. 11, pp. 766-767, 2020.

[16] Centers for Disease Control and Prevention, *Guidance for Risk Assessment and Public Health Management of Healthcare Personnel with Potential Exposure in a Healthcare Setting to Patients with Coronavirus Disease (COVID-19)*, Centers for Disease Control and Prevention, Atlanta, GA, USA, 2020, https://www.cdc.gov/coronavirus/2019-ncov/hcp/guidance-risk-assesment-hcp.html.

[17] Y. Fang, H. Zhang, J. Xie et al., "Sensitivity of chest CT for COVID-19: comparison to RT-PCR," *Radiology*, Article ID 200432, 2020.

[18] T. Ai, Z. Yang, H. Hou et al., "Correlation of chest CT and RT-PCR testing in coronavirus disease 2019 (COVID-19) in China: a report of 1014 cases," *Radiology*, Article ID 200642, 2020.

[19] N. Chen, M. Zhou, X. Dong et al., "Epidemiological and clinical characteristics of 99 cases of 2019 novel coronavirus pneumonia in Wuhan, China: a descriptive study," *The Lancet*, vol. 395, no. 10223, pp. 507–513, 2020.

[20] J. D. Siegel, E. Rhinehart, M. Jackson, and L. Chiarello, *Guideline for Isolation Precautions Preventing Transmission of Infectious Agents in Healthcare Settings*, CDC, Atlanta, GA, USA, 2007.

[21] K. Da Zhuang, B. S. Tan, B. H. Tan, C. W. Too, and K. H. Tay, "Old threat, new enemy: is your interventional radiology service ready for the coronavirus disease 2019?" *CardioVascular and Interventional Radiology*, vol. 43, no. 5, pp. 665-666, 2020.

[22] H. A. Parmar, T. C. C. Lim, J. S.-K. Goh, J. T. Tan, Y. Y. Sitoh, and F. Hui, "Providing optimal radiology service in the severe acute respiratory syndrome outbreak: use of mobile CT," *American Journal of Roentgenology*, vol. 182, no. 1, pp. 57–60, 2004.

[23] L. T. Cheng, L. P. Chan, B. H. Tan et al., "Déjà vu or jamais vu? How the severe acute respiratory syndrome experience influenced a Singapore radiology department's response to the coronavirus disease (COVID-19) epidemic," *American Journal of Roentgenology*, vol. 214, no. 6, pp. 1206–1210, 2020.

[24] A. D. King, A. S. C. Ching, P. L. Chan et al., "Severe acute respiratory syndrome: avoiding the spread of infection in a radiology department," *American Journal of Roentgenology*, vol. 181, no. 1, pp. 25–27, 2003.

[25] W. H. Seto, D. Tsang, R. Yung et al., "Effectiveness of precautions against droplets and contact in prevention of nosocomial transmission of severe acute respiratory syndrome (SARS)," *The Lancet*, vol. 361, no. 9368, pp. 1519-1520, 2003.

[26] A. Bastola, R. Sah, A. J. Rodriguez-Morales et al., "The first 2019 novel coronavirus case in Nepal," *The Lancet Infectious Diseases*, vol. 20, no. 3, pp. 279-280, 2020.

[27] World Health Organization, *Rational Use of Personal Protective Equipment for Coronavirus Disease 2019 (COVID-19)*, World Health Organization, Geneva, Switzerland, 2019, https://apps.who.int/iris/bitstream/handle/10665/331215/WHO-2019-nCov-IPCPPE_use-2020.1-eng.pdf.

[28] Centers for Disease Control and Prevention, *Interim Infection Prevention and Control Recommendations for Patients with Confirmed Coronavirus Disease 2019 (COVID-19) or Persons Under Investigation for COVID-19 in Healthcare Settings*, Centers for Disease Control and Prevention, Atlanta, GA, USA, 2019, https://www.cdc.gov/coronavirus/2019-ncov/infection-control/controlrecommendations.

[29] Centers for Disease Control and Prevention, "Infection control in health care, home, and community settings: public health guidance for community-level preparedness and response to severe acute respiratory syndrome (SARS). Centers for Disease Control and Prevention," Centers for Disease Control and Prevention, Atlanta, GA, USA, 2020, https://www.cdc.gov/sars/guidance/i-infection/index.html.

[30] L. Zhou, Z. Xu, G. M. Castiglione et al., "ACE2 and TMPRSS2 Are expressed on the human ocular surface, suggesting susceptibility to SARS-CoV-2 infection," 2020, https://www.biorxiv.org/content/10.1101/2020.05.09.086165v1.

[31] H. Qing, Z. Yang, M. Shi, and Z. Zhang, "New evidence of SARS-CoV-2 transmission through the ocular surface," *Graefe's Archive for Clinical and Experimental Ophthalmology*, pp. 1-2, 2020.

[32] Centers for Disease Control and Prevention, *Coronavirus (COVID-19)*, Centers for Disease Control and Prevention, Atlanta, GA, USA, 2020, https://www.cdc.gov/coronavirus/2019-ncov/.

[33] S. K. Mirza, T. R. Tragon, M. B. Fukui, M. S. Hartman, and A. L. Hartman, "Microbiology for radiologists: how to minimize infection transmission in the radiology department," *Radiographics*, vol. 35, no. 4, pp. 1231–1244.

[34] Society of Interventional Radiology, *COVID-19 Clinical Notification from the Society of Interventional Radiology*, Society of Interventional Radiology, Fairfax, VA, USA, https://www.sirweb.org/practice-resources/covid-19-resources/covid-19-clinical-notification/.

8

Competency in Chest Radiography Interpretation by Junior Doctors and Final Year Medical Students at a Teaching Hospital

Bashiru Babatunde Jimah,[1] **Anthony Baffour Appiah**,[2] **Benjamin Dabo Sarkodie**,[3] **and Dorothea Anim**[4]

[1]*Department of Medical Imaging, School of Medical Sciences, University of Cape Coast, Cape Coast, Ghana*
[2]*Ghana Field Epidemiology and Laboratory Training Programme, University of Ghana, Accra, Ghana*
[3]*Department of Radiology, University of Ghana, School of Medicine Sciences, Accra, Ghana*
[4]*Department of Radiology, Korle Bu Teaching Hospital, Accra, Ghana*

Correspondence should be addressed to Bashiru Babatunde Jimah; jimah@uccsms.edu.gh

Academic Editor: Lorenzo Faggioni

Background. Chest radiography (CXR) is a widely used imaging technique for assessing various chest conditions; however, little is known on the medical doctors' and medical students' level of skills to interpret the CXRs. This study assessed the residents, medical officers, house officers, and final year medical students' competency in CXRs interpretation and how the patient's clinical history influences the interpretation. *Methods.* We conducted a cross-sectional study in the Cape Coast Teaching Hospital in the Central Region of Ghana among 99 nonradiologists, comprising 10 doctors in residency programmes, 18 medical officers, 33 house officers, and 38 final year medical students. The data collection was done with a semistructured questionnaire in two phases. In phase 1, ten CXRs were presented without patient's clinical history. Phase 2 involved the same ten CXRs presented in the same order alongside the patient's clinical history. Participants were given 3 minutes to interpret each image. Median and interquartile ranges were used to describe continuous variables, while frequencies and percentages were used to describe categorical variables. Test of significant difference and association was conducted using a Wilcoxon rank-sum test/Kruskal–Wallis test and chi-square (X^2) test, respectively. *Results.* The average score for interpreting CXRs was 7.0 (IQR = 5–8) and 4.0 (IQR = 3-4), when CXRs were, respectively, presented with and without clinical history. No significant difference was seen in average scores regarding the levels of formal training. Without clinical history, only 40.0% of residents, 22.2% of medical officers, 24.2% of house officers, and 13.2% of medical students correctly interpreted CXRs, while more than 75% each of all categories correctly interpreted CXRs when presented with clinical history. However, all participants had difficulties in identifying CXR with pneumothorax (27.3% vs. 30.3%), pneumomediastinum or left rib fracture (8.1% vs. 33.3%), and lung collapse (37.4% vs. 37.4%) in both situations, with and without patient clinical history. *Conclusion.* The patient's clinical history was found to greatly influence doctors' competence in interpreting CXRs. We found a gap in doctors' and medical students' ability to interpret CXRs; hence, the development of this skill should be improved at all levels of medical training.

1. Introduction

Evidence-based practice highlights the use of the best available evidence when making clinical decisions about individual patient care [1]. As cited by Andersson et al., "evidence-based medicine is the conscientious, explicit, and judicious use of current best evidence in making decisions about the care of the individual patient" [1]. Medical practice in the tertiary health facility required extensive diversity of skills and competence among various cadre of medical personnel. Medical imaging especially chest radiography is often the first investigation for chest complaints, and the information obtained is key to inform a safe, efficient, and cost-effective intervention for the patients [1–3]. Chest radiography imaging is essential for the diagnosis of several diseases and nonchest-related conditions such as bowel perforation and preoperative assessments of patients [4]. Radiologists are involved in the interpretation of images obtained from computed tomography, magnetic resonance imaging, radiography, ultrasound scan, and others in tertiary hospitals. The inadequate number of radiologists especially in Ghana could hinder a thorough assessment to the overwhelming number of chest radiographs (CXRs). As part of clinical medical training, medical students and junior doctors are endowed with the basic skills to interpret simple radiologic images. However, studies elsewhere indicate poor CXR interpretation skills among medical students and junior doctors [4–7].

Chest radiograph interpretation is less studied worldwide. Miranda et al. assessed the radiological imaging interpretation skills of medical interns in the city of Recife, Pernambuco, Brazil. They observed that both medical interns and final year medical students alike are largely limited in their ability to make radiological diagnoses of simple and commonplace situations [4]. In another study, Christiansen et al. found that Danish junior doctors do not meet the established minimum requirements for radiological diagnostic skills for the use of CXR [7]. These studies suggested formal training for doctors to enhance their skills in interpreting simple radiologic images of their patients. Our search found no published evidence on the competence among various grades of medical doctors and medical students in Ghana. Moreover, this evidence is needed in Ghana to help target interventions among medical doctors in order to maximize the benefit of radiological exams, which is an integral component of our health care delivery. This study, therefore, investigated the competence of residents, medical officers, house officers, and final year medical students in relation to the interpretation of CXR. The study defines a house officer as "a doctor undergoing two-year internship post-medical school," medical officer as "a doctor who has successfully completed two-year internship postmedical school in cape coast teaching hospital," and resident as "a medical officer in residency training in cape coast teaching hospital." This study would provide preliminary data for further assessment and inform effective training of medical practitioners in the interpretation of radiologic images in Ghana.

2. Materials and Methods

2.1. Study Design. We conducted a cross-sectional study in the Cape Coast Teaching Hospital (CCTH) in the Central Region, Ghana, among 99 nonradiologists. The CCTH is a 400-bed teaching hospital with multispecialty departments and serves as main referral Centre for health Facilities in the Central Region and parts of neighboring regions. The study was conducted between the period of April and May 2018. The nonradiologist medical staffs were purposefully sampled, and they comprise 10 residents, 18 medical officers, 33 house officers, and 38 final year medical students of the University Cape Coast Medical School.

2.2. Competence Evaluation. During the study period, one of the investigators was responsible for administering the test to the participants, in small sessions. A semistructured questionnaire contained the professional rank, participation in formal training on radiograph interpretation, and 10 columns for CXR interpretation. Data collection was conducted in two phases. In the first phase, the participants were presented with 10 CXRs without patients' clinical history one at a time, with a time limit of 3 minutes to interpret each image, and to document their interpretations on the questionnaire (Figure 1). Similar to the first phase, the same 10 CXRs were presented to participants in the same order in the second phase with the clinical history of the patients. Interpretations per slide at each phase were marked and scored as a correct answer or wrong answer, the correct answer was scored 1, and the wrong answer was scored 0. The total score was 10 for each phase, and the score ≥5 was considered pass while <5 was rated as fail.

2.3. Data Analysis. Statistical Package for the Social Science (SPSS; IBM Corp, Armonk, NY) version 21 was used to analyze data. The continuous variable was skewed (non-normality distributed) using the Shapiro–Wilk test. Hence, median and interquartile ranges were used to describe the continuous variable, while the Wilcoxon rank-sum test (two levels) and Kruskal–Wallis test (three or more levels) were used to test for significant differences in median scores among groups. Frequencies and percentages were used to describe categorical variables, and comparison of categorical data between subgroups was carried out using the chi-square (X^2) test. All statistical analyses were considered significant at p value ≤0.05.

3. Results

Of the total of 99 participants, 10 were residents, 18 were medical officers, 33 were house officers, and 38 were final year medical students. Majority (62.6%) of the respondents have participated in formal chest radiography training except house officers (30.3%) (Figure 2). There was significant association between the professional rank of participants and their participation in formal training (chi^2 (3) = 32.16, $p < 0.001$).

The median score of CXRs interpretation was 4.0 (IQR = 3-4) with no clinical history and 7.0 (IQR = 5–8) when images were presented with clinical history. Without clinical history, nearly equal median scores were recorded by residents (4.0, IQR = 3–5), medical officers (4.0, IQR = 3-4), and house officer (4.0, IQR = 3-4). The median scores increased across the board when clinical history was presented with CXRs with residents scoring the highest (7.5, IQR = 5–9). Generally, a medical student had the least median score with (5.5, IQR = 5–7) and without (3.0, IQR = 2–4) clinical history. The Kruskal–Wallis test shows a significant difference in median scores obtained by participants when presented with clinical history (p = 0.006). Participants with formal training had lower median scores without any clinical history (3.0, IQR = 3-4) but better when presented with patient's clinical history (7.0, IQR = 5–8) (Table 1).

As shown in Figure 3, majority of the participants correctly interpreted the CXRs when presented with clinical history (83.8%) of patients than those without clinical history (21.2%).

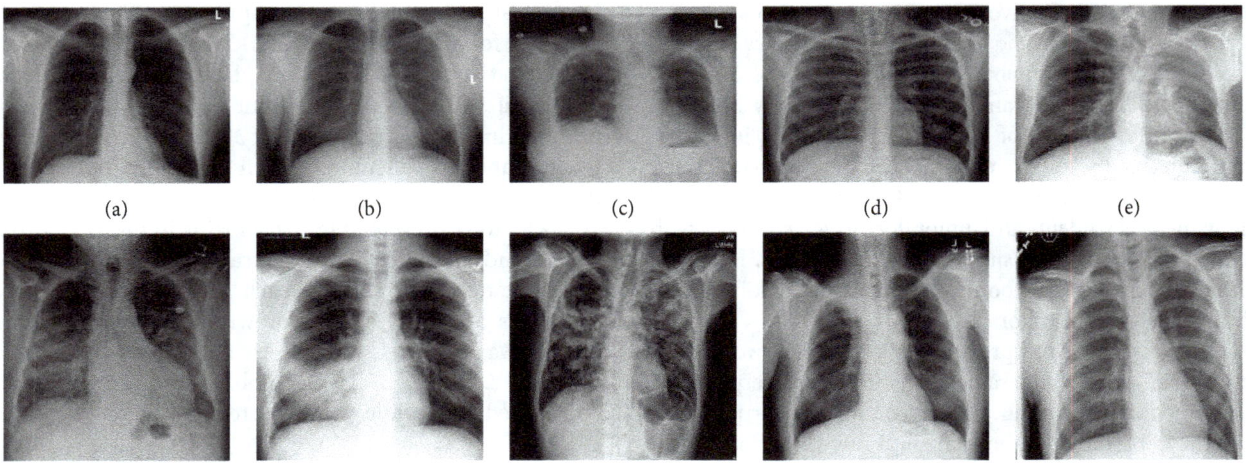

FIGURE 1: Chest radiographs of patients used for the assessment of competence. The expected diagnoses in line with the specialists' interpretations were (a) pneumothorax, (b) normal image, (c) pneumoperitoneum, (d) pneumomediastinum/left rib fracture, (e) lung collapse, (f) pulmonary edema/congestive cardiac failure, (g) pneumonia, (h) tuberculosis/pneumoconiosis/metastasis, (i) Pancoast tumour/*tuberculosis*, and (j) clavicular fracture/acromioclavicular dislocation.

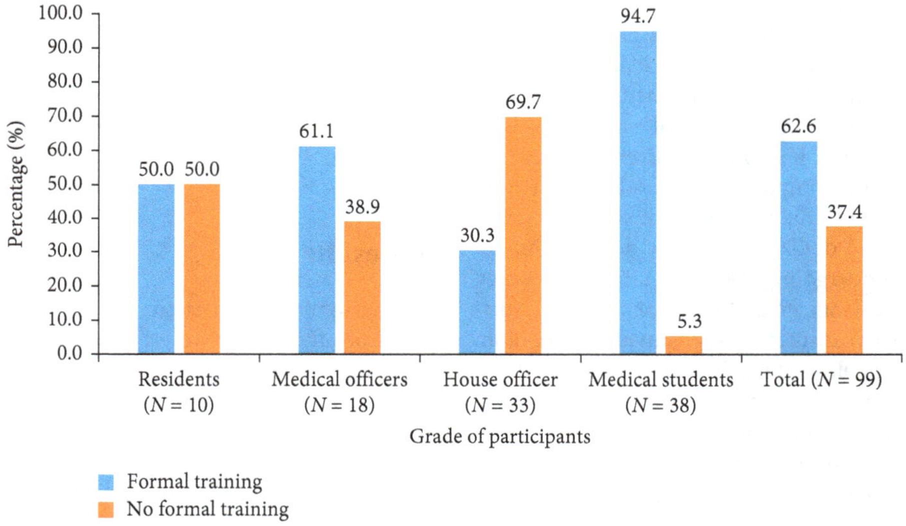

FIGURE 2: Distribution of participants by grade of profession and participation in formal training on interpreting CXRs.

The pass rate for CXRs interpretation was much higher with the presentation of patient clinical history. There was no statistically significant association between participants' performance and their professional rank and participation in formal training (Table 2).

With or without clinical history, few of the participants correctly identified CXR with pneumothorax (30.3% vs. 27.3%), pneumomediastinum/left rib fracture (33.3 vs. 8.1%), and lung collapse (37.4% vs. 37.4%). Only 10% of residents, 16.7% of medical officers, 9.1% of house officer, and 15.8% medical students could correctly identify normal radiographs without clinical history. On the contrary, majority of participants could easily identify CXR with pneumonia (64.7% vs. 92.9%) and tuberculosis/pneumoconiosis (64.7% vs. 83.8%). Correct interpretation of CXR with pneumothorax was significantly higher among house officers and residents when CXR was, respectively, presented without (42.4%, $p = 0.037$) and with (60%, $p < 0.001$) clinical history. Similarly, correct interpretation of CXR with pneumoperitoneum was significantly higher among residents and medical officers when images were presented without (60%, $p = 0.009$) and with (88.9%, $p = 0.037$) clinical history, respectively. The medical officers tend to interpret radiographs with clavicular fracture/acromioclavicular dislocation (55.6%) much better than other counterparts ($p = 0.022$) in the absence of clinical history (Table 3).

4. Discussion

The medical practitioners' ability and competence of interpreting CXRs are vital for patient care [8]. The present study showed that majority (62.6%) of the participants have

Table 1: Summary of CXR interpretation score by grade and formal training.

	Frequency	Overall participants' score (out of 10) No clinical history Median	IQR	Clinical history Median	IQR
Grade					
Resident	10	4.0	3–5	7.5	5–9
Medical officer	18	4.0	3-4	7.0	6–8
House officer	33	4.0	3-4	7.0	6–8
Medical student	38	3.0	2–4	5.5	5–7
Total	99	4.0	3-4	7.0	5–8
Kruskal–Wallis test		$X^2 = 6.647$, $p = 0.084$		$X^2 = 12.448$, $p = 0.006$	
Formal training					
Yes	62	3.0	3-4	7.0	5–8
No	37	4.0	3–5	6.0	6–8
Total	99	4.0	3-4	7.0	5–8
Wilcoxon rank-sum test		$Z = -1.322$, $p = 0.186$		$Z = -0.024$, $p = 0.981$	

IQR, interquartile range.

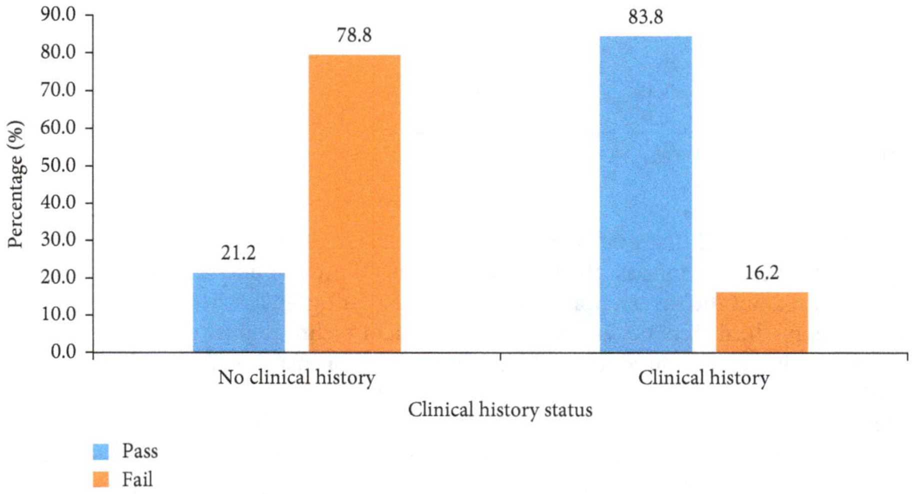

Figure 3: General performance of participant with or without clinical history.

Table 2: Association between the grade of respondents and formal training and CXRs interpretation score.

Variable	No clinical history Pass	Fail	Chi-square p value	Clinical history Pass	Fail	Chi-square p value
Grade						
Resident	4 (40.0)	6 (60.0)		8 (80.0)	2 (20.0)	
Medical officer	4 (22.2)	14 (77.8)		16 (88.9)	2 (11.1)	
House officer	8 (24.2)	25 (75.8)	0.286	29 (87.9)	4 (12.1)	0.679
Medical student	5 (13.2)	33 (86.8)		30 (78.0)	8 (12.1)	
Total	21 (21.2)	78 (78.8)		83 (83.8)	16 (16.2)	
Formal training						
Yes	11 (17.7)	51 (82.3)		61 (84.7)	11 (15.3)	
No	10 (27.0)	27 (73.0)	0.274	22 (81.5)	5 (13.5)	0.696
Total	21 (21.2)	78 (78.8)		83 (83.8)	16 (16.2)	

had formal chest radiography interpretation training. The highest of them was observed among final year medical students (94.7%), while the least was found among house officers (30.3%). At the time of the study, the medical students were in their final stages of clinical training prior to graduation which included chest radiograph interpretation, a possible explanation for the aforementioned. Also, it is entirely possible that many of the house officers trained from institutions outside our studied institution do not recognize their training as formal, rather as a routine lecture. The findings further showed that the professional rank of participants was significantly linked with formal training

Table 3: Proportion of correct CXR interpretation by grade of participants.

Slide number, interpretation	Clinical history	Grade of participants (% correct) Residents ($N = 10$)	Medical officers ($N = 18$)	House officer ($N = 33$)	Medical students ($N = 38$)	Total ($N = 99$)	Chi-square p value
1, pneumothorax	No	40.0	11.1	42.4	18.4	27.3	0.037*
	Yes	60.0	5.6	57.6	10.5	30.3	<0.001**
2, normal image	No	10.0	16.7	9.1	15.8	13.1	0.803
	Yes	70.0	66.7	78.8	57.9	67.7	0.313
3, pneumoperitoneum	No	60.0	27.8	21.2	10.5	22.2	0.009*
	Yes	80.0	88.9	81.8	57.9	73.7	0.039*
4, pneumomediastinum	No	10.0	5.6	6.1	10.5	8.1	0.875
	Yes	50.0	55.6	24.2	26.3	33.3	0.062
5, lung collapse	No	30.0	33.3	54.6	26.3	37.4	0.090
	Yes	30.0	44.4	42.4	31.6	37.4	0.677
6, pulmonary edema	No	40.0	38.9	51.5	47.4	46.5	0.817
	Yes	90.0	88.9	81.8	89.3	86.9	0.848
7, pneumonia	No	70.0	72.2	60.6	63.2	64.7	0.837
	Yes	100.0	94.4	84.9	97.4	92.9	0.155
8, tuberculosis	No	70.0	72.2	75.8	50.0	64.7	0.115
	Yes	90.0	100.0	84.9	73.7	83.8	0.083
9, Pancoast tumour	No	50.0	22.2	48.5	42.1	41.4	0.293
	Yes	60.0	61.1	75.8	47.4	60.6	0.113
10, clavicular fracture	No	30.0	55.6	15.2	39.5	33.3	0.022*
	Yes	50.0	66.7	72.7	65.8	66.7	0.613

**significant at p-value < 0.001 *significant at p-value p-value < 0.05.

($p < 0.001$). This may be misinterpreted that one is likely to be trained on radiographic interpretation as they move higher in their professional rank, but the reverse was seen in this study. As majority of the medical students and medical officers had received formal training compared to residents, house officers were outliners.

Previous studies have shown that training students in radiological imaging interpretation significantly improves their skills and competence on interpreting CXRs [6, 9]. In spite of this, the findings of the present study found no statistically significant association between participants' competence and formal training in interpreting radiographic images. The results show that the average scores for CXRs interpretation was the highest among the residents with (7.5, IQR = 5–9) and without (4.0, IQR = 3–5) clinical history, but mean and median scores did not increase significantly with the level of medical training. Previously, we found that most of the medical students have received some form of radiology training, but they performed the least in CXR interpretation with a median score of 5.5 (IQR = 5–7) (with clinical history) and 3.0 (IQR = 2–4) (without clinical history). In contrast, Eisen et al. [6] found that the median overall score increased with the level of training. The observed differences in findings could be due to the focus of the radiology curriculum, effectiveness of training, and the level of integration in the medical training [9–11]. If training on radiographic interpretation is not effective, CXR interpretation for patients in the outpatient department and emergency will be difficult for medical practitioners. There is the need to focus the radiology course during medical training as well as routine refresher training to improve doctor's confidence and competence [6, 7, 12].

In this study, the competence of residents, medical officers, house officers, and final year medical students in interpreting CXRs heightened the outmost importance of patient's clinical history for doctors to correctly interpret CXRs. For instance, the median score for interpreting CXRs was 4.0 (IQR = 3-4) when no clinical history was presented and 7.5 (IQR = 5–8) when CXRS were presented with clinical history. The observed difference in the median was nearly 2 times when patient's clinical history was available. On the proportion who passed, majority of the participants correctly interpret the CXRs when presented with clinical history (83.8%) while 4 times less was seen when no clinical history (21.2%) was indicated. These findings highlight the relevance of clinical history documentation in medical imaging as well as the physician in interpreting CXRs of their patients. It is, therefore, vital that requesting physicians provide accurate and adequate patient's clinical history when requesting radiographs.

In many teaching hospitals, the frontline staff are predominantly house officers and medical officers. They are expected to request and interpret CXRs and make clinical decisions prior to consultants or senior doctors review. This is particularly important for emergency chest radiographs such as pneumothorax, pneumoperitoneum, pneumomediastinum, lung collapse, pulmonary edema or congestive cardiac failure, pneumonia, *tuberculosis*, clavicular fracture, and acromioclavicular dislocation. The findings indicated that junior doctors and final year medical students alike are limited in their ability to make radiological diagnoses of simple CXRs usually in the absence of clinical history. For instance, both junior doctors and students had difficulties in identifying CXRs with pneumothorax (30.3% vs. 27.3%), pneumomediastinum (33.3% vs. 8.1%), and lung collapse

(37.4% vs. 37.4%) in both situations, i.e., with and without patient clinical history. Pneumothorax and rib fractures are somewhat a very common presentation in the emergency room of this tertiary hospital where this study was conducted. It was the expectation that majority of our doctors will know from experience. Similarly, the medical students performed poorly as only 15.8% could correctly identify normal CXR without being presented with clinical history. A significant limitation of the medical interns and students in relation to competency to interpret similar CXRs was reported by Eisen et al. [6] and Miranda et al. [4]. Our findings suggest that more than 85% of the participants had difficulty in interpreting normal CXRs when no clinical history was presented. The tendency that medical doctors and students would interpret the normal CXR as abnormal has been documented by other investigators [4, 6, 7, 13]. Possibly, interpreting a normal CXR as abnormal could lead to inappropriate decisions which might affect the patient's health and unwarranted cost of treatment.

On the other hand, CXRs with pneumonia (64.7% vs. 92.9%) and tuberculosis (64.7% vs. 83.8%) could easily be identified by the majority of our participants. By stratification, correct interpretation of CXR with pneumothorax was significantly higher among house officers (42.4%) and residents (60%), respectively, when CXR was presented without and with clinical history. Similarly, correct interpretation of CXR with pneumoperitoneum was significantly higher among residents (60%) and medical officers (88.9%) when the images were presented without and with clinical history, respectively. The medical officers tend to interpret CXR with clavicular fracture or acromioclavicular dislocation (55.6%) much better than other counterpart in absence of clinical history. The higher level of competence with interpreting CXRs with pneumonia, tuberculosis, pneumothorax, and clavicular fracture could be attributed to experience in practice and not because they had higher training [7]. Therefore, there is the need to intensify refresher training and coaching for all medical doctors to improve their competence.

The findings of the present study could not be generalized to all health facilities in Ghana since it was conducted in a single tertiary health institution and among few medical practitioners. However, to the best of our knowledge, this is the first-time residents, medical officers, house officers, and final year medical students in Ghana have been evaluated in terms of their competence in interpreting CXRs. This study provides preliminary data for further assessment and to inform scale-up training of medical practitioners and students in the interpretation of radiologic images at the Ghana College of Physicians and Surgeons and Medical schools in Ghana.

The present study is probably the first study of CXR interpretation in Ghana and in terms of categories of medical staff involved. Secondly, participants were from multiple fields of medicine and surgery. Thirdly, this study compared participant performance in two different scenarios (with and without clinical history) that directly confirm the importance of clinical history in medical practice, especially in CXR interpretation.

Meanwhile, our study had some limitations: foremost, a small and somewhat arbitrary sample of CXRs was chosen for the survey which does not represent numerous chest anomalies seen in medical practice and while these were representative of common conditions, and results may have been different with other CXRs. Also, there are over 150 cadre of clinicians and 60 final year medical students working at the CCTH, but only 61 clinicians and 38 final year medical students agreed to participate. Hence, we could not generalize the findings from this study.

5. Conclusion

This study assessed the competence of residents, medical officers, house officers, and final year medical students in relation to the interpretation of CXRs. The competence in interpreting CXRs of common presentations was moderate in residents, medical officers, and house officers but low among final medical students. The presentation of patient's clinical history was found to significantly improve doctors' competence in interpreting CXRs. We found a gap in their ability to interpret CXRs, and hence, development of this skill should be improved. We recommend that medical training and health training institutions in Ghana could attach importance to the development of effective curricular interventions and reliable assessment methods for radiograph interpretation skills. We also recommend a scale-up assessment of clinicians, radiographers, and medical students CXR interpretation skills to help drive timely interventions in our practice.

References

[1] B. T. Andersson, "Radiographers' professional competence: development of a context-specific instrument," Doctoral thesis, Jönköping University, Jönköping, Sweden, 2012.

[2] L. A. Eisen, J. S. Berger, A. Hegde, and R. F. Schneider, "Competency in chest radiography; a comparison of medical students, residents, and fellows," *Journal of General Internal Medicine*, vol. 21, no. 5, pp. 460–465, 2006.

[3] A. Alotaibi and N. Muhyi, "Assessing the radiation protection knowledge among non-radiologists," *International Journal of Medicine in Developing Countries*, vol. 3, pp. 159–162, 2019, https://www.ijmdc.com.

[4] A. C. G. Miranda, C. C. P. Monteiro, M. L. C. Pires, and L. E. C. Miranda, "Radiological imaging interpretation skills of medical interns," *Revista Brasileira de Educação Médica*, vol. 43, no. 3, pp. 145–154, 2019.

[5] V. M. Carneiro da Silva, R. R. Luiz, M. M. Barreto, R. S. Rodrigues, and E. Marchiori, "Competence of senior medical students in diagnosing tuberculosis based on chest X-rays," *The Jornal Brasileiro de Pneumologia*, vol. 36, no. 2, pp. 190–196, 2010.

[6] L. A. Eisen, J. S. Berger, A. Hegde, and R. F. Schneider, "Competency in chest radiography," *Journal of General Internal Medicine*, vol. 21, no. 5, pp. 460–465, 2006.

[7] J. M. Christiansen, O. Gerke, J. Karstoft, and P. E. Andersen, "Poor interpretation of chest X-rays by junior doctors," *Danish Medical Journal*, vol. 61, no. 7, pp. A487–5, 2014.

[8] A. Vanckavičienė, J. Macijauskienė, A. Blaževičienė, A. Basevičius, and B. T. Andersson, "Assessment of radiographers' competences from the perspectives of radiographers and radiologists : a cross-sectional survey in lithuania," *BMC Medical Education*, vol. 17, no. 25, pp. 1–10, 2017.

[9] J. D. Scheiner, R. B. Noto, and K. M. Mccarten, "Importance of radiology clerkships in teaching medical students life-threatening abnormalities on conventional chest radiographs," *Academic Radiology*, vol. 9, no. 2, pp. 217–220, 2002.

[10] B. Petinaux, R. Bhat, K. Boniface, and J. Aristizabal, "Accuracy of radiographic readings in the emergency department," *The American Journal of Emergency Medicine*, vol. 29, no. 1, pp. 18–25, 2011.

[11] S. Kalén, H. Lachmann, M. Varttinen, R. Möller, T. S. Bexelius, and S. Ponzer, "Medical students' experiences of their own professional development during three clinical terms: a prospective follow-up study," *BMC Medical Education*, vol. 17, no. 1, pp. 1–10, 2017.

[12] LCME, LCME Functions and Structure of a Medical School, Standards for Accreditation of Medical Education Programs Leading to the MD Degree, LCME the Association of American Medical Colleges and the American Medical Association, 2020, https://lcme.org/publications/.

[13] C. M. Walsh-Kelly, M. D. Melzer-Lange, H. M. Hennes et al., "Clinical impact of radiograph misinterpretation in a pediatric ED and the effect of physician training level," *The American Journal of Emergency Medicine*, vol. 13, no. 3, pp. 262–264, 1995.

9

Radiologic Mimics of Osteomyelitis and Septic Arthritis: A Pictorial Essay

Wanyin Lim, [1,2] **Christen D. Barras**, [1,2,3] **and Steven Zadow**[1,4]

[1]*Dr Jones and Partners Medical Imaging, Adelaide, South Australia, Australia*
[2]*Department of Radiology, Royal Adelaide Hospital, Adelaide, South Australia, Australia*
[3]*South Australian Health and Medical Research Institute and the University of Adelaide, Adelaide, South Australia, Australia*
[4]*Flinders Medical Centre, Bedford Park, South Australia, Australia*

Correspondence should be addressed to Wanyin Lim; ynyn146@gmail.com

Academic Editor: André Luiz Ferreira COSTA

Various imaging techniques may be employed in the investigation of suspected bone and joint infections. These include ultrasound, radiography, functional imaging such as positron emission tomography (PET) and nuclear scintigraphy, and cross-sectional imaging, including computed tomography (CT) and magnetic resonance imaging (MRI). The cross-sectional modalities represent the imaging workhorse in routine practice. The role of imaging also extends to include assessment of the anatomical extent of infection, potentially associated complications, and treatment response. The imaging appearances of bone and joint infections are heterogeneous and depend on the duration of infection, an individual patient's immune status, and virulence of culprit organisms. To add to the complexity of radiodiagnosis, one of the pitfalls of imaging musculoskeletal infection is the presence of other conditions that can share overlapping imaging features. This includes osteoarthritis, vasculopathy, inflammatory, and even neoplastic processes. Different pathologies may also coexist, for example, diabetic neuropathy and osteomyelitis. This pictorial review aims to highlight potential mimics of osteomyelitis and septic arthritis that are regularly encountered, with emphasis on specific imaging features that may aid the radiologist and clinician in distinguishing an infective from a noninfective aetiology.

1. Introduction

Osteomyelitis is defined as bone inflammation due to infection whilst septic arthritis is defined by infection within a joint [1]. Bone and joint infections have a variable clinical presentation ranging from acute sepsis to insidious onset of pain, with or without fever. Laboratory results such as white cell count, C-reactive protein, and erythrocyte sedimentation rate are often, but not always, abnormal. In some cases, blood cultures are positive. Ultimately, bone biopsy may ultimately be required to identify the offending organism [2].

Imaging plays a crucial role in the diagnosis of infection, assessing disease extent, associated complications, planning biopsy sites, and monitoring treatment response. The various imaging tools employed include radiography, ultrasound, computed tomography (CT), and functional studies including nuclear scintigraphy, white cell scan, and positron emission tomography (PET). Magnetic resonance imaging (MRI), being moderately sensitive and specific, is the imaging modality of choice in the evaluation of suspected osteomyelitis [3, 4].

Understandably, given the heterogeneity of clinical presentations, imaging appearances of infection also vary considerably, being affected by factors such as the virulence of the implicated organism, the site of involvement, the individual's immune status, and the duration of symptoms [1]. To add to the complexity, imaging features for infection are not necessarily specific for osteomyelitis and can also be shared with multiple other conditions [1]. These include degenerative processes, trauma or stress responses, neoplastic processes, vasculopathy, inflammation, neuropathic

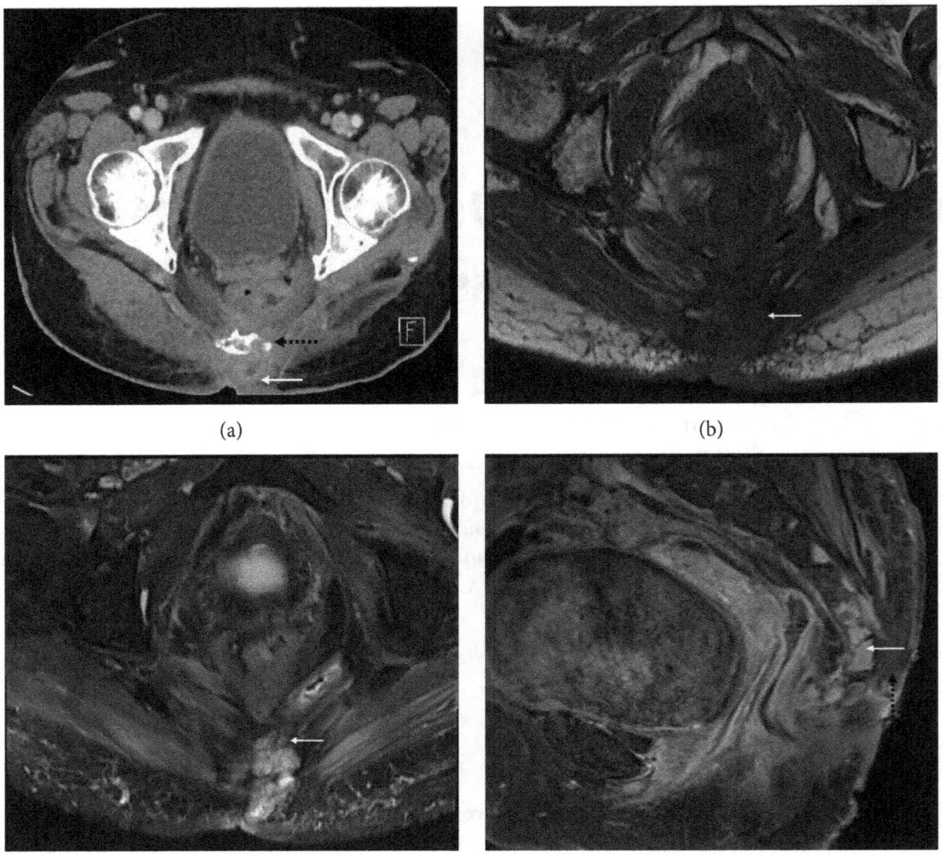

(a) (b) (c) (d)

Figure 1: Osteomyelitis with an ulcer tract arising from a necrotic, infected pressure sore. Axial CT pelvis with intravenous contrast (a) of a 78-year-old bedbound female worked up for sepsis secondary to an infected pressure ulcer showed the ulcer extending to the coccyx in the left parasagittal region (arrow), with bone erosion (dotted line). The affected bone is hypointense on the axial T1 (b) and hyperintense on fluid-sensitive, PDFS (proton density with fat saturation, (c)) sequences. Sagittal T1FS postcontrast image (d) shows enhancement of the coccyx (arrow) and sacrococcygeal joint confirming the diagnosis. The adjacent deep subcutaneous region of nonenhancement is compatible with the area of necrosis (dotted arrow).

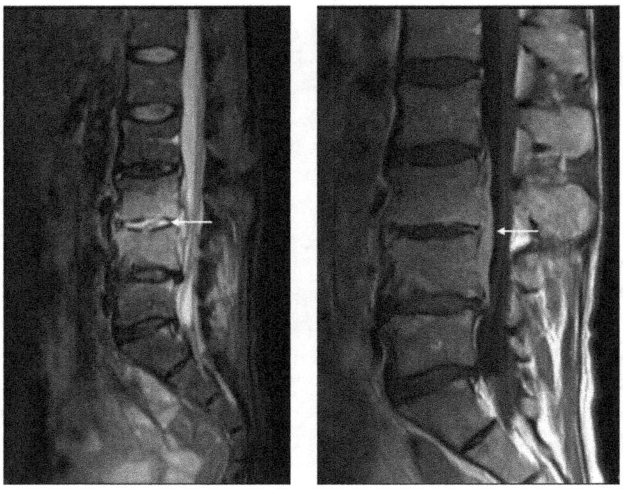

(a) (b)

Figure 2: Discitis-osteomyelitis. (a) Sagittal STIR (short tau inversion recovery) with contiguous marrow oedema signal in the L3 and L4 vertebral bodies with involvement and effusion of the intervening L3/4 disc (arrow). Adjacent diffusely enhancing phlegmon (arrow) on a sagittal T1 postcontrast sequence (b) encroaching on the anterior epidural space, resulting in moderate spinal canal stenosis.

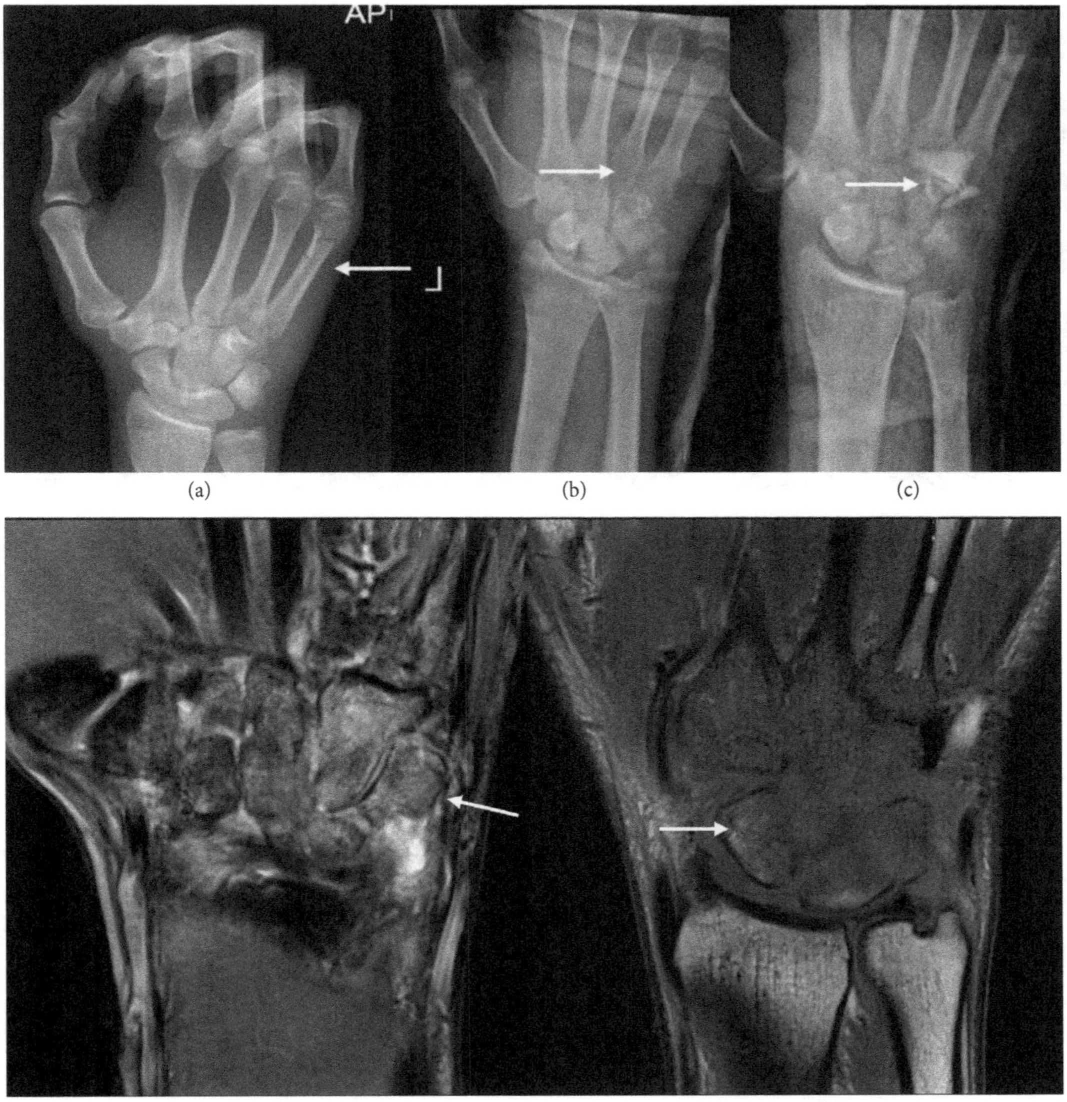

(a) (b) (c) (d) (e)

FIGURE 3: A 45-year-old man involved in a motor vehicle accident sustained an undisplaced 5th metacarpal shaft fracture ((a), arrow). Repeating X-ray 16 days later (b), given the persistent pain, revealed rarefaction of 4th and 5th carpometacarpal (CMC) joints consistent with osteomyelitis and septic arthritis (arrow). X-ray-following washout and introduction of antibiotic-impregnated cement spacer (arrow). Coronal STIR (d) and T1 (e) sequences of the wrist show the extent of the infection involving all carpal bones and base of the 2nd to 5th metacarpals. (c)

arthropathy, iatrogenic processes, and depositional diseases. At times, clinical details may be insufficient to aid image interpretation.

This pictorial review aims to highlight a few of the potential mimics of osteomyelitis and septic arthritis that are commonly encountered, with emphasis on specific MRI features that may aid the radiologist and clinician in distinguishing infection from a noninfective aetiology. Variants of infection/osteomyelitis are also briefly covered.

1.1. Typical Imaging Appearances of Osteomyelitis and Septic Arthritis. To understand the MR imaging appearances of infection mimics, it is first important to know the classic appearances of infection. Pyogenic osteomyelitis is typically T1 hypointense, due to the replacement of normal fatty marrow tissue. The confluent T1-hypointensity usually results in loss of distinction between the cortex and medulla, referred to as the "ghost sign" (Figure 1). On T2-weighted sequences, such as T2 with fat saturation (T2FS) and short tau inversion recovery (STIR), affected areas are fluid-hyperintense. Various terms are applied to this finding, including "marrow oedema," "marrow oedema signal," and "bone marrow lesion (BML)" [5]. Areas of established infection usually demonstrate enhancement following contrast administration.

In peripheral body parts, ancillary features to actively search for include soft tissue inflammation, abscess, and ulceration or sinus tract formation, contiguous with the site of bone signal abnormality. Areas of geographical

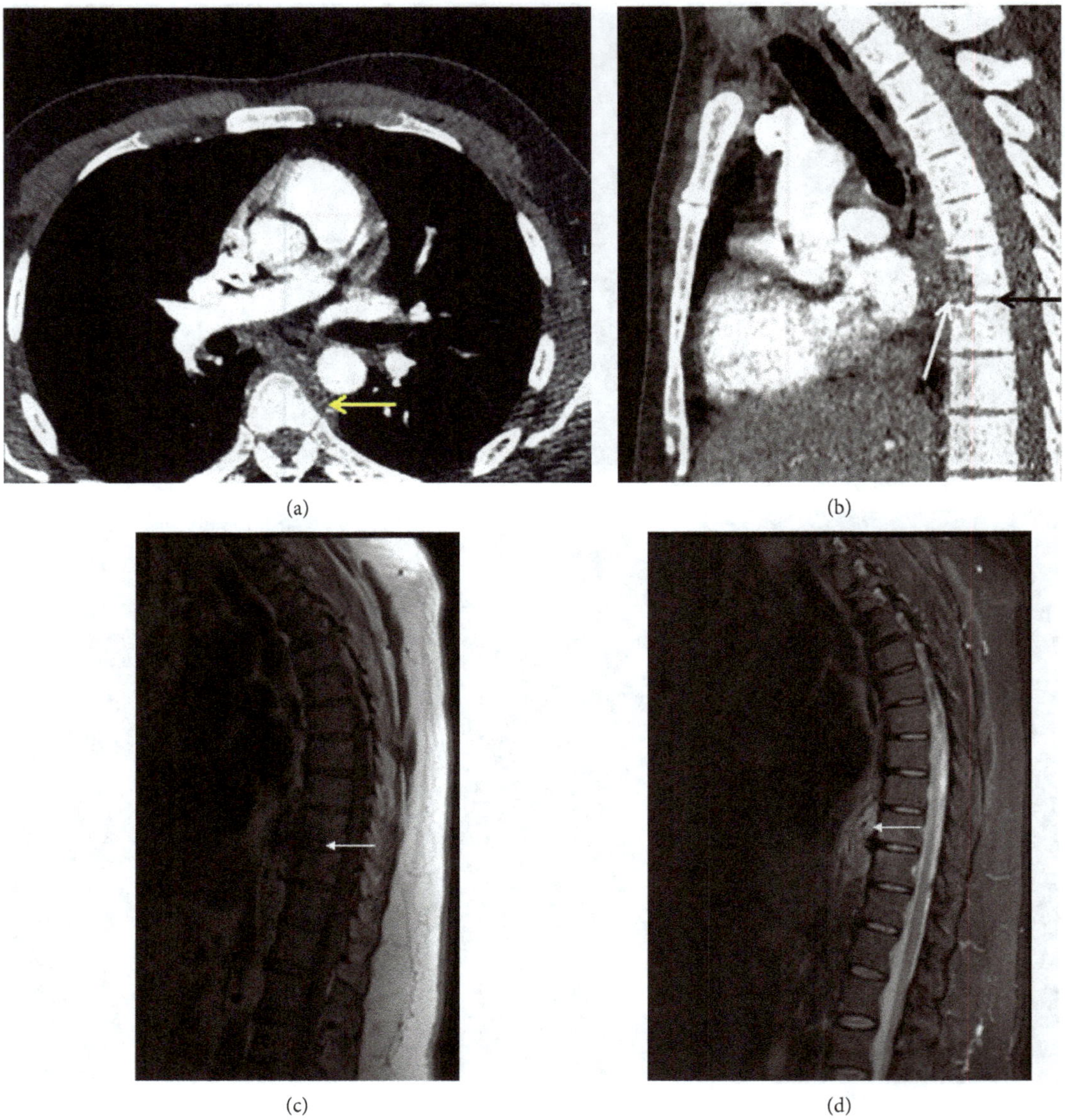

FIGURE 4: Tuberculous osteomyelitis. Postcontrast axial (a) and sagittal (b) chest CT of a 34-year-old patient with biopsy-proven TB discitis-osteomyelitis. There is lytic destruction of the T7 vertebral body anteriorly ((b) white arrow). There is subligamentous soft tissue density extending from T5-T8 (A yellow and B white arrows) with relative sparing of the adjacent T7 end plates (b black arrow). Sagittal T1 (c) and STIR (d) of a different patient with T9/10 osteomyelitis (c arrow) and pronounced subligamentous spread of disease from T8/9-T11 (d arrow). Note the relative sparing of the disc in early disease (c arrow).

nonenhancement, which can indicate necrosis, are also important to note (Figure 1). In the spine, the involvement of two contiguous vertebral bodies and their intervening disc is usually indicative of discitis-osteomyelitis (Figure 2).

The earliest findings of marrow oedema signal can be present within 2 days of symptom onset [1]. In the event of discordant clinical and imaging information, where there is a high clinical index of suspicion for infection despite negative initial imaging results, repeat imaging is important as imaging findings may lag behind clinical manifestations by up to 2 weeks [6] (Figure 3).

With atypical organisms such as tuberculous osteomyelitis, systemic manifestations may not be as florid. Useful features for mycobacterial infection particularly in the spine are the relative sparing of intervertebral disc spaces early in the infective process, the subligamentous spread of infection, and involvement of multiple contiguous levels at once [1] (Figure 4).

Chronic osteomyelitis can occur in the context of incomplete treatment or atypical organisms. Disruption of vascular supply results in necrosis or sequestrum formation which then serves as a nidus for continued infection. To wall off the infection, granulation tissue and new bone, or involucrum, form around the sequestrum. Imaging is characterised by a mixed pattern of lysis and sclerosis [1]. Sinus tracts can form within the involucrum through which pus or sequestrum may be expelled (Figure 5).

Features that are specific for joint infection include lamellated synovial thickening (Figure 6), rapid destruction,

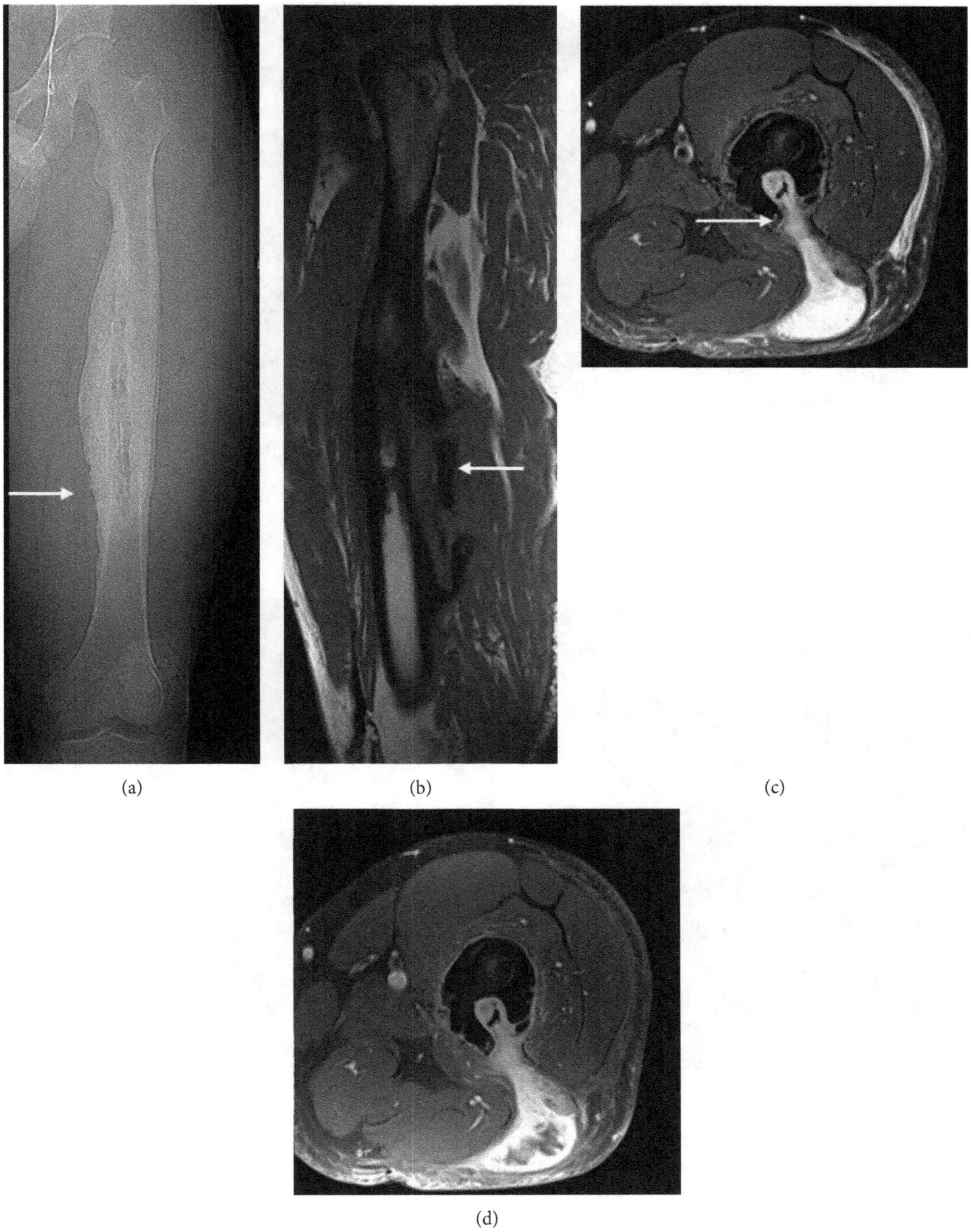

Figure 5: A 30-year-old systemically well man with chronic osteomyelitis who initially presented with an enlarging mass in the posterior thigh. The planning CT (a) showed femoral shaft sclerosis, periosteal thickening, and cortical expansion which is worse medially. A lucent tract at the inferior border of the abnormal bone extends from the medulla to the cortex, consistent with a sinus tract (arrow). Sagittal T1 (b) demonstrating the extent of the osteomyelitis with sequestrum posteroinferiorly (arrow). Axial PDFS (c) and T1FS postcontrast (d) MRI shows the new bone formation or involucrum attempting to envelop the infection. A cloaca or sinus tract involving the posterolateral thigh discharges into the subcutaneous plane, accounting for the presentation (C arrow).

and erosion of the bare areas, where there is less coverage of the bone by hyaline cartilage [7]. Usually, there is a marrow oedema signal on both sides of the articular surface, often with an accompanying joint effusion and synovial enhancement, although these features are not as specific [7] (Figure 3).

1.2. Mimics of Osteomyelitis

1.2.1. Degeneration/Mechanical Type. Degenerative spondyloarthropathy, involving end plate degeneration in the spine, particularly of the inflammatory type (Modic type I), characterised by end plate T1-hypointensity and fluid-

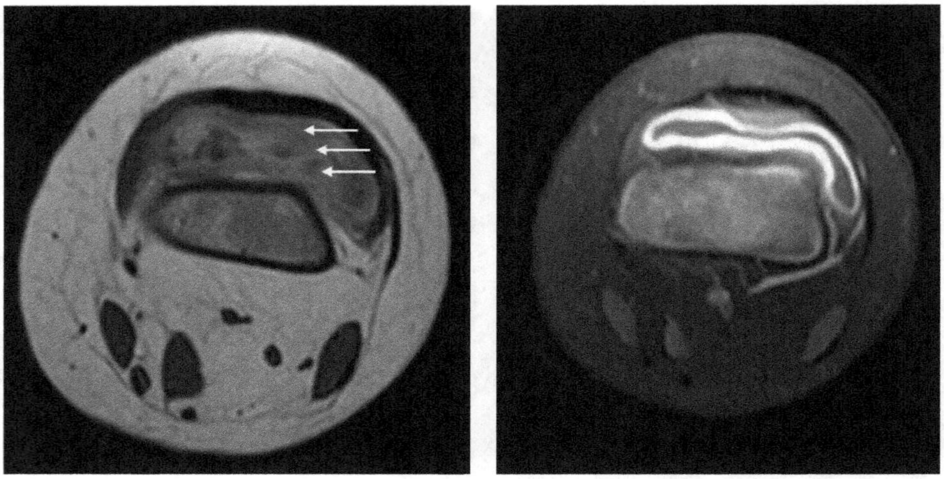

(a) (b)

FIGURE 6: Axial T2 (a) and T1FS postcontrast (b) MRI of the knee in a 6-year-old boy. Lamellated synovial thickening (a) is specific for septic arthritis.

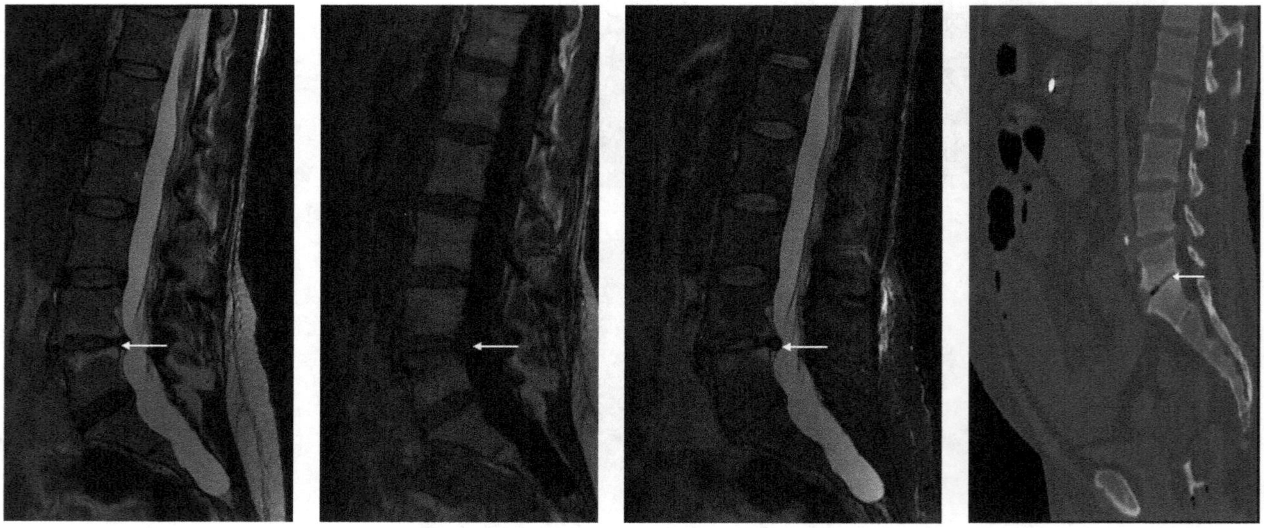

(a) (b) (c) (d)

FIGURE 7: End plate degeneration. Sagittal T2 (a), T1 (b), and STIR (c) lumbar spine of a 40-year-old female presenting with right L5 radiculopathy in the background of low back pain. The fluid-hyperintensity (a, c) and T1 hypointense marrow signal (b) on either side of the L4/5 end plate (arrow), in the context of end plate irregularity and preservation of normal/hypointense disc signal, is consistent with inflammatory or Modic type I degeneration. The radiculopathy was secondary to impingement of the right L5 nerve root from the herniated disc at this level (not shown). Sagittal CT lumbar spine of a different patient (d) shows a vacuum cleft in the L5/S1 disc space with adjacent end plate sclerosis (Modic III degeneration). The vacuum cleft is a useful sign of degeneration.

hyperintensity, can mimic infection. A useful distinguishing feature is end plate irregularity without erosion and presence of gas in the adjacent disc space, hypointense on all MRI sequences (Figure 7). The gas indicates the vacuum phenomenon in the context of degeneration [8, 9] (Figure 7(d)). The disc desiccation that accompanies degeneration is hypointense instead of hyperintense, as demonstrated in discitis [9].

Rapidly destructive osteoarthritis of the hip is a unique condition characterised by rapid cartilage loss [10]. The MR features include joint effusion, bone marrow oedema in the proximal femur and adjacent acetabulum, and hatchet-like deformity or flattening of the femoral head (Figure 8). These changes can mimic septic arthritis. Useful discriminatory features are subchondral geodes and femoral head destruction that is disproportionately advanced relative to the acetabular involvement [10].

1.2.2. Trauma. Fractures or stress responses can sometimes be mistaken for infection on imaging, particularly when a history of trauma is not provided. Both trauma and infection

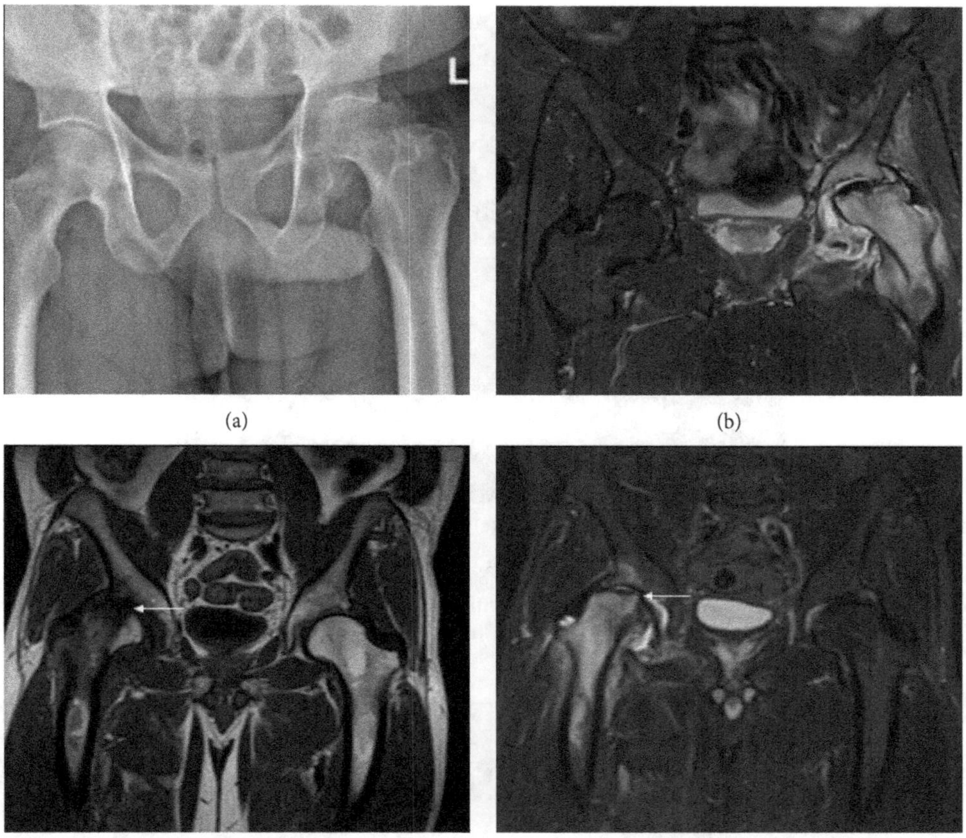

(a) (b) (c) (d)

Figure 8: Two cases of rapidly progressive hip osteoarthritis. X-ray (a) and coronal STIR (b) of a 78-year-old man presenting with an increasingly painful and stiff left hip, demonstrating left hip joint effusion, joint marrow oedema signal, and flattening of the femoral head. Joint aspirate and subsequent washout were negative for infection. Coronal T1 (c) of a second patient with coronal STIR (d) performed 2 months apart shows the rapidly progressive nature of this condition, with hatchet-like deformity of the femoral head in the latter study (d arrow) due to subchondral insufficiency fracture.

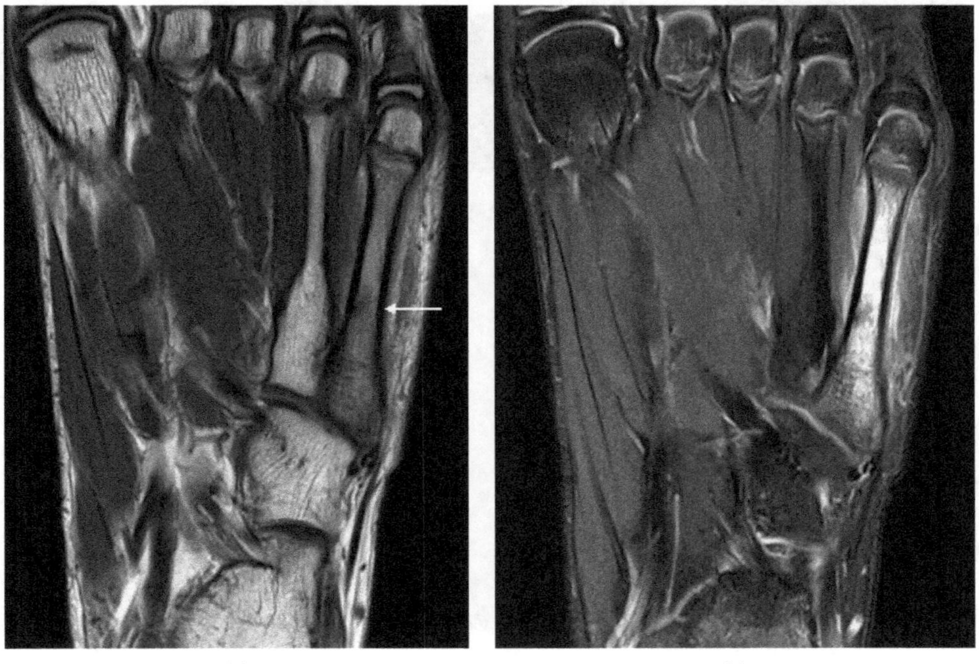

(a) (b)

Figure 9: Continued.

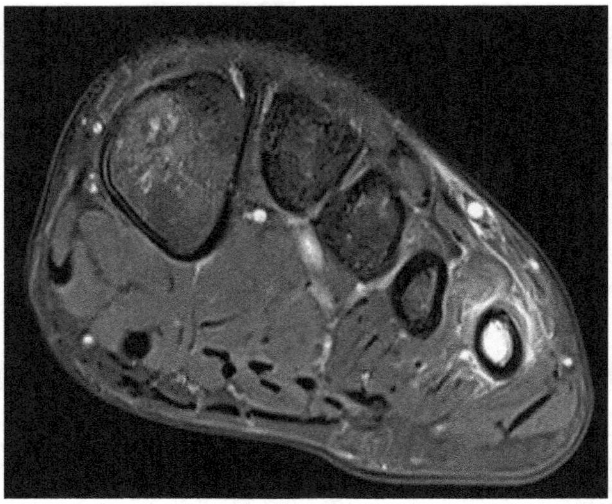

(c)

FIGURE 9: Stress response. Coronal PD (a), coronal (b), and axial PDFS (c) of a 13-year-old soccer player with persistent forefoot pain. There is diffuse marrow oedema signal centred in the 5th metatarsal shaft with surrounding periosteal and soft tissue oedema. The linear signal at the medial border of the metatarsal shaft represents an incomplete fracture (a, arrow).

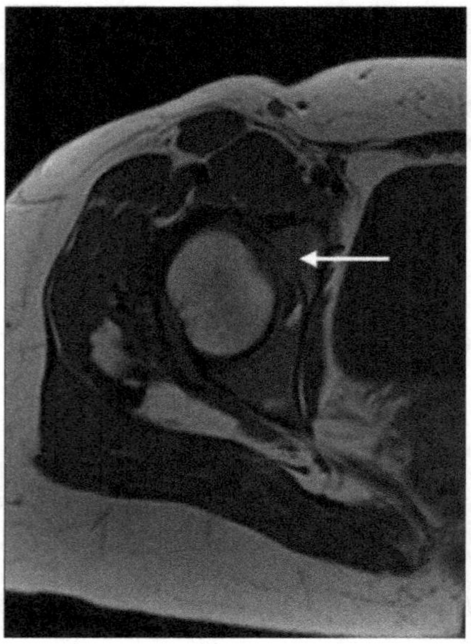

(a)

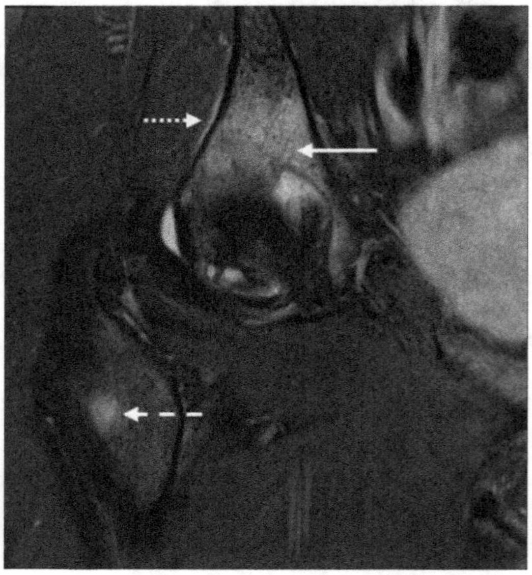

(b)

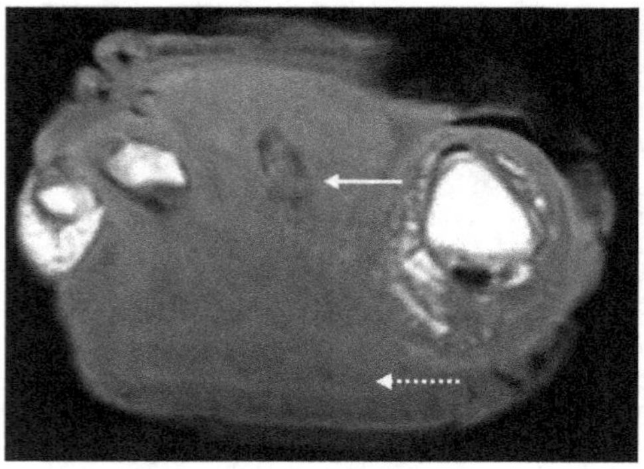

(c)

FIGURE 10: Continued.

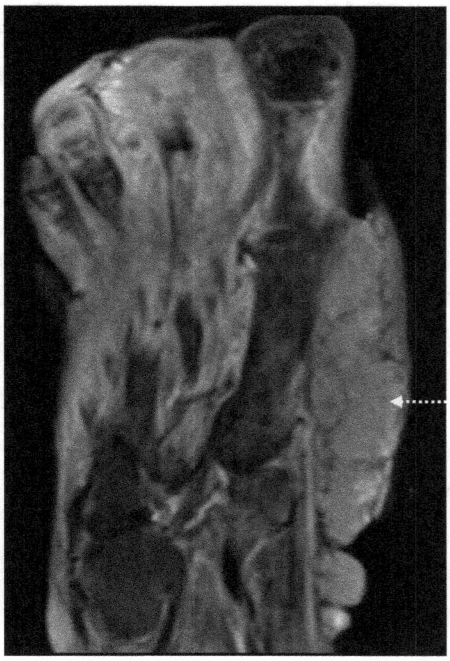

(d)

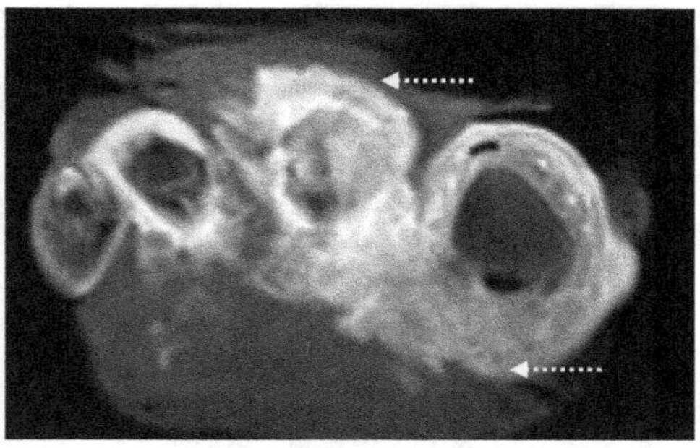

(e)

Figure 10: Metastases. Axial T1 (a) pelvis at the level of the hip joint of a 47-year-old female with metastatic breast cancer involving the right acetabulum. Ill-defined acetabular cortex is consistent with cortical breach of tumour and intraarticular extension (arrow). Tumour exhibits mass-effect that is usually readily apparent on MRI. Tumour is usually hyperintense in fluid-sensitive sequences which can mimic infection. Coronal PDFS (b) at the anterior acetabular margin with fluid-hyperintensity of the tumour breaching the acetabular cortex (arrow). Periosteal extension lateral pelvis (dotted arrow). A separate metastatic deposit also presents in the proximal right femoral shaft which helps clinch the diagnosis (dash). Axial T1 (c) and coronal STIR (d) and axial fat-saturated postcontrast T1 (e) of the right foot of a 38-year-old man with AIDS-related Kaposi sarcoma. The fungating, partially necrotic/enhancing mass (e) is centred in the forefoot, particularly involving the second metatarsal (arrow). The signal intensity of the involved bone mimics that of osteomyelitis, although infection should not be infiltrative and mass-forming (dotted arrows).

can have surrounding the soft tissue oedema signal. The presence of a hypointense fracture line on MRI helps to distinguish a fracture from osteomyelitis (Figure 9). In absence of a clear fracture line, the stress response occurs more commonly at the mid-diaphysis, whilst infection typically occurs in areas of the increased vascular supply, such as at the epiphysis or metaphysis [1]. The location of stress fractures is usually characteristic, such as the tibia, distal fibula, and metatarsal shafts.

1.2.3. Neoplasm. Neoplastic processes, either primary bone tumours or skeletal metastases, can also mimic infection. Tumours are usually mass-forming, and whilst this can be difficult to appreciate on CT or radiographs, this is usually evident on a T1 sequence [11] (Figure 10). It is important to assess for extraosseous extension of tumour and not confuse it with soft tissue inflammation (Figure 10(c)–10(e)).

One specific neoplasm that can be confused with infection is osteoid osteoma. This is a benign osteoblastic neoplasm which is richly innervated and induces a florid host response by means of periostitis and marrow oedema signal [12]. In addition, up to 10% can be intra-articular which can incite marked synovitis and joint effusion (Figure 11). The clue to the correct diagnosis is the detection of a nidus at the epicentre of the marrow oedema signal, which is usually T1 hypointense and T2 hyperintense (Figure 11). The nidus can often be better appreciated on CT and can have a calcified or lucent matrix.

1.2.4. Vasculopathy. Raynaud phenomenon can affect the vasculature of the extremities by vasospasm and vasoconstriction following exposure to various stressors such as cold temperature. This can be associated with an abnormal marrow oedema-like signal limited to the distal phalanges of the hands or feet [13]. Similar changes have also been observed in patients with critical limb ischemia. Although the mechanism remains unclear, the signal changes may be due to tissue damage from ischaemic injury, oedema following reperfusion, or fibrosis from marrow necrosis. In these cases, noncontiguity of the marrow oedema-like signal involving multiple bones and absence of surrounding soft tissue abnormality is the key to accurate diagnosis (Figure 12).

1.2.5. MRI Artefact: Failure of Fat Suppression. The failure of fat suppression on MRI, manifesting as increased fluid-signal towards the extremities of the scan field, or in presence of metalware which can alter the uniformity of the magnetic field, is a potential artefactual pitfall. This can be distinguished

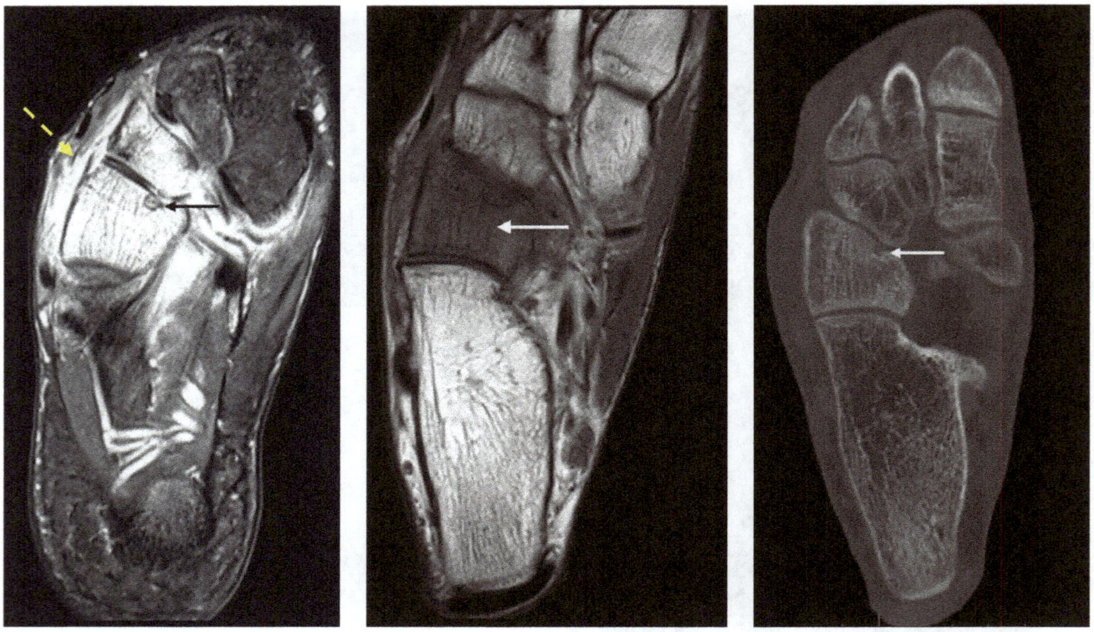

(a) (b) (c)

Figure 11: Cuboid osteoid osteoma in a 17-year-old presenting with a 2-month history of foot pain. Axial PDFS (a) of the foot shows diffuse marrow oedema-signal in the cuboid and lateral cuneiform with adjacent synovitis and soft tissue oedema. There is T1 marrow replacement of the cuboid ((b), arrow). A fluid-hyperintense nidus, best seen on the fluid-sensitive sequence, is noted in the medial border of the cuboid, with extension into the articular surface (arrow), accounting for the effusion and reactive synovitis (A yellow dash). The nidus is confirmed on the CT ((c), arrow), demonstrating central calcification, and distinguishes the diagnosis of osteoid osteoma from infection.

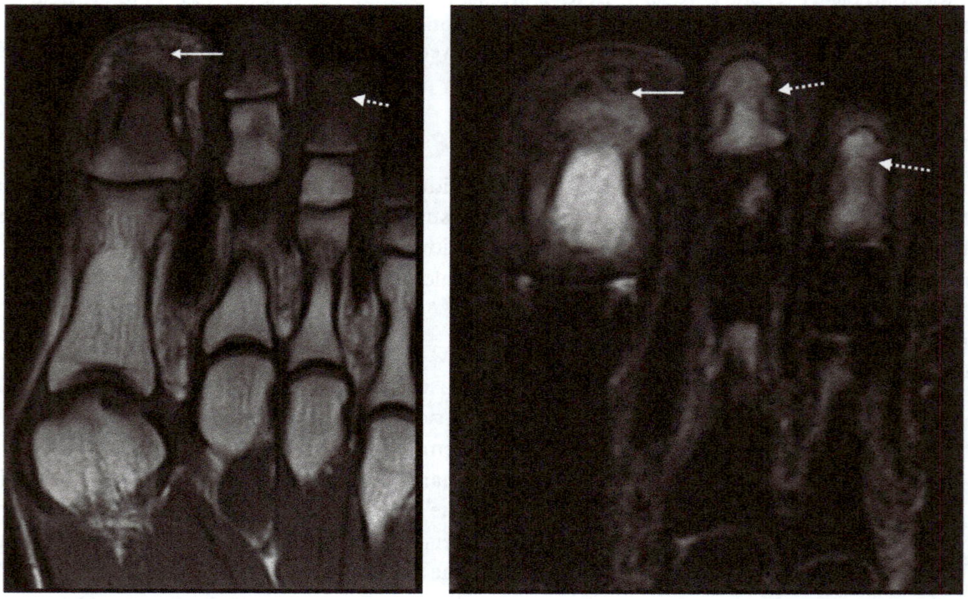

(a) (b)

Figure 12: Coronal forefoot T1 (a) and STIR (b) sequence of a 45-year-old female with Raynaud phenomenon. There is an altered marrow signal (A dotted arrow) with oedema signal (b dotted arrow) in the distal phalanges involving noncontiguous bone. There is an impression of early tuft resorption involving the great toe (arrow), with an ill-defined cortex.

from pathology, as the adjacent subcutaneous fat will also be involved or incompletely suppressed (Figure 13). Various techniques can be employed to minimise these artefacts, although this is beyond the scope of the manuscript [5].

1.2.6. Inflammation. Inflammatory spondyloarthropathy comprises a group of chronic inflammatory rheumatologic conditions with a predilection for the axial skeleton [14, 15]. The sacroiliac joints are usually involved during the early

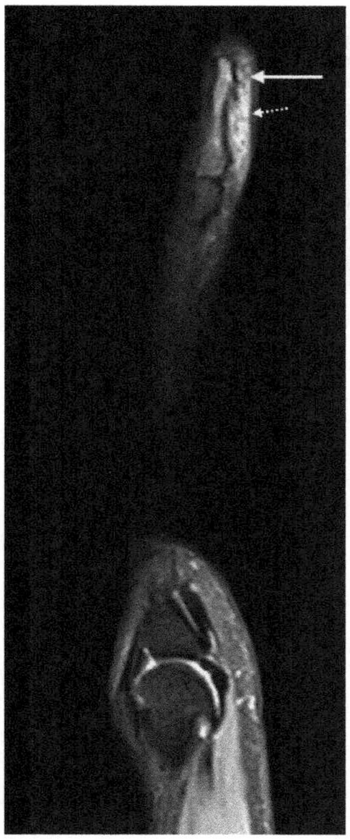

FIGURE 13: Artefact. Sagittal PDFS of the ring finger of a healthy volunteer demonstrating a failure of fat suppression at the tip of the finger resulting in a false impression of marrow hyperintensity in the distal phalanx. The adjacent subcutaneous tissue is also inadequately suppressed (dash).

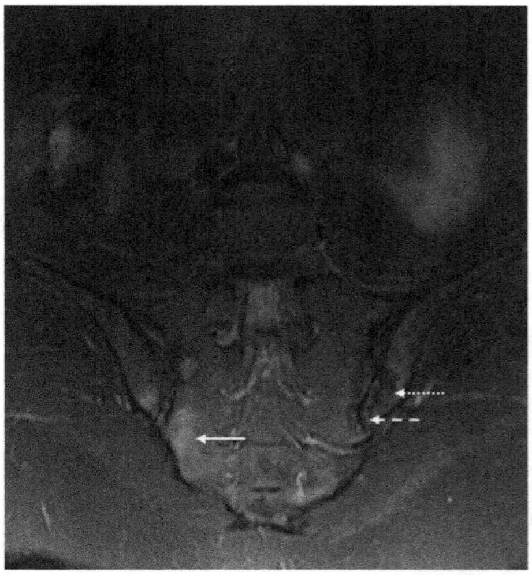

FIGURE 14: Sacroiliitis. Coronal STIR sequence of sacroiliac joints (SIJ) of a 34-year-old male with right acute on chronic and left chronic sacroiliitis. The region of the acute inflammatory process is denoted by the marrow oedema signal in the cartilaginous component of the right SIJ (arrow). Marrow fat infiltration (dotted arrow) adjacent to the left SIJ inferiorly implies prior inflammation. Irregular joint surface (dash) is consistent with erosion.

course of the disease process. Early detection of sacroiliitis using a combination of radiologic and clinical findings is important since the condition usually responds well to disease-modifying therapies, which can prevent or slow the progression to structural damage.

MRI manifestations include marrow oedema on both sides of the sacroiliac joints, usually involving the anteroinferior or cartilaginous articulation. In the early stages of the disease, joint effusion and marrow oedema signal can be more pronounced at the iliac border as the cartilage is thinner here. As the disease progresses, fatty infiltration in adjacent bone, erosion, and ankylosis can be observed (Figure 14). This inflammation, unlike infection, is confined to this space, does not cross anatomical borders, and is not associated with surrounding soft tissue oedema [14].

Chronic recurrent multifocal osteomyelitis (CRMO) is an idiopathic inflammatory disorder and shares similar appearances with subacute/chronic osteomyelitis [16]. Medial clavicular and multifocal involvement in children or adolescents is classically described. In suspected cases of CRMO, a whole-body MRI should be considered to look for other areas of bone involvement (Figure 15). CRMO is a diagnosis of exclusion after excluding other secondary causes for chronic OM.

SAPHO (synovitis, acne, pustulosis, hyperostosis, osteitis) is a rare condition affecting mostly young to middle-aged adults, representing an older demographic than the CRMO subset [17]. It may sometimes mimic osteomyelitis due to its bony involvement and osteitis. This is also usually polyostotic and classically affects the sternoclavicular joints, first rib, sternomanubrial joint, and the anterior aspect of the vertebral bodies (Figure 16).

1.2.7. Iatrogenic Processes. Radiation osteonecrosis can occur following radiotherapy (30–50 Gy) due to a combination of damage to osteoblasts, resulting in unopposed osteoclastic activity, and vascular injury [18]. There is an initial osteopenia or lysis, followed by a delayed and disorganised bony repair at least 3 years following radiotherapy, resulting in trabecular disorganisation and patchy marrow density (Figure 17(a)). On MRI, the initial acute changes can be associated with marrow and soft tissue oedema, and these can be difficult to distinguish from osteomyelitis or tumour recurrence (Figures 17(b) and 17(c)). Radiotherapy treatment timing, duration, dose, and field are useful parameters in this setting along with previous, baseline imaging for comparison, as radiation osteonecrosis will be confined within the field of radiotherapy even when the borders of the abnormal bone are poorly defined [19]. Associated osteolysis, osseous expansion, or fistula formation is usually more indicative of infection than osteonecrosis [19].

Postoperative findings and sterile collections can often be difficult to distinguish from infection and image interpretation can be further complicated by the presence of orthopaedic hardware which can lead to susceptibility and field inhomogeneity artefacts (Figure 13). The presence of metalware reduces the ability to adequately suppress the fat-signal, simulating marrow and soft tissue oedema. Whilst various MRI techniques have been employed for artefact reduction, nuclear medicine studies and, in particular, the

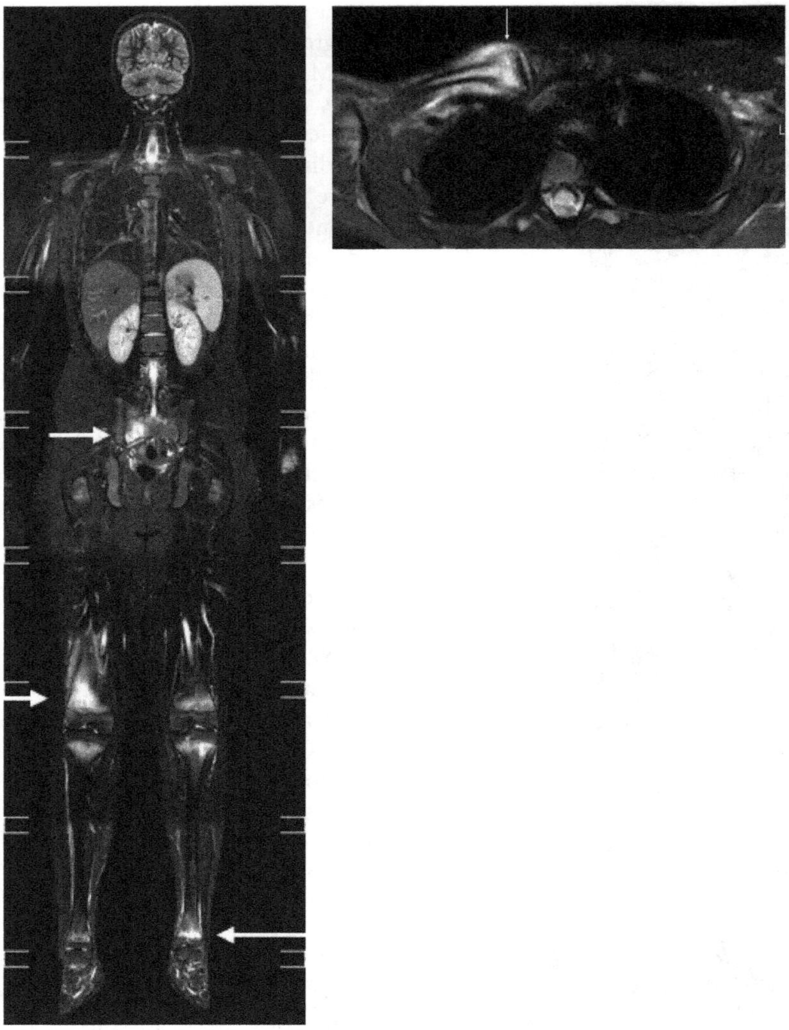

(a) (b)

Figure 15: CRMO. Coronal whole-body MRI of an 8-year-old boy (a) with CRMO initially presenting with right knee pain. Note the multifocal involvement which included both knees, left ankle, and the sacrum (arrow). Axial STIR (b) of a different CRMO patient aged 7, with classic involvement of right medial clavicle with associated hyperostosis (arrow).

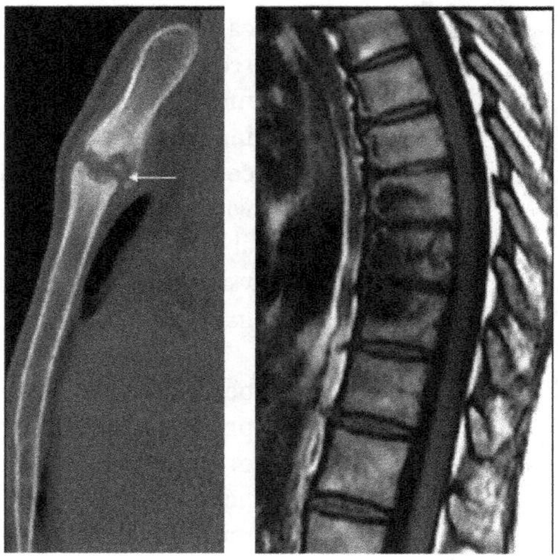

(a) (b)

Figure 16: A 27-year-old female with SAPHO. There is hyperostosis and osteitis of the sternomanubrial junction on the sagittal CT (a). Contiguous involvement of multiple vertebral bodies anteriorly with sparing of the intervening disc space as demonstrated on sagittal T1 thoracic spine is typical of this condition (b).

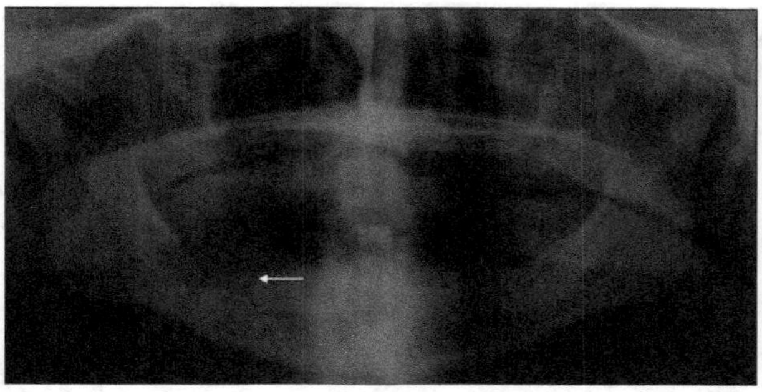

(a)

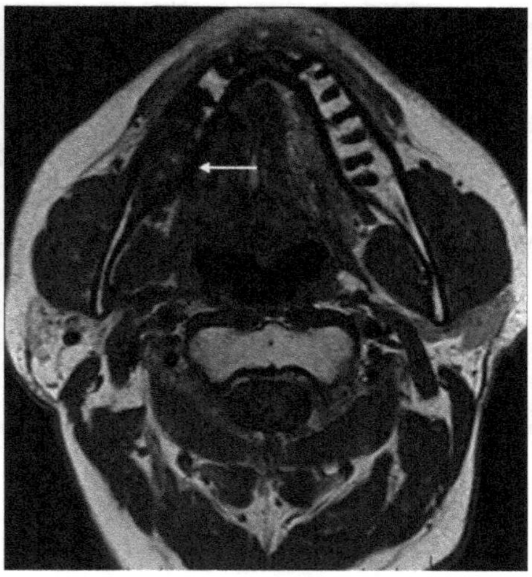

(b)

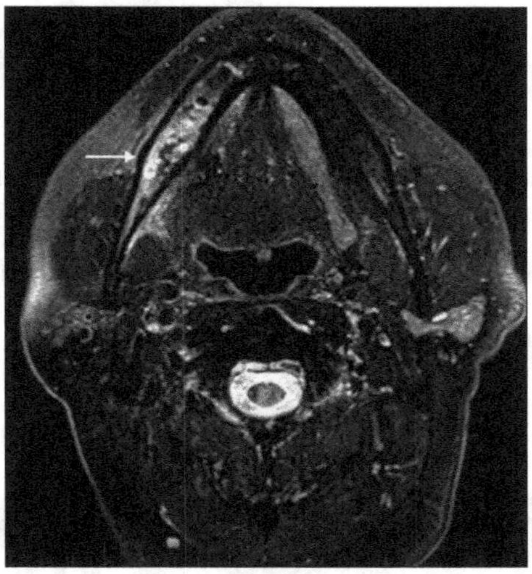

(c)

FIGURE 17: Osteoradionecrosis. Orthopantomogram (OPG, (a)) of a 74-year-old male with a history of T3 oropharyngeal tumour having undergone prior resection and chemoradiotherapy, complicated by osteoradionecrosis. There is ill-defined lytic lucency eroding the right mandibular body with background coarsened trabeculation and patchy sclerosis. Axial T1 (b) and T2FS (c) of a different patient with a previous history of radiotherapy for skin SCC, presenting with a nonhealing ulcer due to osteoradionecrosis. There are T1 hypointensity and fluid-hyperintensity in the body of the right mandible ((a) arrow). Mild surrounding soft tissue oedema ((b) arrow).

white cell scan remains the most valuable imaging modality to assess for infection around a prosthesis [20].

MRI plays a key role in the assessment of delayed-hypersensitivity reactions to arthroplasty-related metal products, known as pseudotumour or adverse reaction to metal debris. This can lead to aggressive soft tissue destruction if untreated. Imaging features include effusion with variable thickness of the synovial lining of synovial proliferation (Figure 18). It can be associated with perisynovial oedema and local nodal enlargement, mimicking infection. Increased synovial thickness and T1 and T2-hypointensity favour pseudotumour over infection [21].

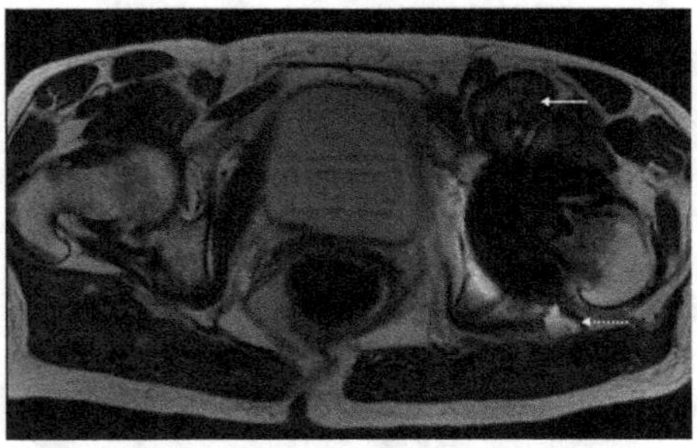

FIGURE 18: Adverse reaction to metallic debris (ARMD). A 70-year-old female with left hip resurfacing complicated by pseudotumour formation. Axial T2 pelvis with metal artefact reduction technique demonstrating distension of the left hip pseudocapsule posteriorly (dotted line) and a larger anterior pseudocapsule defect decompressing into the iliopsoas bursa (arrow). This thickened, T2-hypointense rim with synovial proliferation favours pseudotumour/ARMD over infection.

1.2.8. Neuropathy. Neuropathic arthropathy most commonly occurs in patients with altered pain sensation and proprioception resulting in the accumulation of

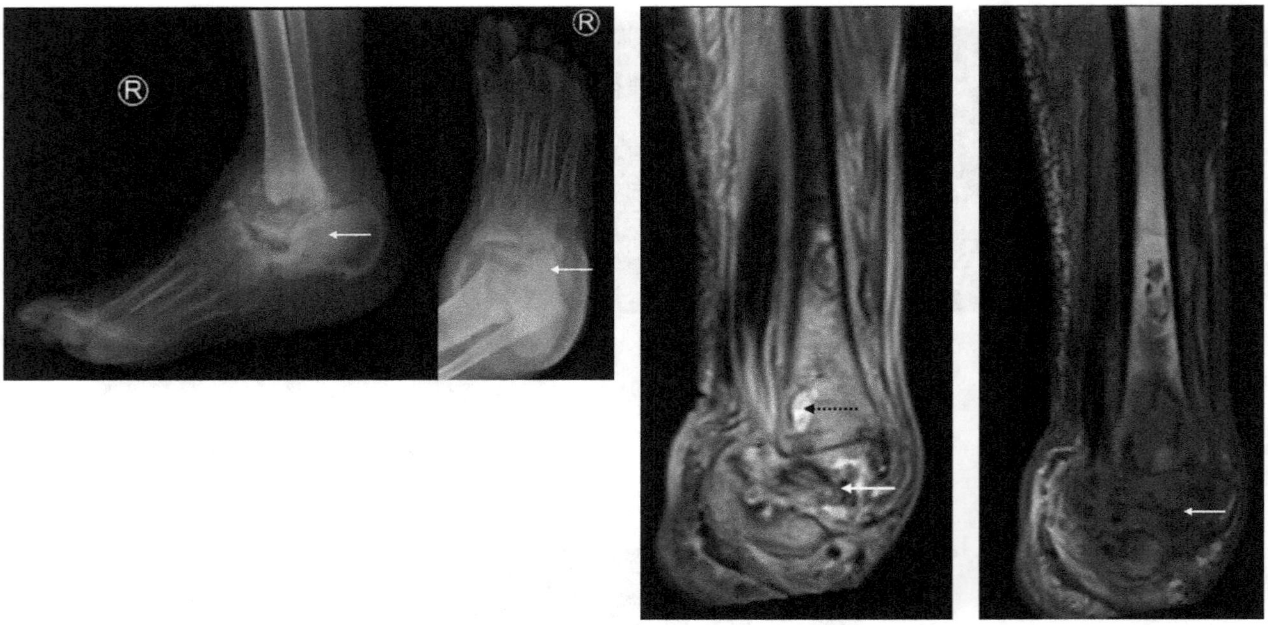

(a) (b) (c)

Figure 19: Lateral and oblique right foot radiographs (a) of a 47-year-old woman with type II diabetes and Charcot arthropathy involving the midfoot. Disorganised hindfoot with joint destruction and disorganisation (arrow). Note the absence of osteopenia that is typically observed in infection. Coronal STIR (b) and T1 (c) of a different patient with Charcot arthropathy with hindfoot destruction, hindfoot valgus, and dislocation. The contrast was not administered due to chronic renal failure. The talus is flattened and sclerotic (arrow). Note the fluid collection in the distal tibial shaft (dotted arrow) and the medial tibiotalar articulation. This patient had both neuropathic arthropathy complicated by chronic osteomyelitis with intraosseous abscess formation. At times, different conditions can preexist, and ultimately, tissue sampling may be required.

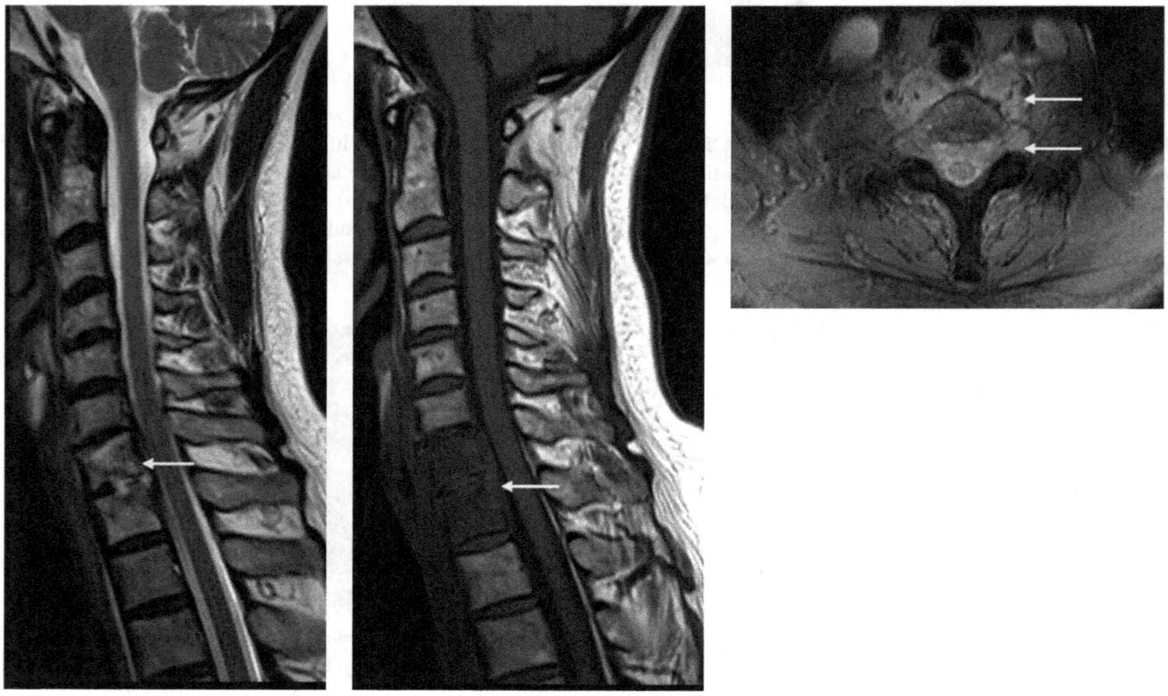

(a) (b) (c)

Figure 20: Continued.

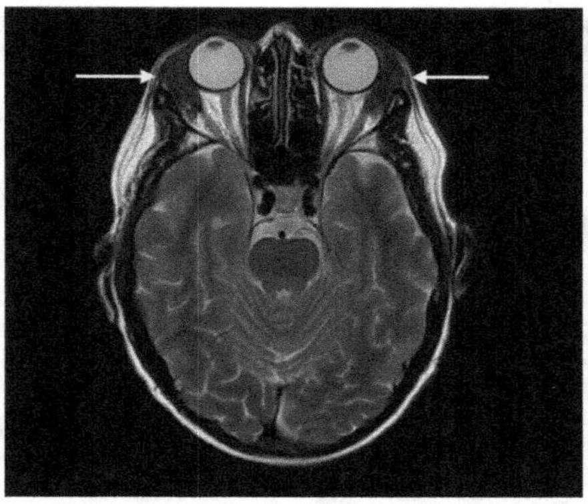

(d)

Figure 20: Primary amyloidosis. A 64-year-old woman with known primary amyloidosis of lacrimal glands, initially presenting with neck pain. Sagittal T2 (a), T1 (b), and axial T2FS (c) spine shows an infiltrative process involving the C7 and T1 vertebrae with an extraosseous extension of soft tissue into the epidural and prevertebral spaces (arrow). End plate irregularity is also present. Axial T2FS (c) at the level of C7 demonstrating epidural and prevertebral soft tissue infiltration (arrow). This case was difficult to distinguish from infection, ultimately requiring a biopsy for the final diagnosis of C7/T1 amyloid deposition. Axial T2 head at the level of the orbits (d) showed bilateral lacrimal gland enlargement secondary to amyloid deposition (arrow).

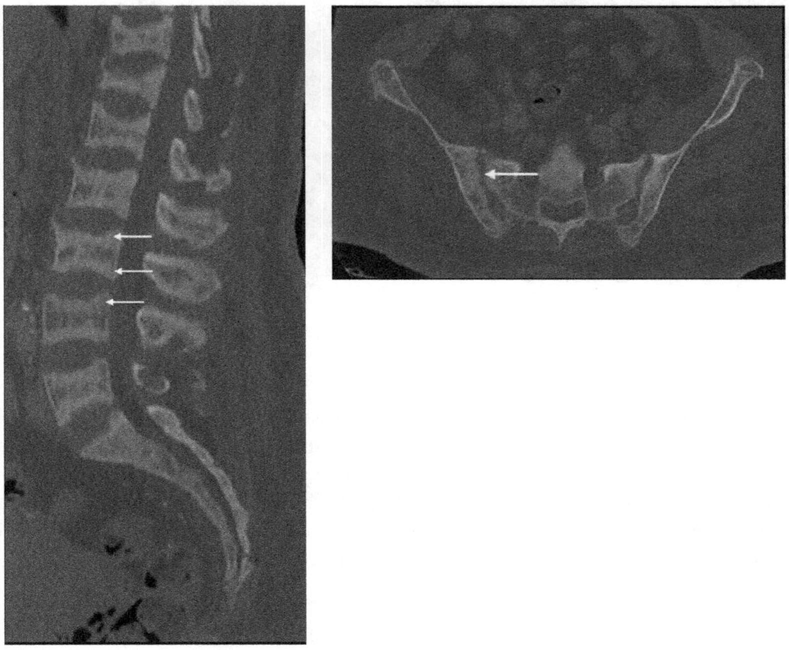

(a) (b)

Figure 21: A 49-year-old female with end stage renal failure and tertiary hyperparathyroidism. Sagittal lumbar spine (a) with bone reconstructions shows rugger-jersey spine with sclerosis adjacent to end plates (arrow) whilst axial pelvis (b) demonstrates subperiosteal resorption of the SIJs (arrow).

microtrauma [22, 23]. It commonly occurs in the feet of diabetic patients. In the acute stage, the foot may be painful and erythematous, followed by bone disorganisation, dislocation, secondary degeneration, and debris formation with preservation of bone density, also known as the "Five Ds" (Figure 19). Features that favour neuropathy over osteomyelitis are periarticular marrow oedema-like signal, joint subluxation, and geode formation, since neuropathy is predominantly an articular process. Sclerosis on radiographs and stability of findings over time favour Charcot neuropathy over infection. On the contrary, the contiguity of the marrow change with any ulcer or collection supports infection (Figures 1, 19(b), and 19(c). The areas affected by osteomyelitis may be more conspicuous on contrast-enhanced sequences. Various new techniques such as the use of diffusion-weighted imaging (DWI), dynamic postcontrast enhancement, and perfusion may provide further useful

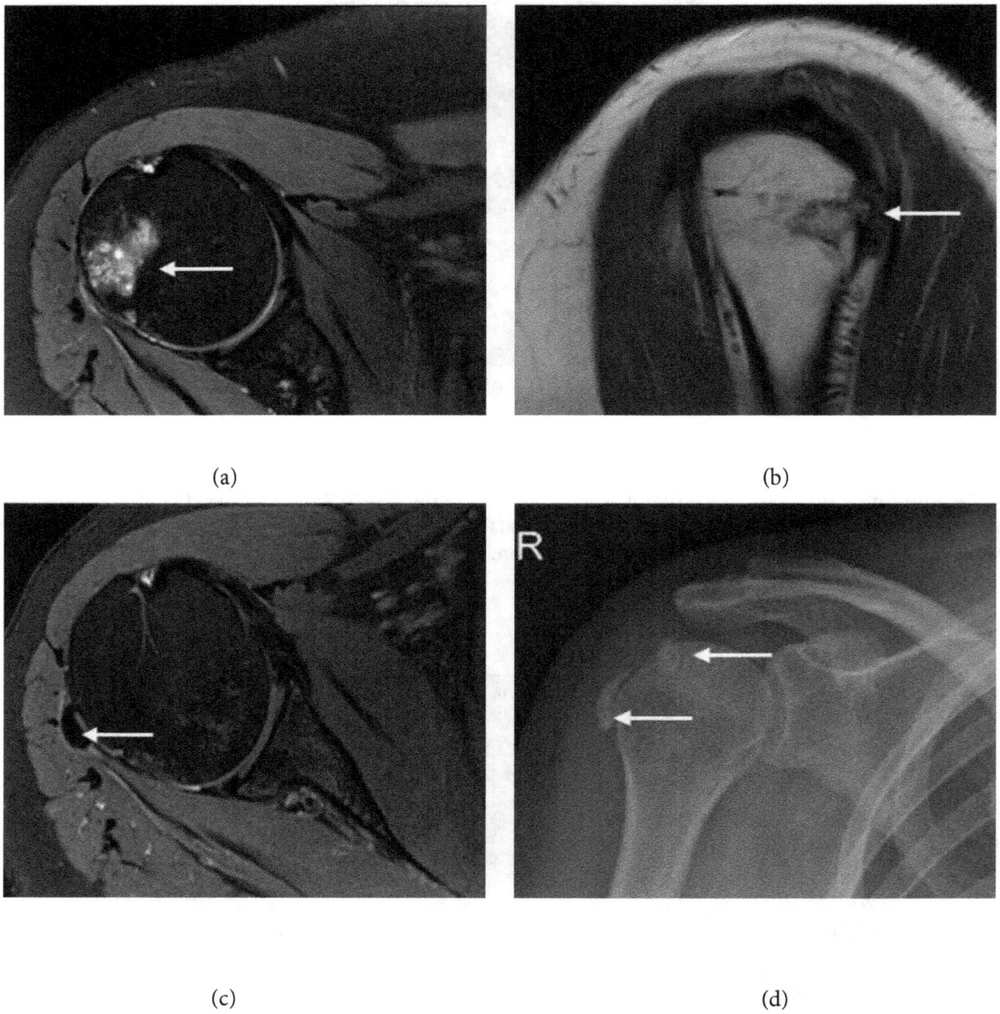

Figure 22: Calcific tendinitis in a 40-year-old female presenting with persistent shoulder pain. Axial PDFS (a) demonstrating marrow oedema signal in the humeral head at the greater tuberosity at teres minor tendon footprint. Sagittal PDFS (b) demonstrating corresponding cortical erosion. The MRI performed 5 months previously at the comparable plane (c) showed globular hypointense structure within the teres minor tendon footprint (arrow), confirming intraosseous migration of the calcific tendinitis in the most recent images. AP radiograph of the right shoulder (d) performed at the time of initial presentation also demonstrated calcium deposition in rotator cuff tendons. The calcium deposit is not well appreciated in the more recent study given the acute resorptive phase.

information although the utility of these more advanced techniques remains to be validated [22].

1.2.9. Depositional Disease. Depositional disease such as amyloidosis can radiologically resemble an infection, ultimately requiring biopsy for diagnosis (Figure 20). In patients with chronic renal insufficiency, aggressive spondylosis can also occur due to amyloid deposition. Features of hyperparathyroidism such as sclerosis adjacent to end plates (rugger-jersey spine) and subperiosteal or subligamentous bone resorption can help clinch the diagnosis [24] (Figure 21).

Microcrystals can deposit in periarticular or intra-articular soft tissue. This includes monosodium urate in gouty arthropathy and calcium hydroxyapatite deposition. Most cases are usually asymptomatic although the crystals can, at times, incite an inflammatory response and result in bone erosion, mimicking infection. In the acute phase, soft tissue swelling and joint effusion can be present. More chronic crystal deposits are usually T1 and T2 hypointense, without significant blooming artefact on susceptibility sequences that may otherwise suggest pigmented villonodular synovitis (PVNS). Calcific phosphate can deposit within tendons and can provoke an acute inflammatory response in the resorptive phase, during which the calcium can migrate into the adjacent bursa or bone, mimicking osteomyelitis (Figure 22). Calcium at this phase may be oedematous and difficult to depict on MRI. A radiograph can be useful for the assessment of soft tissue calcification which may not be apparent on MRI [25]. Dual-energy CT can also be used in distinguishing gout from other calcium deposition (Figure 23).

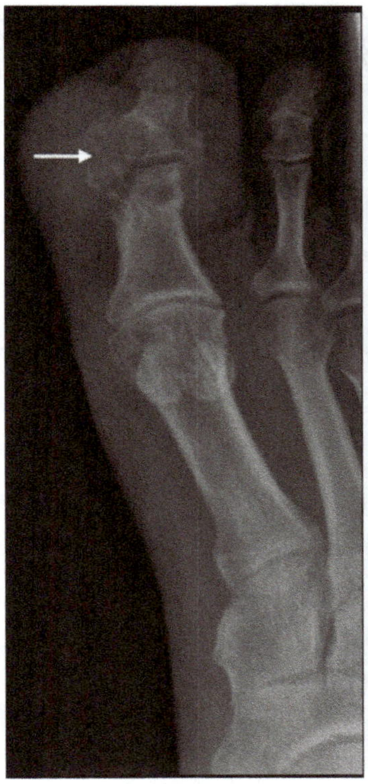

(a)

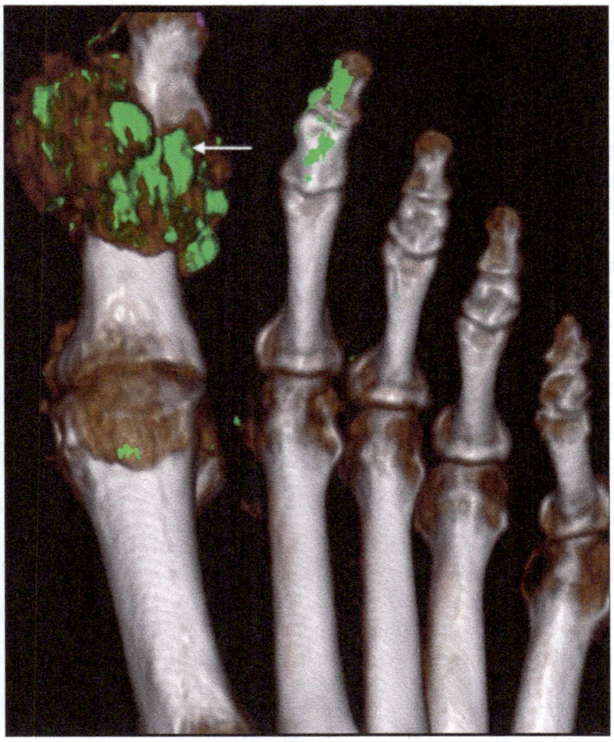

(b)

FIGURE 23: Gouty tophus in a 39-year-old man presenting with a swollen and erythematous toe which was clinically suspected to be an infection. X-ray showed 1st MTPJ erosion at the medial border associated with dense soft tissue swelling (arrow). Dual-energy CT with material decomposition helped differentiate urate crystals (mapped as green, arrowed) from calcium (blue, not present in this case).

2. Conclusion

The imaging appearance of the bone and joint infections may be mimicked by many conditions. It is important to consider other differentials when a specific clinical scenario is discordant from the imaging findings. Whilst it is always important to consider the clinical picture and laboratory findings when interpreting radiologic findings, pertinent information may not always be available. An appreciation of the overlap of these differential diagnoses with infection and key differentiating factors equips the radiologist with the ability to make a significant contribution to diagnosis and appropriate, timely management.

Acknowledgments

The authors would like to thank Dr. Ricky Lu Shi Sheng for his contribution to the earlier version of the manuscript.

References

[1] Y. J. Lee, S. Sadigh, K. Mankad, N. Kapse, and G. Rajeswaran, "The imaging of osteomyelitis," *Quantitative Imaging in Medicine and Surgery*, vol. 6, no. 2, pp. 184–198, 2016.

[2] J. Pupaibool, S. Vasoo, P. J. Erwin, M. H. Murad, and E. F. Berbari, "The utility of image-guided percutaneous needle aspiration biopsy for the diagnosis of spontaneous vertebral osteomyelitis: a systematic review and meta-analysis," *The Spine Journal*, vol. 15, no. 1, pp. 122–131, 2015.

[3] F. D. Beaman, P. F. von Herrmann, M. J. Kransdorf et al., "ACR appropriateness criteria suspected osteomyelitis, septic arthritis, or soft tissue infection (excluding spine and diabetic foot)," *Journal of the American College of Radiology*, vol. 14, no. 5, pp. S326–S337, 2017.

[4] C. Pineda, A. Vargas, and A. V. Rodríguez, "Imaging of osteomyelitis: current concepts," *Infectious Disease Clinics of North America*, vol. 20, no. 4, pp. 789–825, 2006.

[5] W. Lim and A. Saifuddin, "Review article: the differential diagnosis of bone marrow edema on wrist MRI," *Skeletal Radiology*, vol. 48, no. 10, pp. 1525–1539, 2019.

[6] C. Pineda, R. Espinosa, and A. Pena, "Radiographic imaging in osteomyelitis: the role of plain radiography, computed tomography, ultrasonography, magnetic resonance imaging, and scintigraphy," *Seminars in Plastic Surgery*, vol. 23, no. 02, pp. 080–089, 2009.

[7] M. Karchevsky, M. E. Schweitzer, W. B. Morrison, and J. A. Parellada, "MRI findings of septic arthritis and associated osteomyelitis in adults," *American Journal of Roentgenology*, vol. 182, no. 1, pp. 119–122, 2004.

[8] D. Resnick, G. Niwayama, J. Guerra Jr., V. Vint, and J. Usselman, "Spinal vacuum phenomena: anatomical study and review," *Radiology*, vol. 139, no. 2, pp. 341–348, 1981.

[9] R. Rahme and R. Moussa, "The modic vertebral endplate and marrow changes: pathologic significance and relation to low back pain and segmental instability of the lumbar spine," *American Journal of Neuroradiology*, vol. 29, no. 5, pp. 838–842, 2008.

[10] N. Boutry, C. Paul, X. Leroy, D. Fredoux, H. Migaud, and A. Cotten, "Rapidly destructive osteoarthritis of the hip: MR imaging findings," *American Journal of Roentgenology*, vol. 179, no. 3, pp. 657–663, 2002.

[11] M. D. Murphey, L. T. Senchak, P. K. Mambalam, C. I. Logie, M. K. Klassen-Fischer, and M. J. Kransdorf, "From the radiologic pathology archives: ewing sarcoma family of tumors: radiologic-pathologic correlation," *RadioGraphics*, vol. 33, no. 3, pp. 803–831, 2013.

[12] J. W. Chai, S. H. Hong, J.-Y. Choi et al., "Radiologic diagnosis of osteoid osteoma: from simple to challenging findings," *RadioGraphics*, vol. 30, no. 3, pp. 737–749, 2010.

[13] E. Smitaman, B. P. G. Pereira, B. K. Huang, M. M. Zakhary, E. Fliszar, and D. L. Resnick, "Abnormal bone marrow signal intensity in the phalanges of the foot as a manifestation of Raynaud phenomenon: a report of six patients," *American Journal of Roentgenology*, vol. 207, no. 6, pp. 1252–1256, 2016.

[14] M. Navallas, J. Ares, B. Beltrán, M. P. Lisbona, J. Maymó, and A. Solano, "Sacroiliitis associated with axial spondyloarthropathy: new concepts and latest trends," *RadioGraphics*, vol. 33, no. 4, pp. 933–956, 2013.

[15] C. Tsoi, J. F. Griffith, R. K. L. Lee, P. C. H. Wong, and L. S. Tam, "Imaging of sacroiliitis: current status, limitations and pitfalls," *Quantitative Imaging in Medicine and Surgery*, vol. 9, no. 2, pp. 318–335, 2019.

[16] G. Khanna, T. S. P. Sato, and P. Ferguson, "Imaging of chronic recurrent multifocal osteomyelitis," *Radiographics*, vol. 29, no. 4, pp. 1159–1177, 2009.

[17] A. Cotten, R. M. Flipo, A. Mentre, E. Delaporte, B. Duquesnoy, and P. Chastanet, "SAPHO syndrome," *Radiographics*, vol. 15, no. 5, pp. 1147–1154, 1995.

[18] R. Hermans, "Imaging of mandibular osteoradionecrosis," *Neuroimaging Clinics of North America*, vol. 13, no. 3, pp. 597–604, 2003.

[19] P. M. Phal, R. W. T. Myall, L. A. Assael, and J. L. Weissman, "Imaging findings of bisphosphonate-associated osteonecrosis of the jaws," *American Journal of Neuroradiology*, vol. 28, no. 6, pp. 1139–1145, 2007.

[20] C. J. Palestro, "Nuclear medicine and the failed joint replacement: past, present, and future," *World Journal of Radiology*, vol. 6, no. 7, pp. 446–458, 2014.

[21] J. Fritz, B. Lurie, T. T. Miller, and H. G. Potter, "MR imaging of hip arthroplasty implants," *RadioGraphics*, vol. 34, no. 4, pp. E106–E132, 2014.

[22] T. M. Noguerol, A. L. Alcalá, L. S. Beltrán, M. G. Cabrera, J. B. Cabrero, and J. C. Vilanova, "Advanced MR imaging techniques for differentiation of neuropathic arthropathy and osteomyelitis in the diabetic foot," *RadioGraphics*, vol. 37, no. 4, pp. 1161–1180, 2017.

[23] E. A. Jones, B. J. Manaster, D. A. May, and D. G. Disler, "Neuropathic osteoarthropathy: diagnostic dilemmas and differential diagnosis," *RadioGraphics*, vol. 20, pp. S279–S293, 2000.

[24] M. J. Cobby, R. S. Adler, R. Swartz, and W. Martel, "Dialysis-related amyloid arthropathy: MR findings in four patients," *American Journal of Roentgenology*, vol. 157, no. 5, pp. 1023–1027, 1991.

[25] P. Omoumi, P. Zufferey, J. Malghem, and A. So, "Imaging in gout and other crystal-related arthropathies," *Rheumatic Disease Clinics of North America*, vol. 42, no. 4, pp. 621–644, 2016.

10

Computed Tomography (CT) Imaging Features of Patients with COVID-19

Ephrem Awulachew, Kuma Diriba, Asrat Anja, Eyob Getu, and Firehiwot Belayneh

Dilla University, College of Health Science and Medicine, Dila, Ethiopia

Correspondence should be addressed to Ephrem Awulachew; efriye@gmail.com

Academic Editor: Paul Sijens

Introduction. Severe acute respiratory syndrome coronavirus 2 (SARS-CoV-2) is a highly contagious disease, and its first outbreak was reported in Wuhan, China. A coronavirus disease (COVID-19) causes severe respiratory distress (ARDS). Due to the primary involvement of the respiratory system, chest CT is strongly recommended in suspected COVID-19 cases, for both initial evaluation and follow-up. *Objective.* The aim of this review was to systematically analyze the existing literature on CT imaging features of patients with COVID-19 pneumonia. *Methods.* A systematic search was conducted on PubMed, Embase, Cochrane Library, Open Access Journals (OAJ), and Google Scholar databases until April 15, 2020. All articles with a report of CT findings in COVID-19 patients published in English from the onset of COVID-19 outbreak to April 20, 2020, were included in the study. *Result.* From a total of 5041 COVID-19-infected patients, about 98% (4940/5041) had abnormalities in chest CT, while about 2% have normal chest CT findings. Among COVID-19 patients with abnormal chest CT findings, 80% (3952/4940) had bilateral lung involvement. Ground-glass opacity (GGO) and mixed GGO with consolidation were observed in 2482 (65%) and 768 (18%) patients, respectively. Consolidations were detected in 1259 (22%) patients with COVID-19 pneumonia. CT images also showed interlobular septal thickening in about 691 (27%) patients. *Conclusion.* Frequent involvement of bilateral lung infections, ground-glass opacities, consolidation, crazy paving pattern, air bronchogram signs, and intralobular septal thickening were common CT imaging features of patients with COVID-19 pneumonia.

1. Introduction

Severe acute respiratory syndrome coronavirus 2 (SARS-CoV-2) is a highly contagious disease, and its first outbreak was reported in Wuhan, China [1]. On January 30, 2020, the World Health Organization (WHO) declared it a pandemic disease [2]. Currently, the disease has been reported in more than 212 countries worldwide [3]. As of May 01, a total of 3,325,620 cases and 234,496 deaths due to COVID-19 were reported worldwide [4]. The most common diagnostic tool for coronavirus disease 2019 (COVID-19) infection is real-time polymerase chain reaction (RT-PCR), which is regarded as the reference standard [5, 6].

COVID-19 causes severe respiratory distress (ARDS). Due to the primary involvement of the respiratory system, chest computed tomography (CT) is strongly recommended in suspected COVID-19 cases, for both initial evaluation and follow-up [7]. Recent studies addressed the importance of chest CT examination in COVID-19 patients with false-negative RT-PCR results [8] and reported the CT sensitivity as 98% [9]. Additionally, CT examinations also have great significance in monitoring disease progression and evaluating therapeutic efficacy.

The SARS-CoV-2 has four major structural proteins: the spike surface glycoprotein, small envelope protein, matrix protein, and nucleocapsid protein [10]. The spike protein binds to host receptors via the receptor-binding domains (RBDs) of angiotensin-converting enzyme-2 (ACE2) [11]. The ACE2 protein has been identified in various human organs, including the respiratory system, GI tract, lymph nodes, thymus, bone marrow, spleen, liver, kidney, and brain. SARS-CoV-2 was reported to utilize angiotensin-converting enzyme-2 (ACE2) as the cell receptor in humans [12], firstly causing pulmonary interstitial damage and subsequently with parenchymal changes. Reportedly, chest CT images could manifest different imaging features or patterns in COVID-19 patients with different time course and disease severity [13, 14].

Studies suggest that routine chest CT is a useful tool in the early diagnosis of COVID-19 infection, especially in settings of limited availability of reverse-transcriptase polymerase chain reaction (RT-PCR [15]. Imaging is critical in assessing severity and disease progression in COVID-19 infection. Radiologists should be aware of the features and patterns of imaging manifestations of the novel COVID-19 infection. A variety of imaging features have been described in similar coronavirus-associated syndromes. Due to an alarming spread of COVID-19 outbreak throughout the world, a comprehensive understanding of the importance of evaluating chest CT imaging findings is essential for effective patient management and treatment. Individual literature published is required to be summarized. Thus, a comprehensive systematic review has to be performed. Therefore, this study systematically reviewed CT imaging features of patients with COVID-19 pneumonia.

2. Methods

2.1. Search Strategy. A systematic search was conducted on PubMed, Embase, Cochrane Library, Open Access Journals (OAJ), and Google Scholar databases until April 15, 2020. Keywords used to search eligible studies were "severe acute respiratory syndrome 2," "SARS CoV 2," "2019-nCoV," "COVID-19," "computed tomography," "CT," and "radiology." All identified keywords and mesh terms were combined using the "OR" operator and "AND" operator for searching literatures. We simultaneously searched the reference lists of all recovered articles for potentially eligible studies.

2.2. Eligibility Criteria. All articles with a report of CT findings in COVID-19 patients published in English from the onset of COVID-19 outbreak to April 20, 2020, were included in the study. Case studies and case series reported on chest CT imaging findings of patients with COVID-19 were included with caution. Studies pertaining to other coronavirus-related illnesses were excluded.

2.3. Assessment of Study Quality. Studies selected for inclusion were assessed for methodological quality by two teams of independent reviewers using the standard critical appraisal instruments of the Joanna Briggs Institute Meta-Analysis of Statistics Assessment for the Review Instrument (JBI-MAStARI) [16]. Disagreements were resolved by consensus.

2.4. Data Extraction and Synthesis. Data were extracted by two teams of the investigators using a standardized data extraction form. In addition, eligible case studies and case series studies were extracted carefully. Then the extracted data were merged for systematic analysis. The main outcomes extracted from each study were study design, country, patient demographics, and chest CT findings. Additional findings extracted were the patient's clinical characteristics. Disagreements were discussed with other reviewers and subsequently resolved via consensus.

2.5. Data Analysis and Data Synthesis. Systematic reviews and meta-analyses were carried out using R software version 3.6.1 with user-contributed commands for meta-analyses: metaprop, metan, metainf, metabias, and metareg. The effect sizes and SEs of the studies were pooled using a random-effects model to calculate the pooled estimates of CT findings among COVID-19 patients. A meta-analysis was also planned to assess the association of various imaging findings with demographic data.

2.6. Risk of Bias and Sensitivity Analysis. Evidence for statistical heterogeneity of the results was assessed using the Cochrane Q *x2* test and *I2* statistic. A significance level of $P < 0.10$ and *I2* >50% was interpreted as evidence of heterogeneity [17]. A potential source of heterogeneity was investigated by subgroup analysis and meta-regression analysis [18]. Where statistical pooling was not possible, the findings were presented in a narrative form including tables and figures to aid in data presentation where appropriate.

Sensitivity analyses were conducted to weigh up the relative influence of each individual study on the pooled effect size using a user-written function, metainf. The presence of publication bias was assessed informally by visual inspection of funnel plots [19].

3. Result

3.1. Study Selection. Following the initial search, 241 studies were identified from the electronic databases (Figure 1). After the removal of 67 duplicates, 17 noneligible studies, and six studies with unclear population, 78 studies were retrieved for full-text review. Of this, 18 studies were of poor quality that did not meet the eligibility criteria. Following methodological quality assessment, 60 articles were included in the meta-analysis. In the included studies, a total of 5041 patients with COVID-19 were assessed for CT imaging features. All papers were published in English.

3.2. Study Characteristics. In this review, 60 papers were eligible and a total of 5041 patients had CT imaging findings [8, 12–14, 19–72]. From a total of 5401 participants, about half of them were male 2710 (50.2%), while 2693 (49.8%) were female. The mean age of the participants was 49 years with a standard deviation of 11.6 years.

3.2.1. Clinical Features of Patients with COVID-19. From a total of 60 included studies, only 48 studies had reported the clinical features of COVID-19 infected patients. According to the report of 48 studies, the main clinical features of

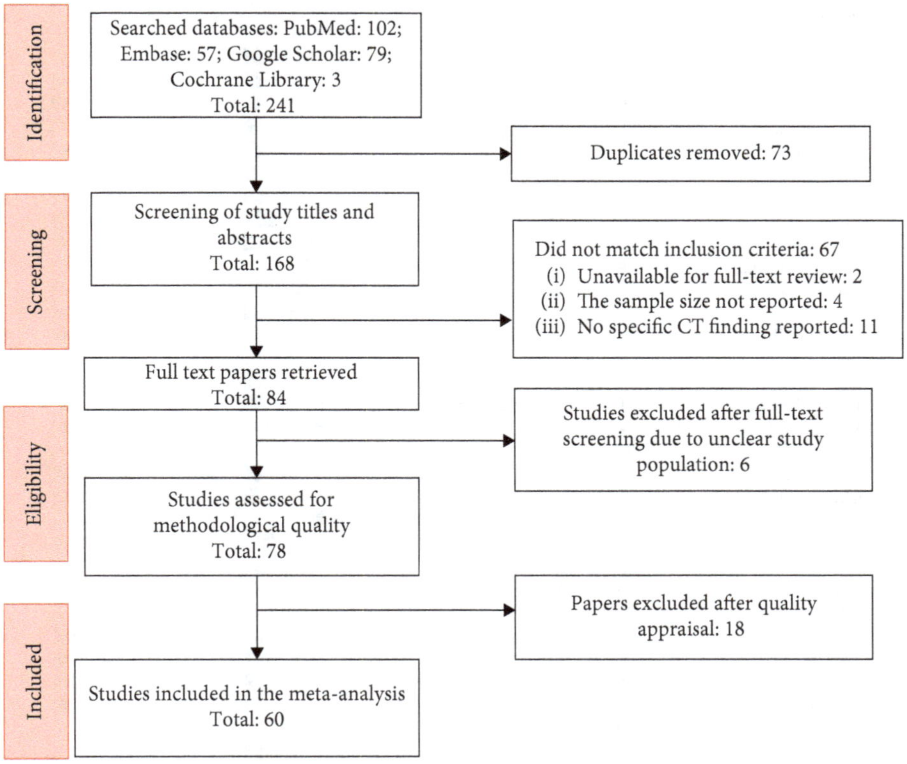

FIGURE 1: Flow chart of the search and study inclusion.

COVID-19 infected patients were fever and dry cough, which accounted for 80% (2954/3800) and 56.2% (2137/3800), respectively, while about 2.3% (86/3800) patients with COVID-19 infection are asymptomatic. The total white blood cell count was decreased in about 24% (410) of patients with COVID-19, while about 2% [43] had increased white blood cells. Decreased lymphocyte count was detected in about 442 (43%) patients with COVID-19, and only 1% had increased lymphocyte count. Markers like C-reactive protein were found to be increased in about 87% (458) patients, while only 13% (254) had normal C-reactive protein (Table 1).

TABLE 1: Review of clinical features of patients with COVID-19.

Clinical features	Number of studies	Number of patients (%)
Sign and symptoms		
Fever	48	2954 (80%)
Dry cough	48	2137 (56.2%)
Respiratory distress	29	462 (15%)
Pharyngeal pain	48	381 (13%)
Fatigue	32	481 (27%)
Total WBC count		
Normal	22	1195 (68%)
Decreased	22	410 (24%)
Increased	22	45 (2%)
Lymphocyte count		
Normal	22	566 (56%)
Decreased	22	442 (43%)
Increased	22	2 (1%)
C-reactive protein		
Normal	15	254 (13%)
Decreased	15	0 (0%)
Increased	15	458 (87%)

3.2.2. Chest CT Imaging Features of COVID-19-Infected Patients. We performed meta-analyses of primary outcome data and secondary outcomes with available data. From a total of 5041 COVID-19-infected patients, about 98% (4940/5041) had abnormalities in chest CT, while about 2% had normal chest CT findings (Figure 2). Among COVID-19 patients with abnormal chest CT findings, 80% (3952/4940) had bilateral lung involvement. About 20% (641/3206) patients had exclusively unilateral lung involvement. When a single lobe was involved, the right lung was most often affected (62%) and 38% of them had only left lung involvement. In the right lung, the lower lobe was frequently involved (74% (784)), while the middle lobe was less frequent (38% (326)). In the left lung, the upper lobe was frequently involved (74% (731)).

Regarding the patterns of lung lesions in patients with COVID-19, ground-glass opacity (GGO) and mixed GGO with consolidations were observed in 2482 (65%) and 768 (18%) patients, respectively. Consolidation, which is defined as denser opacities and blurred margins of pulmonary blood vessels and bronchial tubes, was detected in 1259 (22%) patients with COVID-19 pneumonia. CT images also showed interlobular septal thickening in about 691 (27%) patients. CT showed that 11 (21.6%) patients had discrete pulmonary nodules. Crazy paving patterns of lesions were observed in 575

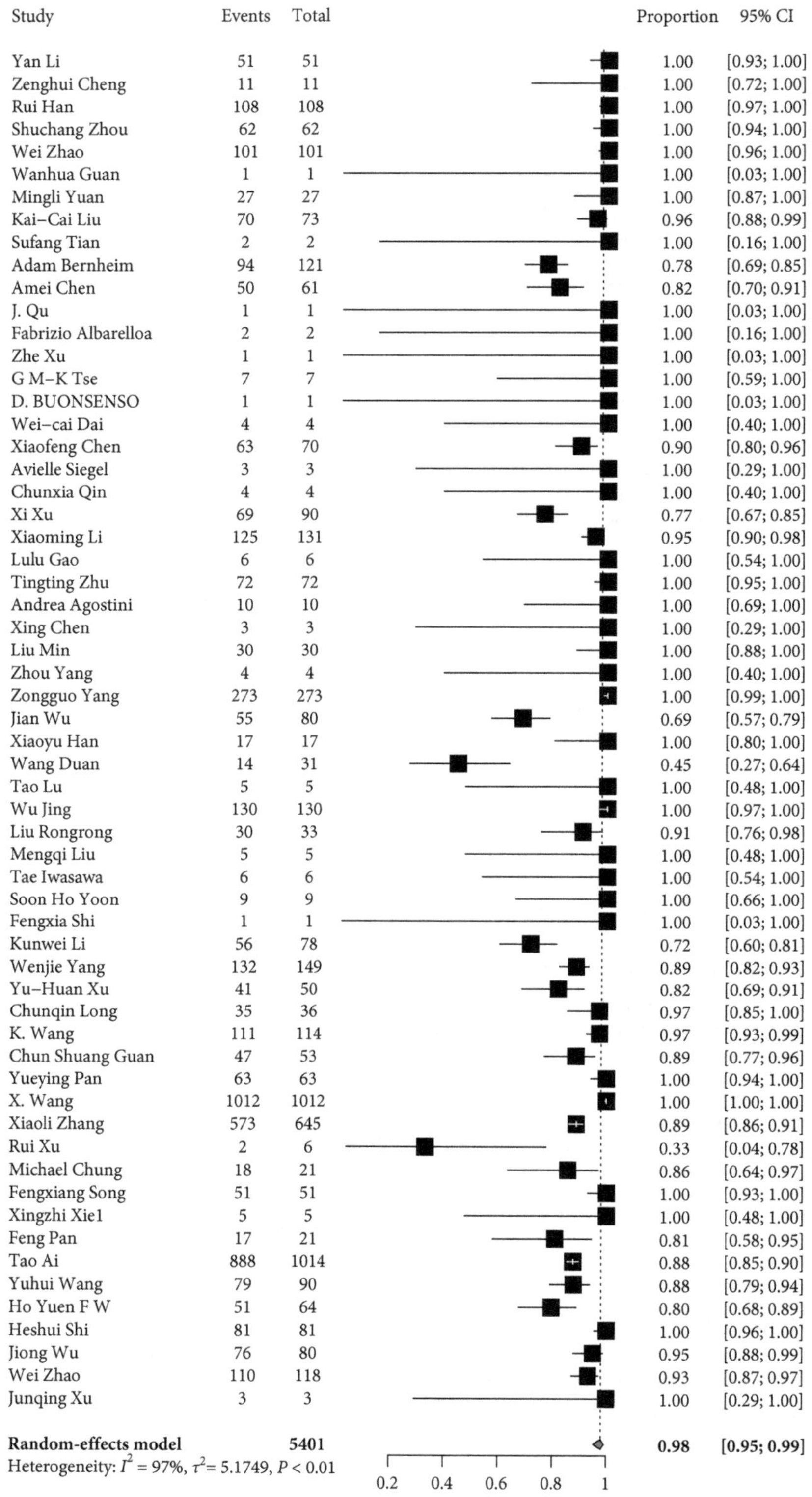

Figure 2: Magnitude of abnormal chest CT finding of patients with COVID-19.

(12%) patients. Five hundred thirty-one (18%) patients had an air bronchogram sign. Pleural effusion and lymphadenopathy were observed in 94 (1.6%) and 21 (0.7%) patients with COVID-19 pneumonia, respectively. Pulmonary nodules were reported in 262 (9%) patients (Table 2).

3.3. Additional Analysis. We also gathered data to demonstrate if there is a difference in the CT findings related to infection time course. In the included studies, the mean time between initial chest CT and follow-up was about 6.5 days (range, 0–21 days). According to the report of 9 included studies, 43% (95 CI: 26%–61%) patients have improved

TABLE 2: CT imaging features of patients with COVID-19.

CT findings	Number of studies	Number of patients (%)
Patterns of the lesion		
Ground-glass opacity with consolidation	60	768 (18%)
Ground-glass opacity	60	2482 (65%)
Consolidation	60	1259 (22%)
Crazy paving pattern	24	575 (12%)
Reversed halo sign	24	146 (1%)
Other signs in the lesion		
Interlobular septal thickening	23	691 (27%)
Air bronchogram sign	23	531 (18%)
Distribution		
Bilateral	48	3952 (80%)
Unilateral	48	641 (20%)
Right lung	8	48 (62%)
Left lung	8	29 (38%)
Number of lobes involved		
One lobe	13	278 (14%)
Two lobes	13	299 (11%)
Three lobes	13	250 (13%)
Four lobes	13	212 (15%)
Five lobes	14	384 (34%)
More than one lobe	14	1145 (76%)
Lobe of lesion distribution		
Left upper lobe	14	731 (74%)
Left lower lobe	20	504 (46%)
Right upper lobe	19	455 (40%)
Right middle lobe	15	326 (38%)
Right lower lobe	17	784 (74%)
Other findings		
Pleural effusion	60	94 (1.6%)
Lymphadenopathy	60	21 (0.7%)
Pulmonary nodules	22	262 (9%)

follow-up chest CT findings, while 30% (95 CI: 18%–46%) have advanced chest CT findings [40, 43, 44, 50, 52, 57, 64–66]. Our findings demonstrated pure ground-glass opacity in early disease, followed by the development of crazy paving, and finally increasing consolidation latter in the disease course. GGO density increased and transformed into consolidation; consolidation edges were flat or contracted; and fibrous cord shadow appeared. GGO with consolidation was higher in the advanced stage than in the early stage of the disease (OR 3.2, 95% CI: 2.2–4.7, $P = 0.013$). A crazy paving pattern and a reverse halo sign were all rare in the early sign, but were present in the late stage of the disease. In terms of distribution of disease, bilateral involvements were prominent in the later stage than in the early stage ($P < 0.001$). According to the report of two included studies, pure GGO was the common imaging feature of mild and moderate stages of the disease course, while consolidation and GGO with consolidation increased by 64% and 79% in the critical stage of the disease, respectively [57, 58].

3.4. Heterogeneity and Risk of Bias. Subgroup analysis was conducted to justify the cause of heterogeneity. Subgroup analysis of the included studies showed that the possible cause of heterogeneity was sample size (P value < 0.01). Funnel plots did not suggest a publication bias for the majority of the parameters. We demonstrated no publication bias (P value $= 0.1947$).

4. Discussion

4.1. Summary of Evidence. In this review, we have demonstrated that the main signs and symptoms of hospital admission of patients with COVID-19 pneumonia were fever, dry cough, fatigue, pharyngeal pain, and respiratory distress. About 24% of the patients had reduced total leukocyte count and 43% had reduced lymphocyte count. Although the laboratory findings are not specific for viral pneumonia, leukopenia and lymphocytopenia may be helpful to distinguish COVID-19 from common bacterial infections. The majority of the patients had increased C-reactive protein.

In this study, common CT imaging features in patients with COVID-19 pneumonia included bilateral involvement, ground-glass opacities, consolidation, crazy paving pattern, air bronchogram signs, and intralobular septal thickening. At a later stage of the disease, mixed GGO with consolidation was the more frequent finding. Pulmonary consolidation was mainly found in the severe and progressive late stages of the disease, which can coexist with ground-glass and fibrotic changes. The pathological basis of these changes could be due to inflammatory cell infiltration and interstitial thickening, cell exudation, and hyaline membrane formation.

In the present study, the increased frequency of GGO, consolidation, bilateral disease, intralobular septal thickening, a crazy paving pattern of the lesion, and appearance of reverse halo sign lesions over more than one lobe of the lung could represent the pathophysiology of the disease process as it organizes and it could also probably explain chest CT hallmark of COVID-19 infection. CT imaging findings can be correlated with the severity of the disease and disease progression after efforts of treatment.

The majority of the patients (76%) had multilobar involvement, and lesions were more frequent in the right lung. Pleural effusion, lymphadenopathy, and pulmonary nodules were less common imaging findings in these patients. About 2% of the patients had normal initial CT findings. When a single lobe was involved, the right lung was most often affected and more than half of the patients with COVID-19 had multiple lobe infections. In the right lung, the lower lobe is frequently involved while the middle lobe was less frequent. In the left lung, the upper lobe was frequently involved. This might indicate the virus tends to disseminate all over all lobes of both lungs as the disease progress. Chest CT imaging features may avoid repeated laboratory testing and may be helpful in a resource-limited country.

According to the present study, chest CT imaging showed similar characteristics in the majority of patients, including predominantly bilateral and multilobe involvement. The pattern of ground-glass and consolidative pulmonary opacities, often with a bilateral lung distribution, is somewhat similar to that described in earlier coronavirus outbreaks such as SARS and MERS, which was known to cause ground-glass opacities that may coalesce into dense consolidative lesions [73, 74].

According to the report of 9 included studies, 43% (95 CI: 26%–61%) patients have improved follow-up chest CT findings, while 30% (95 CI: 18%–46%) have advanced chest CT findings. Our findings demonstrated pure ground-glass opacity in early disease, followed by the development of crazy paving and finally increasing consolidation latter in the disease course. According to the report of two included studies, pure GGO was the common imaging feature of mild and moderate stages of the disease course, while consolidation and GGO with consolidation increased by 64% and 79% in the critical stage of the disease, respectively.

4.2. Limitation. This systematic review and meta-analysis came up with CT imaging features of patients with COVID-19; we acknowledge a few limitations of the present systematic review and meta-analysis, which may affect the results. First of all, two relevant studies which were identified through our literature search were excluded due to unavailability for full-text review. The other limitation of the present study was that it was limited to articles published in English.

5. Conclusions

The present study showed that common CT imaging features of COVID-19 pneumonia included frequent involvement of bilateral lung infections, ground-glass opacities, consolidation, crazy paving pattern, air bronchogram signs, and intralobular septal thickening. Bilateral involvement was common while single lobe involvement was rare. This sign of CT imaging might be an important tool for diagnosis and monitoring disease progression in patients with COVID-19 infection.

Abbreviations

ACE2: Angiotensin-converting enzyme-2
ARDS: Acute respiratory distress
CT: Computed tomography imaging
COVID-19: Coronavirus disease 2019
GGO: Ground-glass opacity
2019-nCoV: Novel coronavirus
SAR CoV 2: Severe acute respiratory syndrome coronavirus 2.

Authors' Contributions

E. A, K. D, A. A, E.G, and F. B designed the study, extracted, critically reviewed, and analyzed the data, and wrote the first draft of the manuscript and approved the manuscript.

References

[1] N Zhu, D. Zhang, and W. Wang, "A novel coronavirus from patients with pneumonia in China, 2019," *New England Journal of Medicine*, vol. 382, no. 8, pp. 727–733, 2020.

[2] World Health Organization, *Coronavirus Disease 2019 (COVID-19) Situation Report–39*, World Health Organization, Geneva, Switzerland, 2020, https://www.who.int/docs/default-ource/coronaviruse/situation-eports/20200228-itrep-covidpdf?sfvrsnbf3e7d_2.

[3] W. Wang, J. Tang, and F. Wei, "Updated understanding of the outbreak of 2019 novel coronavirus (2019nCoV) in Wuhan, China," *Journal of Medical Virology*, vol. 92, no. 4, pp. 441–447, 2020.

[4] World Health Organization, *Update on the Situation Regarding the New Coronavirus*, World Health Organization, Geneva, Switzerland, 2020.

[5] K. McIntosh, *Coronavirus Disease 2019 (COVID-19): Epidemiology, Virology, Clinical Features, Diagnosis, and Prevention*, Practice changing updates, Riverwoods, IL, USA, 2020.

[6] World Health Organization, *Laboratory Testing for Coronavirus Disease 2019 (COVID-19) in Suspected Human Cases*, World Health Organization, Geneva, Switzerland, 2020.

[7] Y. H. Jin, L. Cai, and Z. S. Cheng, "A rapid advice guideline for the diagnosis and treatment of 2019 novel coronavirus (2019-nCoV) infected pneumonia (standard version)," *Military Medical Research*, vol. 7, no. 4, 2020.

[8] X. Xie, Z. Zhong, W. Zhao et al., "Chest CT for typical 2019-nCoV pneumonia: relationship to negative RT-PCR testing," *Radiology*, p. 200343. In press, 2020.

[9] Y. Fang, H. Zhang, and J. Xie, "Sensitivity of chest CT for COVID-19: comparison to RT-PCR," *Radiology*, In press, 2020.

[10] A. Wu, Y. Peng, B. Huang et al., "Genome composition and divergence of the novel coronavirus (2019-nCoV) originating in China," *Cell Host & Microbe*, vol. 27, no. 3, pp. 325–328, 2020.

[11] J. Lan, J. Ge, J. Yu et al., "Crystal structure of the 2019-nCoV spike receptor-binding domain bound with the ACE2 receptor," *bioRxiv*, In press, 2020.

[12] X. Xu, P. Chen, J. Wang et al., "Evolution of the novel coronavirus from the ongoing Wuhan outbreak and modeling of its spike protein for risk of human transmission," *Science China Life Sciences*, vol. 63, no. 3, pp. 457–460, 2020.

[13] H. Shi, X. Han, N. Jiang et al., "Radiological findings from 81 patients with COVID-19 pneumonia in Wuhan, China: a descriptive study," *The Lancet Infectious Diseases*, vol. 20, no. 4, pp. 425–434, 2020.

[14] F. Pan, T. Ye, P. Sun et al., "Time course of lung changes on chest CT during recovery from 2019 novel coronavirus (COVID-19) pneumonia," *Radiology*, vol. 295, no. 3, pp. 715–721, 2020.

[15] V. M. Corman, O. Landt, M. Kaiser et al., "Detection of 2019 novel coronavirus (2019-nCoV) by real-time RT-PCR," *Euro Surveillance*, vol. 25, no. 3, 2020.

[16] R. Armstrong, E. Waters, N. Jackson et al., *Guidelines for Systematic Reviews of Health Promotion and Public Health Interventions: Version 2*, Melbourne University Australia, Melbourne, Australia, 2007.

[17] S. G. Thompson and S. J. Sharp, "Explaining heterogeneity in meta-analysis: a comparison of methods," *Statistics in Medicine*, vol. 18, no. 20, pp. 2693–2708, 1999.

[18] W. G. Cochran, "The comparison of percentages in matched samples," *Biometrika*, vol. 37, no. 3-4, pp. 256–266, 1950.

[19] M. Egger, G. D. Smith, M. Schneider, and C. Minder, "Bias in meta-analysis detected by a simple, graphical test," *British Medical Journal*, vol. 315, no. 7109, pp. 629–634, 1997.

[20] A. Bernheim, X. Mei, M. Huang et al., "Chest CT findings in coronavirus disease-19 (COVID-19): relationship to duration of infection," *Radiology*, vol. 295, no. 3, p. 200463, 2020.

[21] T. Ai, Z. Yang, H. Hou et al., "Correlation of Chest CT and RT-PCR testing in coronavirus disease 2019 (COVID-19) in China: a report of 1014 cases," *Radiology*, vol. 20, p. 200642, 2020.

[22] A. Chen, J. Huang, Y. Liao et al., "Differences in clinical and imaging presentation of pediatric patients with COVID-19 in comparison with adults," *Cadiology: Cardiothoracic Imaging*, vol. 2, no. 2, Article ID e200117, 2020.

[23] A. Agostini, C. Floridi, A. Borgheresi et al., "Proposal of a low-dose, long-pitch, dual-source chest CT protocol on third-generation dual-source CT using a tin filter for spectral shaping at 100 kVp for coronavirus disease 2019 (COVID-19) patients: a feasibility study," *La Radiologia Medica*, vol. 125, no. 4, pp. 365–373, 2020.

[24] A. Siegel, P. J. Chang, Z. J. Jarou et al., "Lung base findings of coronavirus disease (COVID-19) on abdominal CT in patients with predominant gastrointestinal symptoms," *American Journal of Roentgenology*, vol. 215, pp. 1–3, 2020.

[25] Z. Chengl, Y. Lu, Q. Cao et al., "Clinical features and chest CT manifestations of coronavirus disease 2019 (COVID-19) in a single-center study in Shanghai, China," *American Journal of Roentgenology*, vol. 215, no. 1, pp. 121–126, 2020.

[26] C. S. Guan, Z. B. Lv, S. Yan et al., "Imaging features of coronavirus disease 2019 (COVID-19): evaluation on thin-section CT," *Academic Radiology*, vol. 27, no. 5, pp. 609–613, 2020.

[27] C. Longb, H. Xuc, Q. Shend et al., "Diagnosis of the coronavirus disease (COVID-19): rRT-PCR or CT?" *European Journal of Radiology*, vol. 126, p. 108961, 2020.

[28] C. Qin, F. Liu, T.-C. Yen, and X. Lan, "^{18}F-FDG PET/CT findings of COVID-19: a series of four highly suspected cases," *European Journal of Nuclear Medicine and Molecular Imaging*, vol. 47, no. 5, pp. 1281–1286, 2020.

[29] D. Buonsenso, A. Piano, F. Raffaelli, N Bonadia, K. de Gaetano Donati, and F Franceschi, "Point-of-Care Lung Ultrasound findings in novel coronavirus disease-19 pnemoniae: a case report and potential applications during COVID-19 outbreak," *European Review for Medical and Pharmacological Sciences*, vol. 24, no. 5, pp. 2776–2780, 2020.

[30] F. Albarelloa, E. Pianuraa, F. D. Stefanoa et al., "2019-novel coronavirus severe adult respiratory distress syndrome in two cases in Italy: an uncommon radiological presentation," *International Journal of Infectious Diseases*, vol. 93, pp. 192–197, 2020.

[31] F. Shi, Q. Yu, W. Huang, and C. Tan, "2019 novel coronavirus (COVID-19) pneumonia with hemoptysis as the initial symptom: CT and clinical features," *Korean Journal of Radiology*, vol. 21, no. 5, pp. 537–540, 2020.

[32] F. Song, N. Shi, F. Shan et al., "Emerging 2019 novel coronavirus (2019-nCoV) pneumonia," *Radiology*, vol. 295, no. 1, pp. 210–217, 2020.

[33] L. Gao and J. Zhang, "Pulmonary high-resolution computed tomography (HRCT) findings of patients with early-stage coronavirus disease 2019 (COVID-19) in Hangzhou, China," *Medical Science Monitor*, vol. 26, Article ID e923885, 2020.

[34] H. Y. F. Wong, H. Y. S. Lam, A. Ho-Tung Fong et al., "Frequency and distribution of chest radiographic findings in COVID-19 positive patients," *Radiology*, p. 201160. In press, 2020.

[35] J. Qu, R. Yang, L. Song, and I. R. Kamel, "Atypical lung feature on chest CT in a lung adenocarcinoma cancer patient infected with COVID-19," *Annals of Oncology*, vol. 31, no. 6, pp. 825-826, 2020.

[36] J. Wu, J. Liu, X. Zhao et al., "Clinical characteristics of imported cases of COVID-19 in Jiangsu province: a multicenter descriptive study," *Infectious Diseases Society of America*, vol. 20, 2020.

[37] J. Wu, X. Wu, W. Zeng et al., "Chest CT findings in patients with coronavirus disease 2019 and its relationship with clinical features," *Investigative Radiology*, vol. 55, no. 5, 2020.

[38] J. Xu, R. Wu, H. Huang et al., "Computed tomographic imaging of 3 patients with coronavirus disease 2019 pneumonia with negative virus real-time reverse-transcription polymerase chain reaction test," *Clinical Infectious Diseases*, vol. 20, 2020.

[39] K. Wang, S. Kang, R. Tian, X. Zhang, X. Zhang, and Y. Wang, "Imaging manifestations and diagnostic value of chest CT of coronavirus disease 2019 (COVID-19) in the Xiaogan area," *Clinical Radiology*, vol. 75, no. 5, pp. 341–347, 2020.

[40] K.-C. Liu, P. Xu, W.-F. Lv, J.-L. Yao, J.-F. Gu, and W. Wei, "CT manifestations of coronavirus disease-2019: a retrospective analysis of 73 cases by disease severity," *European Journal of Radiology*, vol. 126, p. 108941, 2020.

[41] K. Li, Y. Fang, W. Li et al., "CT image visual quantitative evaluation and clinical classification of coronavirus disease (COVID-19)," *European Radiology*, vol. 30, 2020.

[42] M. Liu, P. He, H. Liu et al., "Analysis of clinical characteristics of 30 new coronavirus pneumonia in medical staff," *Chinese Journal of Tuberculosis and Respiratory Diseases*, vol. 43, no. 3, pp. 209–214, 2020.

[43] M. Liu, Z. Song, and K. Xiao, "High-resolution computed tomography manifestations of 5 pediatric patients with 2019 novel coronavirus," *Journal of Computer Assisted Tomography*, vol. 44, no. 3, pp. 311–313, 2020.

[44] M. Chung, A. Bernheim, X. Mei et al., "CT imaging features of 2019 novel coronavirus (2019-nCoV)," *Radiology*, vol. 295, no. 1, pp. 202–207, 2020.

[45] M. Yuan, Y. Wen, Z. Tao, W. Tan, and Y. Hu, "Association of radiologic findings with mortality of patients infected with 2019 novel coronavirus in Wuhan, China," *PLoS One*, vol. 15, no. 3, Article ID e0230548, 2020.

[46] L. Rongrong, Z. Yi, W. Minyu et al., "CT imaging analysis of lungs in 33 patients with new coronavirus infection," *Chinese Medical Journal*, vol. 100, no. 13, 2020.

[47] H. Rui, H. Lu, J. Hong, J. Dong, H. Peng, and D. Zhang, "Early clinical and CT manifestations of coronavirus disease 2019 (COVID-19) pneumonia," *American Journal of Roentgenology*, 2020, In press.

[48] S. Zhou, Y. Wang, T. Zhu, and L. Xia, "CT features of coronavirus disease 2019 (COVID-19) pneumonia in 62 patients in Wuhan, China," *American Journal of Roentgenology*, vol. 214, pp. 1287–1294, 2020.

[49] S. H. Yoon, K. H. Lee, J. Y. Kim et al., "Chest radiographic and CT findings of the 2019 novel coronavirus disease (COVID-19): analysis of nine patients treated in Korea," *Korean Journal of Radiology*, vol. 21, no. 4, pp. 494–500, 2020.

[50] S. Tian, W. Hu, L. Niu, H. Liu, H. Xu, and S.-Y. Xiao, "Pulmonary pathology of early-phase 2019 novel coronavirus (COVID-19) pneumonia in two patients with lung cancer," *Journal of Thoracic Oncology*, vol. 15, no. 5, pp. 700–704, 2020.

[51] I. Tae, M. Sato, T. Yamaya et al., "Ultra high resolution computed tomography can demonstrate alveolar collapse in novel coronavirus (COVID-19) pneumonia," *Japanese Journal of Radiology*, vol. 38, no. 5, pp. 394–398, 2020.

[52] T. Lu and H. Pu, "Computed tomography manifestations of 5 cases of the novel coronavirus disease 2019 (COVID-19) pneumonia from patients outside Wuhan," *Journal of Thoracic Imaging*, vol. 35, no. 3, pp. 90–93, 2020.

[53] T. Zhu, Y. Wang, S. Zhou, N. Zhang, and L. Xia, "A comparative study of chest computed tomography features in young and older adults with corona virus disease (COVID-19)," *Journal of Thoracic Imaging*, vol. 35, no. 4, pp. 97–101, 2020.

[54] D. Wang, X. Ju, F. Xie et al., "Clinical analysis of 31 cases of 2019 new coronavirus infection in children from six provinces (autonomous regions) in Northern China," *Chinese Journal of Pediatrics*, vol. 58, 2020.

[55] W. Guan, J. Liu, and C. Yu, "CT findings of coronavirus disease (COVID-19) severe pneumonia," *American Journal of Roentgenology*, vol. 214, no. 5, pp. 85-86, 2020.

[56] W. Xia, J. Shao, Y. Guo, X. Peng, Z. Li, and D. Hu, "Clinical and CT features in pediatric patients with COVID-19 infection: different points from adults," *Pediatric Pulmonology*, vol. 55, no. 5, pp. 1169–1174, 2020.

[57] W. Zhao, Z. Zheng, X. Xie, Q. Yu, and J. Liu, "Relation between chest CT findings and clinical conditions of coronavirus disease (COVID-19) pneumonia: a multicenter study," *American Journal of Roentgenology*, vol. 214, no. 5, pp. 1072–1077, 2020.

[58] W.-C. Dai, H.-W. Zhang, J. Yu et al., "CT imaging and differential diagnosis of COVID-19," *Canadian Association of Radiologists' Journal*, vol. 71, no. 2, pp. 195–200, 2020.

[59] W. Yang, Q. Cao, L. Qin et al., "Clinical characteristics and imaging manifestations of the 2019 novel coronavirus disease (COVID-19): a multi-center study in Wenzhou city, Zhejiang, China," *Journal of Infection*, vol. 80, no. 4, pp. 388–393, 2020.

[60] J. Wu, F. Cailian, X. Xian et al., "CT distribution characteristics and signs of 130 cases of novel coronavirus pneumonia," *Chinese Journal of Tuberculosis and Respiratory Diseases*, vol. 43, 2020.

[61] X. Wang, Y. J. Fang, Y Zhu et al., "Clinical characteristics of non-critically ill patients with novel coronavirus infection (COVID-19) in a Fangcang Hospital," *Clinical Microbiology and Infection*, 2020, In press.

[62] X. Chen, Y. Tang, Y. Mo et al., "A diagnostic model for coronavirus disease 2019 (COVID-19) based on radiological semantic and clinical features: a multi-center study," *European Radiology*, 2020, In press.

[63] X. Zhang, H. Cai, J. Hu et al., "Epidemiological, clinical characteristics of cases of SARS-CoV-2 infection with abnormal imaging findings," *International Journal of Infectious Diseases*, vol. 94, pp. 81–87, 2020.

[64] X. Li, W. Zeng, X. Li et al., "CT imaging changes of corona virus disease 2019(COVID-19): a multi-center study in Southwest China," *Journal of Translational Medicine*, vol. 18, no. 1, p. 154, 2020.

[65] X. Han, Y. Cao, N. Jiang et al., "Novel coronavirus pneumonia (COVID-19) progression course in 17 discharged patients: comparison of clinical and thin-Section CT features during recovery," *Infectious Diseases Society of America*, In press, 2020.

[66] X. Chen, S. Liu, C. Zhang et al., "Dynamic chest CT evaluation in three cases of 2019 novel coronavirus pneumonia," *Archives of Iranian Medicine*, vol. 23, no. 4, pp. 277–280, 2020.

[67] Y. Li and L. Xia, "Coronavirus disease 2019 (COVID-19): role of chest CT in diagnosis and management," *American Journal of Roentgenology*, vol. 214, no. 6, pp. 1280–1286, 2020.

[68] Y. Pan, H. Guan, S. Zhou et al., "Initial CT findings and temporal changes in patients with the novel coronavirus pneumonia (2019-nCoV): a study of 63 patients in Wuhan, China," *European Radiology*, vol. 30, no. 6, pp. 3306–3309, 2020.

[69] Y.-H. Xu, J.-H. Dong, W.-M. An et al., "Clinical and computed tomographic imaging features of novel coronavirus pneumonia caused by SARS-CoV-2," *Journal of Infection*, vol. 80, no. 4, pp. 394–400, 2020.

[70] Y. Wang, C. Dong, Y. Hu et al., "Temporal changes of CT findings in 90 patients with COVID-19 pneumonia: a longitudinal study," *Radiology*, p. 200843, 2020, In press.

[71] Y. Zhou, L. Yang, M. Han et al., "Case report on early diagnosis of COVID-19," *Disaster Medicine and Public Health Preparedness*, pp. 1–4, , 2020, In press.

[72] Z. Yang, S Jia, H. Zhang et al., "Predictors for imaging progression on chest CT from coronavirus disease 2019 (COVID-19) patients," *Aging*, vol. 12, no. 7, 2020.

[73] Y. Ding, H. Wang, H. Shen et al., "The clinical pathology of severe acute respiratory syndrome (SARS): a report from China," *The Journal of Pathology*, vol. 200, no. 3, pp. 282–289, 2003.

[74] D. L. Ng, F. Al Hosani, M. K. Keating et al., "Clinicopathologic, immunohistochemical, and ultrastructural findings of a fatal case of middle east respiratory syndrome coronavirus infection in the United Arab Emirates, April 2014," *The American Journal of Pathology*, vol. 186, no. 3, pp. 652–658, 2016.

11

Verification of the Dose Reduction Effect via Diluted Injection in Dual-Energy Computed Tomography Using a Human Blood Flow Phantom

Hironobu Tomita [1,2] **and Koichi Shibata** [1]

[1] *Graduate School of Healthcare Science, Suzuka University of Medical Science, 1001-1, Kishioka-cho, Suzuka, Mie 510-0293, Japan*
[2] *Department of Radiology, Saiseikai Kawaguchi General Hospital, 5-11-5, Nishikawaguchi, Kawaguchi, Saitama 332-0021, Japan*

Correspondence should be addressed to Hironobu Tomita; ae861600@js7.so-net.ne.jp

Academic Editor: Paul Sijens

Purpose. We sought to examine the possibility of reducing the contrast medium dosage in dual-energy imaging using a saline-mixed injection with a virtual monochromatic energy method of dual-source computed tomography (CT). *Methods*. An X-ray CT (SOMATOM Definition Flash: Siemens, Nurnberg, Germany) was employed. The mixing ratio of contrast medium and saline was gradually changed by 10%, followed by a mixed injection into a dynamic blood flow phantom (Nemoto Kyorindo, Japan) which is a hemodynamic simulation phantom to obtain time-enhancement curves (TECs). Exactly 64 TECs were prepared for each mixing ratio by changing the energy from 40 to 75 keV for monoenergetic imaging. The relationship between the image standard deviation (SD) and the energy of the virtual monochromatic image was determined. Combinations of the mixing ratio and energy (keV), which can maintain high CT numbers and low image SDs for 3D imaging, were tested, and the reduction rate of the contrast medium was calculated. *Results*. The TECs for the mixed injection method changed linearly with the dilution rates. The mixing ratios were strongly correlated with the maximum CT number of the TEC (R^2 = 0.98). Contrast CT numbers and image SDs increased by approximately 20% and 25%, respectively, as the energy decreased by 5 keV. The optimal conditions for reducing the contrast medium dose were a mixing ratio of 6:4 and 55 keV of energy. *Conclusion*. The virtual monochromatic energy method reduced the contrast medium dosage by up to 40% for three-dimensional CT-angio (3DCTA) tests.

1. Introduction

Computer tomography (CT) technology has recently made marked advances, providing various imaging methods. Currently, three-dimensional CT-angio (3DCTA) is widely used in clinical settings. In clinical contrast CT tests, a reduced contrast medium dose is beneficial for patients with renal impairment (particularly for the elderly or repeated tests) because dosage is a risk factor for the development of contrast-induced nephropathy (CIN), and its reduction minimizes the risk of CIN development [1]. Not all patients who undergo contrast CT tests have normal renal function. In Japan, approximately 13.3 million people (one-eighth of all Japanese adults) suffer from chronic kidney disease (CKD). Renal impairment can become end-stage renal failure if it is left untreated. Contrast CT testing is an effective imaging modality for patients with pulmonary infarction who must be treated rapidly. In the PIOPED II study [2], however, a contrast CT test was not indicated for 18.5% of patients suspected of having a pulmonary embolism due to high serum creatinine levels. Thus, renal impairment is common in clinical practice. However, CT tests using a reduced dose of contrast medium are useful in clinical settings because their application range is increased, and the risk of CIN development after the test is likely to decrease. A reduced contrast medium dose for CT tests is beneficial for patients.

3DCTA generates a high-intensity contrast in blood vessels, with differences in CT numbers of several hundred HU. Thus, the effects of image quality (noise) do not need to be considered in 3DCTA tests, unlike with the imaging of solid organs such as the liver. Therefore, the contrast

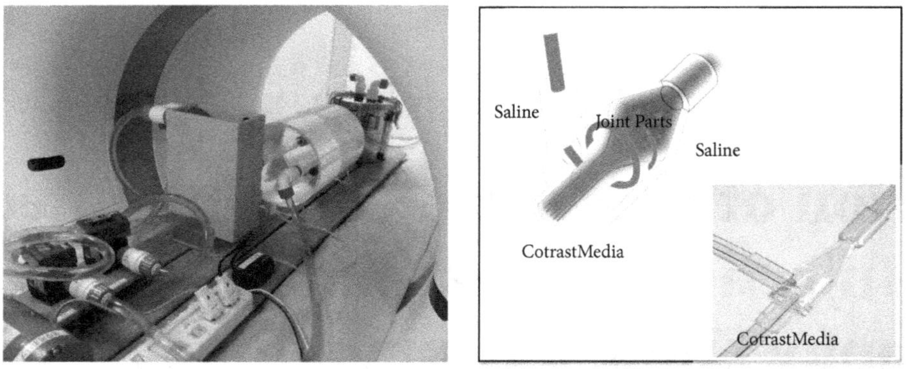

(a) (b)

FIGURE 1: Verification system. (a) Human blood flow phantom and X-ray CT; (b) spiral flow tube.

medium dose can be markedly reduced because dual energy can maintain high CT numbers.

In previous studies, imaging with low contrast medium doses was conducted by enhancing the contrast medium sensitivity with low-tube-voltage imaging [3, 4]. However, not all patients can undergo low-tube-voltage imaging because of the tube capacity of the device in use and the shortage of mA that occurs with larger patients. In a recent study, the contrast medium dose was reduced by approximately 30% via dual-energy imaging in clinical cases [5]. However, stable CT numbers cannot always be obtained because of differences in physical constitution, difficulties in maintaining the upper extremity venous route, and reductions in cardiac function. When the contrast medium was adjusted based on the patient's body weight, the desired CT numbers were obtained from a time-enhancement curve (TEC) by optimizing the injection rate and volume of the contrast medium [6]. However, it is difficult to adjust these factors for each test. Various methods to reduce the contrast medium dose have been examined in clinical cases to obtain the most basic rationale; however, blood flow dynamics and injection methods via phantom simulation have not been investigated. Given the aforementioned situation, we applied dual-energy CT, which enhances contrast media sensitivity, to reduce the contrast media dose in a clinical setting.

The injection volume of contrast media can be reduced in two ways: one is to use contrast media at low concentrations; the other is to lower the contrast injection rate to reduce the total amount of iodine. However, only a few formulations are commercially available at low concentrations, precluding modified concentrations. When injection rates are changed, the TEC is also changed during imaging, demanding a revision of the entire imaging protocol. In the present study, a diluted contrast medium was developed using a mixture of saline and contrast medium, enabling injection at arbitrary concentrations. In addition, images with stable contrast medium concentrations were obtained by adjusting energy (keV) after imaging. The purpose of the present study was to reduce the contrast medium dose using a mixed injection method. However, no research has demonstrated the validity of dual-energy imaging. In the present physical study, a reduction in the contrast medium dose was examined using a human blood flow phantom in actual clinical settings [6].

2. Materials and Methods

2.1. Verification System. The human blood flow phantom (Nemoto Co. Ltd, Tokyo, Japan), which can reproduce TECs in human arteries as reported in a previous paper [7], was used to measure TECs (Figure 1). The human blood flow phantom was established by assuming a 60-kg body weight, 5-L circulating water, and an intra-arterial CT angiography. The contrast medium injection rate was 3.5 mL/sec, and 42 mL of Isohexol contrast medium (350 mgI/mL) was administered. An acrylic cylinder with a diameter of 200 mm in a phantom imaging unit was filled with water. Acrylic tubes, simulating arteries and veins, were placed on both sides of the cylinder to simulate arterial and venous blood flows, through which the contrast medium was circulated.

An X-ray CT (SOMATOM Definition Flash: Siemens, Nurnberg, Germany) and spiral tube (Spiral Flow Tube DS-017: Nemoto Co. Ltd, Tokyo, Japan) [8] were used for the dilution of contrast media and saline (Figure 1).

2.2. Verification Procedure

2.2.1. Comparison between DIC and VMI. Dual imaging on CT can be achieved using two methods. One is the dual-energy imaging composition (DIC) method that generates images by mixing two images of different tube voltages at an arbitrary ratio. The other is the virtual monoenergetic imaging (VMI) method that generates a monoenergetic image of arbitrary energy by calculating a virtual monoenergetic image from two images of different tube voltages. To determine which imaging technique is more advantageous for contrast media reduction, we investigated the imaging characteristics of the contrast media using both DIC and VMI.

For this investigation, we performed dual-energy imaging using the human blood flow dynamic phantom. The tube voltages were 100 kV and 140 kV with a Sn filter. To adjust image quality and image standard deviation (SD), we set

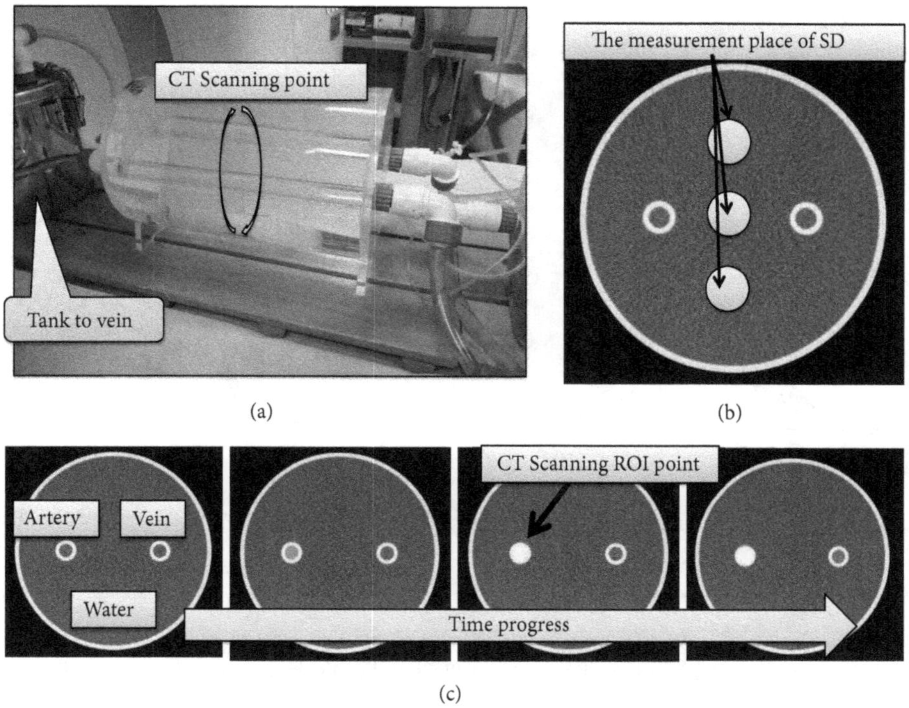

FIGURE 2: Blood circulation mock phantom. (a) CT scanning point; (b) the measurement location of the image SD; (c) CT scanning region of interest (ROI).

the image SD to 11 under 100 kV and the mAs to 180 mAs ($CTDI_{VOL}$ of 12 mGy).

(1) The contrast media Isohexol, at 350 mg/mL of the total 42 mL volume, was injected into the human blood flow phantom at rate of 3.5 mL/s. The total injection time was 12 s. The ROI was set at the arterial region of the phantom (see Figure 2), and the images were acquired temporarily. Image acquisitions were performed every 3.25 s after the contrast media injection for 12 acquisitions. The total acquisition time was 39 s.

(2) We reconstructed the dual-energy images using the DIC and VMI methods and created graphs showing the temporary TEC changes at each imaging energy. The longitudinal axis of the graphs represents time, and the vertical axis represents the CT number. Using these graphs, we investigated the difference in the TECs at 100 kVp, which is used in conventional CT angiography, and at the other imaging energies mentioned below. For example, M0.2 indicates a mixed image comprising 20% of a 100-kVp image and 80% of a 100-kVp image.

Acquired images: 100 kVp, 140 kVp,

DIC images: M0.2 (100 kVp 20% 140 kVp 80%), M0.5 (100 kVp 50% 140 kVp 50%) M0.7 (100 kVp 70% 140 kVp 30%), M0.9 (100 kVp 90% 140 kVp 10%),

VMI images: 40 keV 45 keV 50 keV 55 keV 60 keV 65 keV.

2.2.2. Change in Energy via VMI and CT Number. We created graphs to show the changes in the CT number of the contrast media, water, and fat (from a pig) for every 5 keV from 40 to 190 keV using VMI. The longitudinal axis of the graphs shows the virtual monoenergetic energy, and the vertical axis shows the CT numbers. We used 300 HU, 200 HU, and 100 HU of diluted contrast media at 12 kVp. The acquisition conditions for the CT were 100 kV and 140 kV (using a Sn filter).

2.2.3. The Optimization of the Monoenergetic Imaging Conditions. We investigated the optimum dilution rate, monoenergetic energy, and CT number for the contrast media reduction. The experimental procedures are described below.

Contrast medium: the saline ratio was changed by 10% from 2:8 to 10:0, and a mixture of contrast medium and physiological saline was injected into the human blood flow phantom. The arterial portion of the phantom (Figure 2) was imaged to record the time course of the CT numbers. The imaging conditions were 100 kV and 140 kVp (using an Sn filter). Image quality and SD were adjusted at 180 mAs ($CTDI_{VOL}$ of 12 mGy) to achieve an SD of 11 with a 1-mm slice thickness at 100 kV. Images were obtained every 3.25 s (12 times for 39 s) after the start of contrast medium injection. The CT numbers were plotted over time to create a TEC. For the TEC data from 2:8 to 10:0, the energy was changed by 5 keV from 40 to 75 keV to create VMI images. Thus, 64 TECs were prepared under the various mixture injection conditions. We determined the relationship between the temporal changes of the CT numbers and the monoenergetic energy of VMI by created TEC graphs in which the longitudinal axis represents time, and the vertical axis represents the CT numbers.

2.2.4. The Relationship between Maximum CT Numbers and Mixing Rate. We investigated the relationship between the

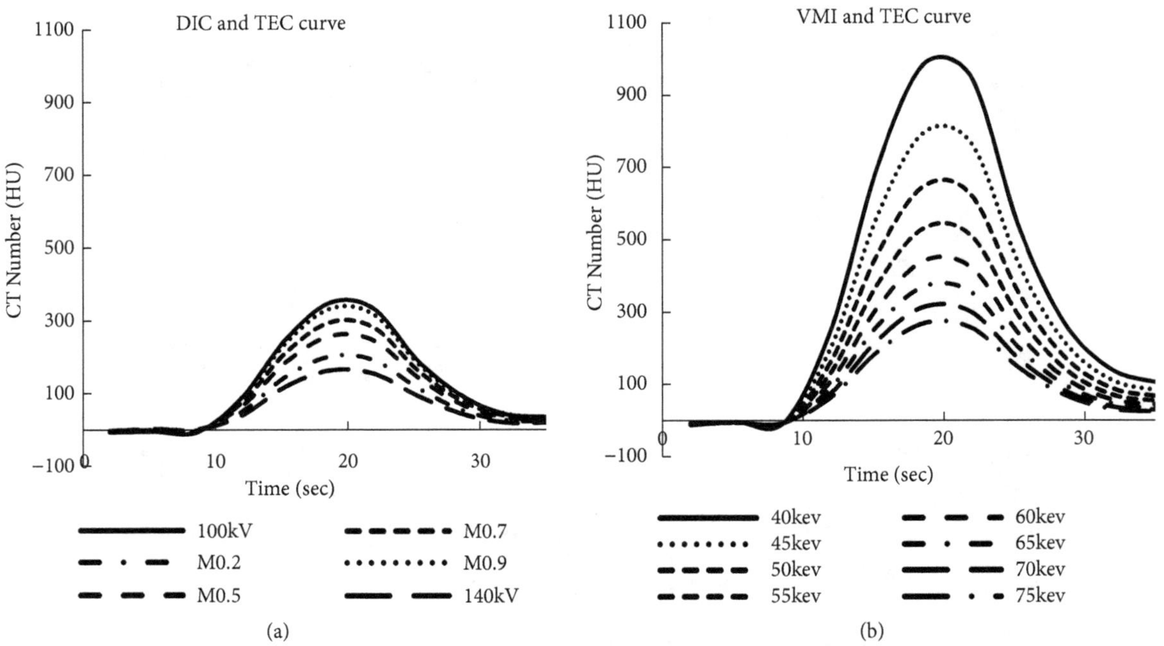

FIGURE 3: The DIC and VMI of the contrast media sensitivity. (a) The TECs of the DIC images, which show the differences among the mixing ratios of 100 kVp and 140 kVp. (b) The TECs of the VMI images, which show the differences among the monoenergetic energies. Injection condition: saline : contrast media, 0 : 10.

maximum number of TECs at each monoenergetic energy and the mixing ratio of contrast media and saline. The maximum CT numbers were obtained from the TECs ranging from 40 to 75 keV, as indicated on the graphs in which the longitudinal axis shows the monoenergetic energy, and the vertical axis shows the CT numbers.

2.2.5. SD Characteristics of Monoenergetic Image. Mean SDs at three water positions in the blood flow phantom (Figure 2) were determined for each monoenergetic energy.

2.2.6. Determination of Optimal Imaging Conditions. A tube voltage of 100 kVp, which is routinely applied for imaging at our hospital, was used as a reference. Combinations that were able to maintain a CT number of > 300 HU and an image SD of 15 or below (a TH of 1 mm and a reconstruction function of D30) were determined to calculate the contrast medium reduction rates [1]. These numbers are the minimum requirements needed to prepare 3DCTA.

3. Results and Discussion

3.1. Comparison between DIC and VMI. Figure 3(a) shows the TECs of the DIC images, revealing the differences among the mixing ratios of the 100 kVp and 140 kVp images. Figure 3(b) shows the TECs of the VMI images and the differences among the monoenergetic energies. The 100-kVp curve had the maximum CT number for DIC, and (compared with DIC) VMI showed a higher increase in the CT number. VMI was superior to DIC under 65 keV, exceeding the maximum number of 300 HU of DIC.

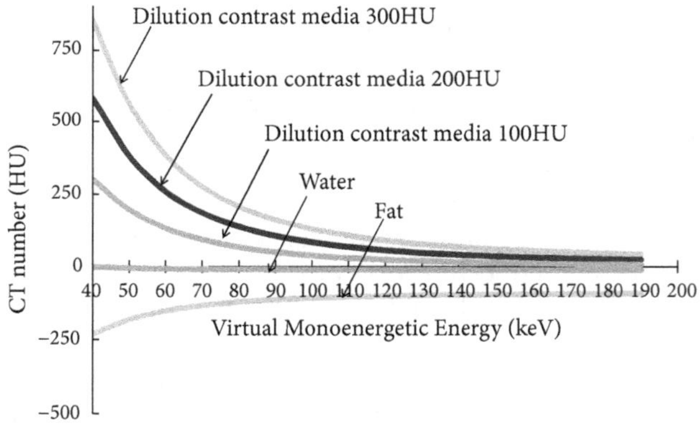

FIGURE 4: Changes in the energy with regard to VMI and CT number.

3.2. Change in the Energy Regarding VMI and CT Number. The changes in the contrast media, water, and fat (from a pig) with regard to the monoenergetic energy in VMI were more obvious when the density of the contrast media was higher or the monoenergetic energy was lower. For example, the CT number of the contrast media, which was diluted to 300 HU, more than doubled to 851 HU at 40 keV. On the other hand, a small change in the CT number was observed for water, and the CT number decreased for fat, which might have opposing characteristics to those of the contrast media. (Figure 4)

3.3. The Optimization of the Monoenergetic Imaging Conditions. Figures 5 and 6 show the TEC results obtained using VMI by changing the dilution rate as well as the relationships among dilution rate, monoenergetic energy, and

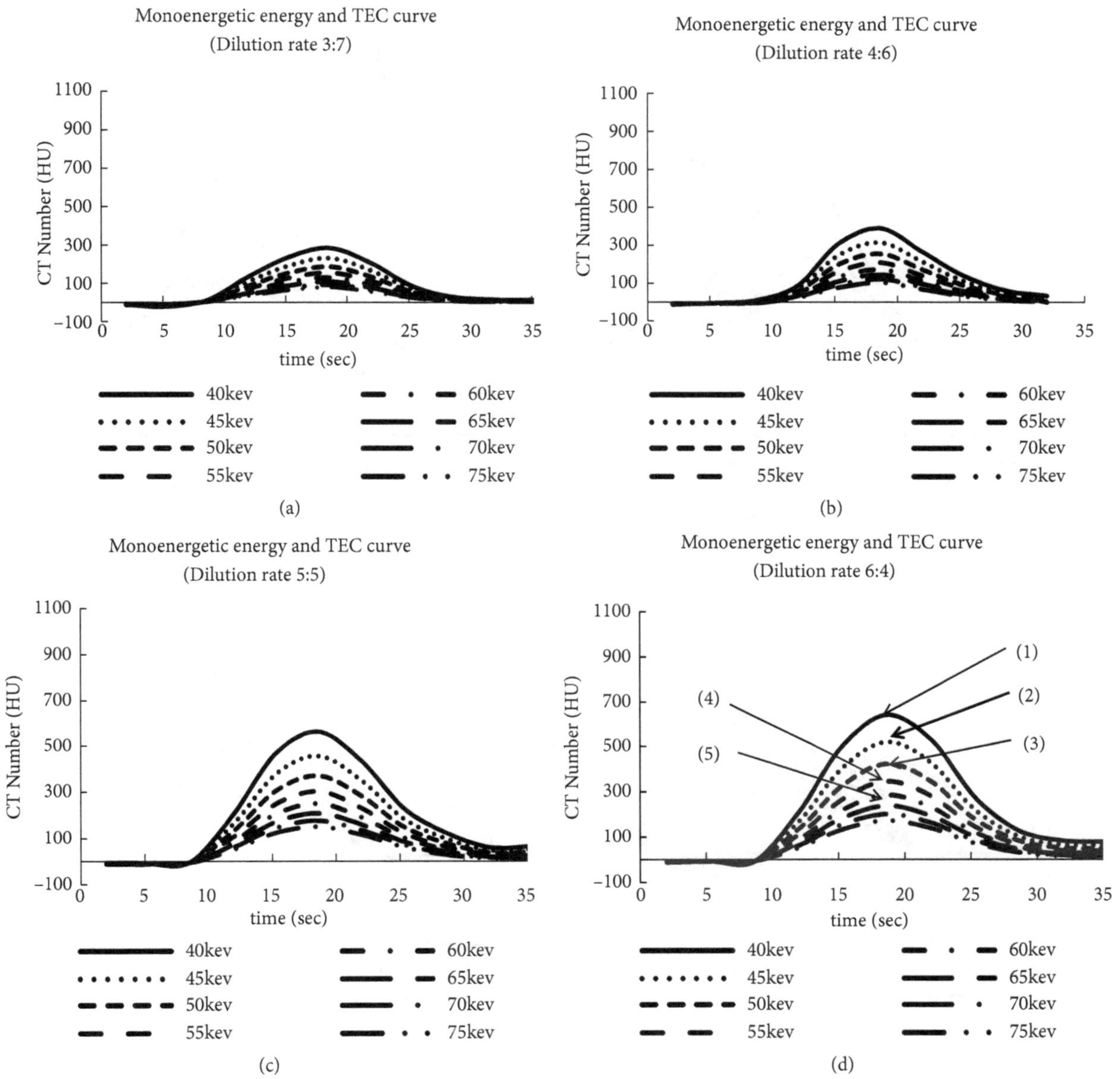

FIGURE 5: Monoenergetic energy and TEC. (a) Dilution rate 3:7; (b) dilution rate 4:6; (c) dilution rate 5:5; (d) dilution rate 6:4.

CT number. The vertical and horizontal axes show the CT number and time (s), respectively, and each TEC ranges from 40 to 75 keV monoenergetic energy. The difference between Figures 5(a)–5(d) and Figures 6(a)–6(d) is the dilution rate. For example, the TECs started to increase approximately 10 s after the start of the injection, reached a peak at approximately 18 s, and gradually decreased by 30 s for a dilution rate of 6:4 (Figure 5(d)). The TEC at 40 keV had the highest peak compared with the other TECs, and its maximum CT number was 642 HU (Figure 5(d) {1}). When the monoenergetic energy increased, the maximum CT numbers decreased (e.g., 518 HU at 45 keV [2], 345 HU at 50 keV [3], and 285 HU at 55 keV [4]). The same tendency was observed in the other figures (i.e., Figures 5(a)–5(c) and Figures 6(a) and 6(b)). The maximum CT numbers increased linearly by approximately 20%, following a decrease of 5 keV for the monoenergetic energy at any dilution rate using VMI.

Figure 7 shows the relationship between the dilution rate and the maximum CT number of the TECs of Figures 5 and 6 at 60 keV of monoenergetic energy. The shapes of the TECs prepared using the diluted injection method changed linearly with the dilution rate. The maximum CT number was strongly correlated with the dilution rate ratio of the contrast medium and saline (R^2 = 0.98), demonstrating a linear rise in the CT numbers with the increase in the dilution rate.

3.4. The Relationship between Maximum CT Number and Dilution Rate. Figure 8 shows the change in the maximum CT number per each dilution rate following the change in monoenergetic energy. The maximum CT numbers for the TEC at each energy increased when the dilution rate of the contrast medium or virtual energy decreased, reaching 1,000 HU at 10:1 and 40 keV.

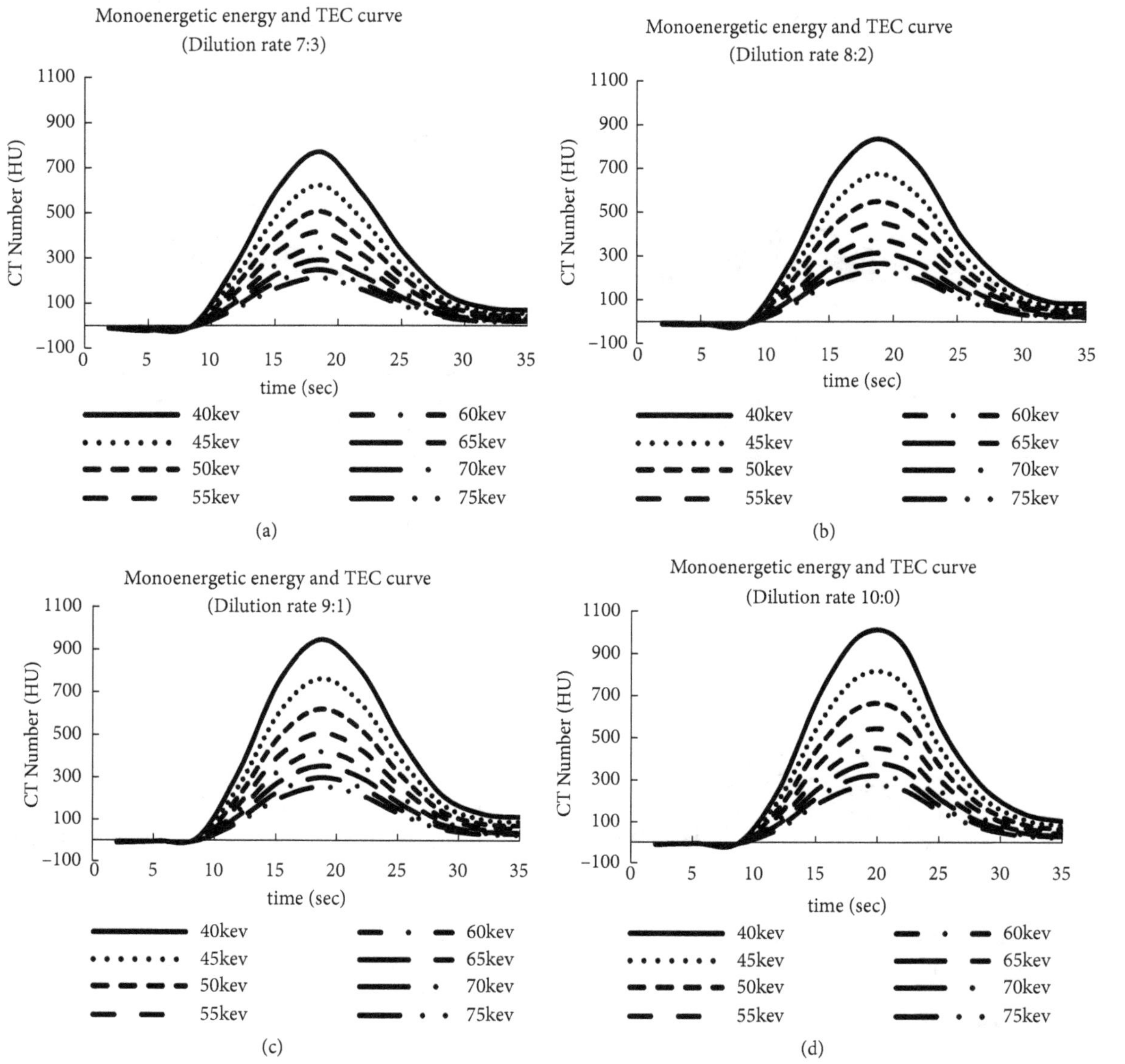

FIGURE 6: Monoenergetic energy and TEC. (a) Dilution rate 7:3; (b) dilution rate 8:2; (c) dilution rate 9:1; (d) dilution rate 10:0.

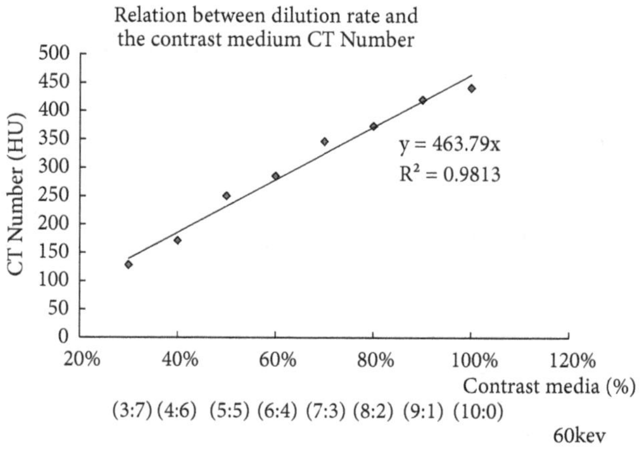

FIGURE 7: The dilution rate of contrast media and saline, exhibiting a strong correlation ($R^2 = 0.98$).

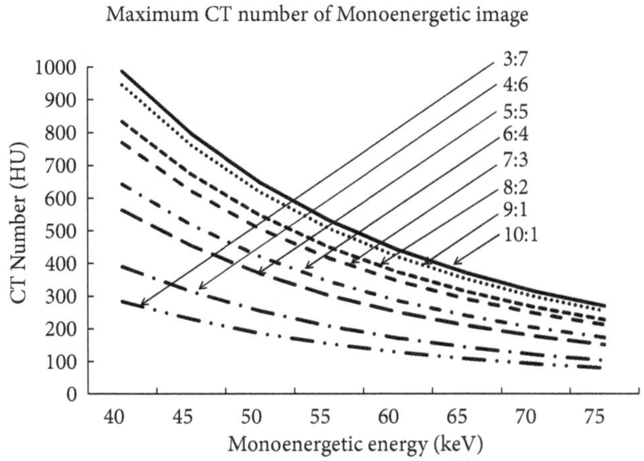

FIGURE 8: The maximum CT number per dilution rate. The maximum CT number per each keV resulted in a higher number if the diluted ratio was higher. If keV was lower, the maximum CT number was higher. Finally, for 100% contrast (0% saline) at 40 kV, the CT number reached 1000 HU.

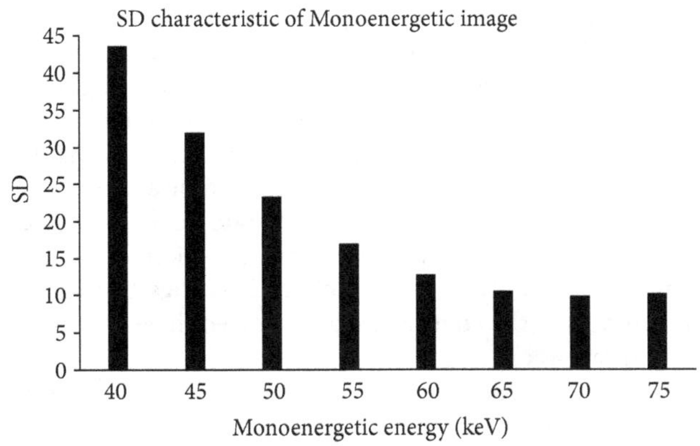

FIGURE 9: The SD characteristic of a monoenergetic image. Image SD increased by 25% for each reduction of 5 kV between 40 and 65 kV; it did not increase and maintained a consistent level for energies higher than 65 kV.

3.5. *SD Characteristics of Monoenergetic Images.* Figure 9 shows the results of the change in image SD with regard to the change in monoenergetic energy. Image SD increased by approximately 25% for every 5-keV decrease between 40 and 65 keV and remained approximately constant above 65 keV. We confirmed that image SD changes with monoenergetic energy, and an increase in image SD of 40 - 50 keV was clearly realized with relatively higher CT numbers.

3.6. *Determination of Optimal Imaging Conditions.* The combinations capable of maintaining the CT number above 300 HU for the 5-s acquisition time [9] were 10:0 and 65 keV, 4:6 and 40 keV, 5:5 and 45 keV, 6:4 and 55 keV, 7:3 and 60 keV, 8:2 and 60 keV, and 9:1 and 65 keV (Figure 10). Of these combinations, the dilution rate of 6:4 and a monoenergetic energy of 55 keV maintained the image at an SD of 15 or below (TH of 1 mm and a reconstruction function of D30).

We confirmed that VMI is able to obtain higher CT numbers than DIC by adjusting the monoenergetic energy

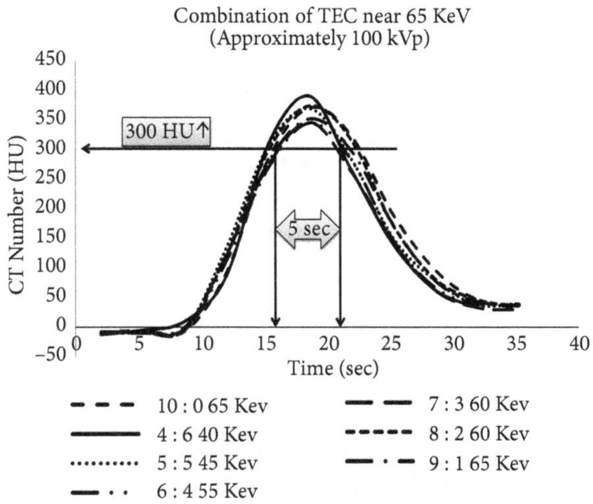

FIGURE 10: Determination of the best combination of dilution rate and monoenergetic energy using VMI. The combinations that maintained enhancement above 300 HU were 10:0 at 65 kV, 4:6 at 40 keV, 5:5 at 45 keV, 6:4 at 55 keV, 7:3 at 60 keV, 8:2 at 60 keV, and 9:1 at 65 keV. In addition, the dilution ratio of 6:4 at 55 keV only provided an enhancement level of 300 HU for 5 s, which corroborates the TEC using single-energy scanning at 100 kV.

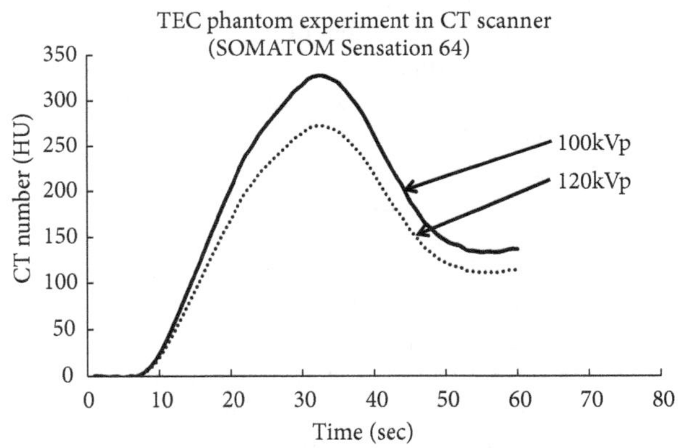

FIGURE 11: TECs of 120 kV and 100 kV obtained from conventional CT images with low kVp imaging. At an injection rate of 3.0 mL/s, 75 mL (60 kg) was injected for 25 s, and the amount of the circulation was set by assumption. Under low kVp imaging, lower kVp (100 kVp) provides higher CT numbers for the contrast material.

(see Figure 3). This result indicates that VMI is a more effective method for reducing the contrast media dose.

Figure 11 shows the experimental results that demonstrate the increase in CT number acquired from the conventional CT image with low kVp imaging. This TEC was created by injecting the total 75-mL volume of contrast media at 3.0 mL/s (for 25 s) into the human blood flow phantom to simulate a human body of 60 kg at 100 and 120 kVp. Low kVp imaging at 100 kVp can obtain relatively higher CT numbers but does not achieve the increases in CT number obtained using the VMI method.

As Table 1 shows, the tube voltage and sensitivity ratio of the contrast medium can be easily measured. Thus, a mixed injection based on sensitivity ratios should facilitate imaging.

TABLE 1: Sensitivity for contrast media under conventional CT. CT numbers were measured from the images acquired under various kVp with diluted contrast media of 5-20 mgI/mL via conventional scans. The sensitivity was calculated by normalizing each CT number with the CT number at 120 kVp (100% at 120 kVp).

Contrast media	Tube voltage				
	70kVp	80kVp	100kVp	120kVp	140kVp
5mgI/mL	1.9	1.6	1.2	1.0	0.9
10mgI/mL	1.9	1.6	1.2	1.0	0.9
15mgI/mL	2.0	1.6	1.2	1.0	0.9
20mgI/mL	2.0	1.6	1.2	1.0	0.8

SIEMENS SOMATOM Definition Flash

CT numbers were measured from the images acquired under various kVp with diluted contrast media of 5-20 mgI/mL via conventional scan. The sensitivity was calculated by normalizing each CT number with the CT number at 120 kVp (100% at 120 kVp).

The present study simulated the examination of vessels, which have relatively high image contrast on dual-energy CT. For examinations with normal image contrast, Albrecht et al. reported the advantages of the VMI method based on a study that compared monoenergetic images at 55 and 70 keV and DIC image of M0.3 (80 kVp 30% and 140 kVp 70%) obtained from 44 patients who were diagnosed with head and neck squamous cell carcinoma.

Hardie AD1 reported that a monoenergetic image at 55 keV showed better results for image noise reduction and diagnostic capability using the VMI method compared with a conventional CT image at 120 kVp. That result was obtained in an angiographic study of pancreas cancer (12 cases of adenocarcinoma, 5 cases of neuroendocrine, and 7 cases of cystic tumors). Although Hardie did not test a contrast media reduction, we also obtained similar results in which 55 keV was the best monoenergetic energy for maintaining less image noise and an appropriate CT number. We confirmed that the VMI method can be applied to diagnose cancer and image other organs that have a rich blood flow.

Depending on the CT numbers of the original images, 1,000 HU or above can be achieved using 40 keV for a virtual monochromatic image. However, this setting is impractical because an image SD of 40 or above is obtained in clinical settings, which is approximately four times greater than single-energy imaging at 100 kVp. Given the commonly used dosage range, the limit is approximately 55 keV. In addition, the combination of 6:4 and 55 keV (see Figure 11) might be suitable for maintaining 300 HU or above for approximately 5 s (imaging time) and obtaining the same 3D image quality (an SD of 15 or less) for the TEC at 100 kV during single-energy imaging (Figure 1).

The present study, performed using a SOMATOM Definition Flash system (Siemens), found that the combination of 6:4 and 55 keV was the optimum condition for VMI. However, the relationship between keV and image SD might differ with imaging devices, limiting this study to the present system. With the development of new devices, the contrast medium dosage might be further reduced.

The contrast medium dose can be reduced in dual-energy imaging, and any CT number can be obtained by adjusting the energy to modify the contrast CT numbers, thereby generating stable 3DCT images. Reliability is critical for CT tests. For example, the same images can be generated even with a fixed threshold number of volume rendering during the preparation of 3DCTA images, as long as the blood CT numbers are constant.

The diluted injection of saline and contrast medium enables energy adjustment for each test case by changing the mixing ratios with the same contrast and imaging timing, and it is easily introduced to clinical settings. Using this method, highly reliable 3DCTA images can be acquired, and the contrast medium dosage reduction rate can be calculated.

In the present study, the diluted injection of contrast medium was highly reliable in clinical settings because the CT numbers of the contrast media changed linearly with the dilution rate as expected.

Currently, a 180- to 300-mg range of iodine is administered as a contrast medium (24-50 mL of 300 mgI/mL) to visualize the arteries on CT angiography [7]. Based on the results of the present study, this dose can be reduced by approximately 30% for imaging in our hospital.

In recent years, there are various types of devices, such as dual source, fast kV switching, dual layer detector, and split-filter types, that can be used for clinical dual energy imaging. Jacobsen [10] et al. have reported variations in VMI sensitivity, as a result of experiments, between these different device types. Washio [11] et al. also compared VMI sensitivity of fast kV switching to that of dual layer detector. But they found only slight differences (less than 10%).

Here, we studied 3DCTA. Since it has a high contrast region of 300 HU or more, which is within the acceptable range of error, we consider that research can be diverted towards sensitivity and infusion dilution ratio of the contrast agent in all methods.

However, since changes in VMI image quality (such as SD) due to energy changes depend on CT (dual source, high-speed kV switching, dual layer detector, and split filter type), we assume that some consideration such as dose is required.

In addition, X-ray CT devices capable of multi-kVp settings will be widely used in clinical practice. The diluted injection method, combined with low-tube-voltage imaging, will reduce both radiation and contrast medium doses in the clinical field.

4. Conclusions

The present phantom experiment demonstrated that vascular CT numbers changed with the mixing ratios and generated stable TECs using the diluted injection method. In addition, the contrast medium dosage was reduced up to approximately 40% in 3DCTA tests using the VMI method of dual-energy CT. This method can be easily applied to clinical practice using mixed angiography and dual-energy CT without changing the imaging and acquisition timing. Furthermore, contrast CT numbers can be finely adjusted via VMI, providing stable 3D images.

Acknowledgments

The authors acknowledge Professor Shigeki Kuzuhara, Professor Yasuo Chinzei, and Professor Masahiro Irimoto at the Graduate school of Healthcare Science, Suzuka University of Medical Science.

References

[1] "Japanese Society of Nephrology Guideline".

[2] P. D. Stein, A. Beemath, F. Matta et al., "Clinical characteristics of patients with acute pulmonary embolism: data from PIOPED II," *American Journal of Medicine*, vol. 120, no. 10, pp. 871–879, 2007.

[3] F. Pontana, J. Pagniez, A. Duhamel et al., "Reduced-dose low-voltage chest ct angiography with sinogram-affirmed iterative reconstruction versus standard-dose filtered back projection," *Radiology*, vol. 267, no. 2, pp. 609–618, 2013.

[4] L. Faggioni, E. Neri, P. Sbragia et al., "80-kV pulmonary CT angiography with 40 mL of iodinated contrast material in lean patients: Comparison of vascular enhancement with iodixanol (320 mg I/mL)and iomeprol (400 mg I/mL)," *American Journal of Roentgenology*, vol. 199, no. 6, pp. 1220–1225, 2012.

[5] M.-A. Delesalle, F. Pontana, A. Duhamel et al., "Spectral optimization of chest CT angiography with reduced iodine load: Experience in 80 patients evaluated with dual-source, dual-energy CT," *Radiology*, vol. 267, no. 1, pp. 256–266, 2013.

[6] K. Terasawa and A. Hatcho, "Contrast enhancement technique in brain 3D-CTA studies: optimizing the amount of contrast medium according to scan time based on TDC," *Nippon Hoshasen Gijutsu Gakkai zasshi*, vol. 64, no. 6, pp. 681–689, 2008.

[7] K. Awai, A. Hatcho, Y. Nakayama et al., "Simulation of aortic peak enhancement on MDCT using a contrast material flow phantom: feasibility study," *American Journal of Roentgenology*, vol. 186, no. 2, pp. 379–385, 2006.

[8] M. Kidoh, T. Nakaura, K. Awai et al., "Novel connecting tube for saline chaser in contrast-enhanced CT: the effect of spiral flow of saline on contrast enhancement," *European Radiology*, vol. 23, no. 11, pp. 3213–3218, 2013.

[9] M. Tanikake, T. Shimizu, I. Narabayashi et al., "Three-dimensional CT angiography of the hepatic artery: use of multi-detector row helical CT and a contrast agent," *Radiology*, vol. 227, no. 3, pp. 883–889, 2003.

[10] M. C. Jacobsen, D. Schellingerhout, C. A. Wood et al., "Intermanufacturer comparison of dual-energy CT iodine quantification and monochromatic attenuation: a phantom study," *Radiology*, vol. 287, no. 1, pp. 224–234, 2018.

[11] H. Washio, S. Ohira, T. Karino et al., "Accuracy of quantification of iodine and hounsfield unit values on virtual monochromatic imaging using dual-energy computed tomography: comparison of dual-layer computed tomography with fast kilovolt-switching computed tomography," *Journal of Computer Assisted Tomography*, vol. 42, no. 6, pp. 965–971, 2018.

12

Dosimetry and Comparison between Different CT Protocols (Low Dose, Ultralow Dose and Conventional CT) for Lung Nodules' Detection in a Phantom

Cleverson Alex Leitão,[1] Gabriel Lucca de Oliveira Salvador,[1] Priscilla Tazoniero,[1] Danny Warszawiak,[1] Cristian Saievicz,[1] Rosangela Requi Jakubiak,[2] and Dante Luiz Escuissato[1]

[1]*Department of Radiology, Universidade Federal do Paraná, Curitiba, Paraná, Brazil*
[2]*Universidade Tecnológica Federal do Paraná, Curitiba, Paraná, Brazil*

Correspondence should be addressed to Gabriel Lucca de Oliveira Salvador; glucca11@gmail.com

Academic Editor: Daniele La Forgia

Background. The effects of dose reduction in lung nodule detection need better understanding. *Purpose.* To compare the detection rate of simulated lung nodules in a chest phantom using different computed tomography protocols, low dose (LD), ultralow dose (ULD), and conventional (CCT), and to quantify their respective amount of radiation. *Materials and Methods.* A chest phantom containing 93 simulated lung nodules was scanned using five different protocols: ULD (80 kVp/30 mA), LD A (120 kVp/20 mA), LD B (100 kVp/30 mA), LD C (120 kVp/30 mA), and CCT (120 kVp/automatic mA). Four chest radiologists analyzed a selected image from each protocol and registered in diagrams the nodules they detected. Kruskal–Wallis and McNemar's tests were performed to determine the difference in nodule detection. Equivalent doses were estimated by placing thermoluminescent dosimeters on the surface and inside the phantom. *Results.* There was no significant difference in lung nodules' detection when comparing ULD and LD protocols ($p = 0.208$ to $p = 1.000$), but there was a significant difference when comparing each one of those against CCT ($p < 0.001$). The detection rate of nodules with CT attenuation values lower than −600 HU was also different when comparing all protocols against CCT ($p < 0.001$ to $p = 0.007$). There was at least moderate agreement between observers in all protocols (κ-value >0.41). Equivalent dose values ranged from 0.5 to 9 mSv. *Conclusion.* There is no significant difference in simulated lung nodules' detection when comparing ULD and LD protocols, but both differ from CCT, especially when considering lower-attenuating nodules.

1. Introduction

Lung cancer represents the main cause of cancer-related deaths in the world [1]. Conventional chest radiographs used to be a screening tool for early diagnosis [2], but low-dose computed tomography (LDCT) proved to be superior [3]. The National Lung Screening Trial (NLST) was the first large multicentric study to show a reduction of 20% in lung cancer mortality in patients enrolled in a screening program using LDCT [4]. Nowadays, the American Cancer Society defends lung cancer screening using LDCT in smokers or former smokers who quit smoking in the last 15 years, aged between 55 and 74, with at least 30 pack-years smoking history [5].

The main issue regarding lung cancer screening is the systematic exposition of patients to ionizing radiation, which is potentially carcinogenic [6]. Patients submitted to annual LDCT have an additional risk of induced major cancers of 0.05% [7].

The pursuit for lower doses led to the creation of ultralow-dose (ULD) protocols, performed in modern CT equipment with iterative reconstruction [8] which expose the patient to amounts of X-rays as low as chest radiography [9].

This study aims to quantify the amount of radiation the patients are exposed to during a specific ultralow-dose protocol and different low-dose protocols and to determine how those doses impact the detection of simulated lung nodules in a phantom.

2. Materials and Methods

2.1. Phantom. The Alderson Rando radiotherapy phantom (RSD phantoms, Long Beach, USA) simulates a male patient (5 ft. 9 in. tall and weighing 162 lb.). It is composed of 2.5 cm thick slices, which contain pins that can be replaced by thermoluminescent dosimeter holders. It is molded of tissue-equivalent material, with lungs made from synthetic foam with a specific gravity of 0.30 g/cc. The pins in each slice have different CT Hounsfield values, which we used to simulate solid and ground-glass lung nodules.

The phantom contains a total of 105 simulated nodules, each one measuring 5 mm. Twelve of those were excluded from analysis due to their interface with the chest wall or mediastinum. The remaining 93 nodules were divided into columns and rows and named in accordance with their position. Three pinholes were left empty (positions E2, E11, and F9), so that they produced negative images (air density) that would help the participants count rows and columns.

We evaluated the mean attenuation coefficient in Hounsfield Units of each lung nodule in all the protocols by placing a 20 mm^2 region of interest inside them, in order to verify if the ones with lower densities (ground-glass nodules) would have lower rates of detection in lower-dose protocols. The nodules attenuation coefficient ranged from −707 to −435 HU. The nodules were divided into three groups: density lower than −600 HU, density between −600 and −500 HU, and density higher than −500 HU. Thirty-two nodules (35%) had attenuation values lower than −600 HU, 48 (51%) between −600 and −500 HU, and 13 (14%) higher than −500 HU.

2.2. CT Protocols. All chest CT examinations were acquired using 256-slice multidetector CT (GE Revolution; General Electric Healthcare, Milwaukee, USA). We first used a usual high-resolution chest CT (CCT) protocol to obtain reference images: 0.5 s gantry rotation time, 120 kVp, 0.984 : 1 beam pitch, 40 mm table feed for gantry rotation, and *z*-axis tube current modulation.

To obtain LD and ULD acquisitions, the automatic tube current modulation was replaced by manually chosen values of mA, while the other parameters were maintained. For the ULD protocol, kVp was lowered to 80 and mA was set to 30. We decided to experiment with different low-dose protocols to verify how reductions in kV and mA affect the dose and nodule detection, since previous studies show that CT performed for other reasons, like pulmonary embolism, can be performed with lower doses and similar detection rates when those parameters are modified [10]. For LD protocol A, (lower mA) mA was lowered to 20 and, for LD protocol B (lower kVp), kVp was lowered to 100. LD protocol C (conventional LDCT) followed the AAPM recommendations for lung cancer screening [11]. Table 1 specifies the protocols used.

Images were reconstructed at 0.625 mm thickness, 512 × 512 matrix, using iterative reconstruction (ASiR-V™ General Electric Healthcare, Milwaukee, USA).

2.3. Image Evaluation. The resulting images were analyzed on a Picture Archiving and Communication System (CARESTREAM Vue PACs; Carestream Health, Inc., Rochester, USA) by four radiologists with at least 10 years of experience in chest radiology over the course of five weeks. The participants received a printed diagram in which the lung nodules were represented in columns and rows (Figure 1). Radiologists were asked to register in which locations they were confident enough to report the presence of a lung nodule. Images were displayed with a lung window setting, the same one used when the radiologists interpret clinical patient images (window level: −800/window width 1300). The radiologists were allowed to change the window settings as they pleased. Images were evaluated in a 3-megapixel, 500 cd/m^2 maximum-luminance monitor (Barco Medical Displays, Duluth, USA).

2.4. Radiation Dose Assessment. Dosimetry was performed by placing lithium-fluoride thermoluminescent dosimeters (TLDs) over the surface of and inside the phantom (5 centimeters under the surface, at the level of the second row of nodules in the right lung), to estimate both entrance surface dose and dose delivered to the lung in each protocol. Since a single scan exposed the dosimeters to a very small amount of radiation, TLDs were scanned five times each and the mean dose for a single exposure was calculated. TLDs were previously calibrated with the aid of an ionizing chamber, being exposed to a specific amount of kV (80, 100, or 120) according to the protocol in which they would be used.

The mean dose absorbed by the dosimeters was converted to equivalent dose using the weighting factor (wR) value of 1 [12].

2.5. Statistical Analysis. Since nodules detection is a qualitative dataset (detection/no detection), thus, not normally distributed, we used nonparametric methods to estimate the significance interval. The comparisons of lung nodules detection with all five protocols were performed using the Kruskal–Wallis test [13]. Furthermore, McNemar's test was used in relation to the factor levels pairs to confirm which of the pairs were not similar, thereby causing a difference. The p value for statistical significance was $p < 0.05$.

In order to rate interobserver agreement, we calculated the κ-values for each pair of readers and for each pair of protocols (κ-value 0–0.2: poor; 0.21–0.4: fair; 0.41–0.6: moderate; 0.61–0.8: substantial; 0.8–1: almost perfect).

All statistical tests (Kruskal–Wallis, McNemar's, and the Kappa statistical analysis) were performed using MedCalc® software, version 19.1.3 (MedCalc software, Mariakerke, Belgium) [14].

Table 1: Protocol specifications.

	ULD	LD (lower mA)	LD (lower kV)	Conventional LDCT	HRCT
Gantry rotation time (s)	0.5	0.5	0.5	0.5	0.5
Beam collimation (mm)	40	40	40	40	40
Pitch	0.984	0.984	0.984	0.984	0.984
kV	80	120	100	120	120
mA	30	20	30	30	Auto/smart mA

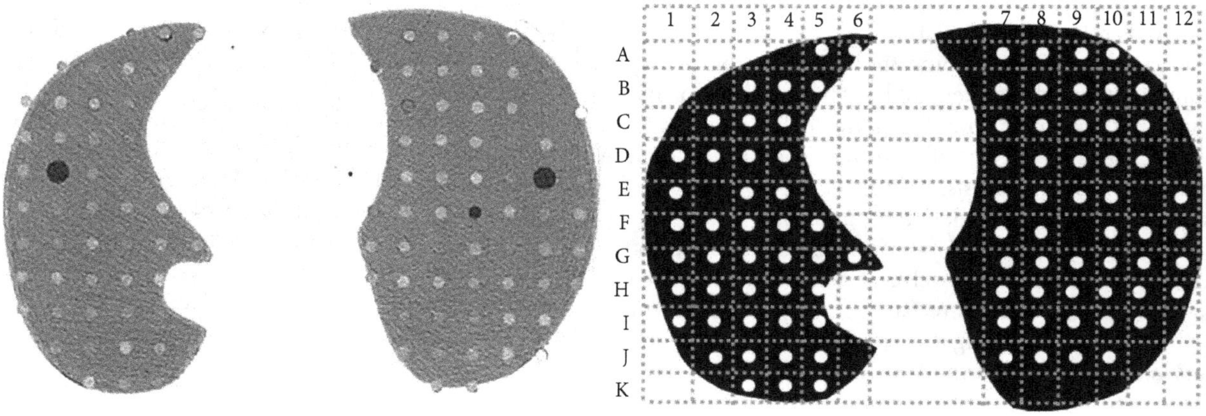

Figure 1: Example of the selected CT slice the radiologists analyzed and the printed diagram in which they registered the nodules they detected. Peripheral nodules such as A3, A4, and B2 were excluded from analysis because of their interface with the chest wall. Positions E2, E11, and F9 had no simulated nodules and served as reference to count columns and rows.

3. Results

3.1. Dosimetry. The estimated equivalent entrance surface dose was 0.5 mSv for ULD acquisition and 9.0 mSv for conventional CT. The equivalent entrance dose for conventional LDCT was 1.8 mSv. The reductions made in kV and mA had a small impact over the equivalent dose. The estimated entrance dose for LDCT protocol A (lower mA) was 1.32 mSv and for LDCT protocol B (lower kV) was 1.34 mSv. Estimated equivalent dose to the lung ranged from 0.6 mSv (ULD) to 9.0 mSv (CCT). Table 2 summarizes the equivalent dose in each protocol and their respective uncertainty values.

3.2. Nodule Detection. Nodule detection rate was 65.6% (±2.5% standard deviation) for ULD protocol, 68.5% (±5.5% standard deviation) for LD protocol A, 66.4% (±5.9% standard deviation) for LD protocol B, 68.5% (±7.6% standard deviation) for conventional LDCT, and 85.8% (±2.8% standard deviation) for conventional CT. Figure 2 summarizes the number of nodules detected in each protocol by all radiologists.

For protocol 1 (ULDCT), 52 simulated nodules (56%) were detected by all radiologists, 8 nodules (10%) were detected by three radiologists, 4 nodules (4%) were detected by two radiologists, 4 nodules (4%) were detected by only one radiologist, and 25 nodules (26%) were missed by all radiologists.

For protocol 2 (LDCT—lower mA), 53 simulated nodules (57%) were detected by all radiologists, 9 nodules (10%) were detected by three radiologists, 6 nodules (6%) were detected by two radiologists, 4 nodules (4%) were detected by only one radiologist, and 21 nodules (23%) were missed by all radiologists.

For protocol 3 (LDCT—lower kV), 58 simulated nodules (62%) were detected by all radiologists, 3 nodules (3.5%) were detected by three radiologists, 3 nodules (3.5%) were detected by two radiologists, 10 nodules (11%) were detected by only one radiologist, and 19 nodules (20%) were missed by all radiologists.

For protocol 4 (conventional LDCT), 54 simulated nodules (58%) were detected by all radiologists, 8 nodules (9%) were detected by three radiologists, 7 nodules (7.5%) were detected by two radiologists, 6 nodules (6%) were detected by only one radiologist, and 18 nodules (19.5%) were missed by all radiologists.

For protocol 5 (CCT), 73 simulated nodules (79%) were detected by all radiologists, 5 nodules (5%) were detected by three radiologists, 2 nodules (2%) were detected by two radiologists, 8 nodules (9%) were detected by only one radiologist, and 5 nodules (5%) were missed by all radiologists.

The comparison between all five protocols revealed that protocols 1, 2, 3, and 4 showed no statistically significant difference in lung nodules detection rate ($p > 0.05$). However, each one of those protocols was statistically different from protocol 5 ($p < 0.001$). Table 3 shows the p values obtained when comparing all protocols. Forty-three simulated nodules (46%) were detected by all radiologists in all protocols and only 3 nodules (3%) were not detected by any radiologist in any protocol. Six nodules (6%) were detected by one or more radiologists only in protocol 5. When comparing detection rates according to CT attenuation values, we detected that for

Table 2: Estimated equivalent doses.

Protocol	kV	mA	Equivalent entrance skin dose/uncertainty (mSv)	Equivalent dose to the lung/uncertainty (mSv)
Ultralow dose	80	30	0.5/0.06	0.6/0.06
Low dose (lower mA)	120	20	1.32/0.26	1.32/0.12
Low dose (lower kV)	100	30	1.34/0.3	1.5/0.3
Conventional low dose	120	30	1.8/0.36	2.0/0.16
Conventional HRCT	120	Automatic	9.0/0.8	9.0/0.58

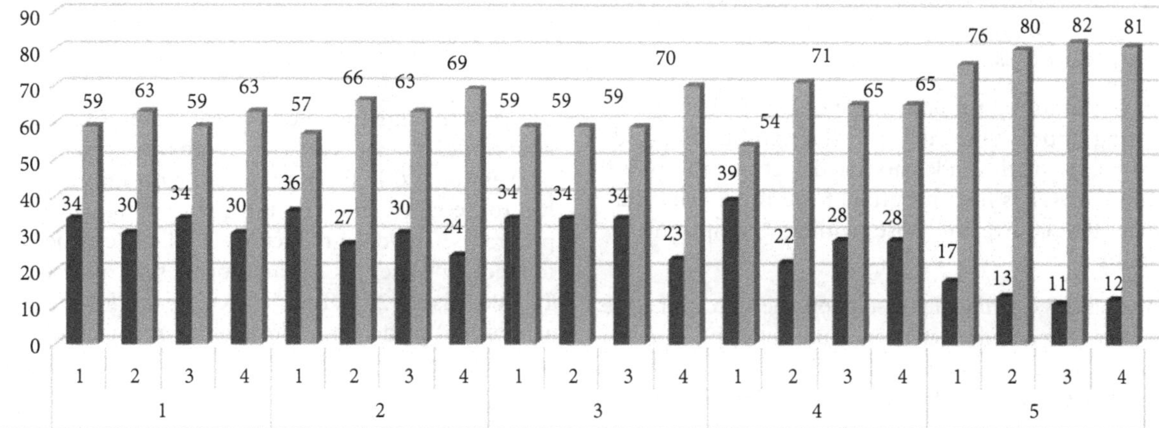

	1				2				3				4				5			
	1	2	3	4	1	2	3	4	1	2	3	4	1	2	3	4	1	2	3	4
0	34	30	34	30	36	27	30	24	34	34	34	23	39	22	28	28	17	13	11	12
1	59	63	59	63	57	66	63	69	59	59	59	70	54	71	65	65	76	80	82	81

Figure 2: The number of nodules detected (gray columns, number 1) and missed (black columns, number 0) in each protocol (numbers 1 to 5, lower row) for every radiologist (numbers 1 to 4, upper row). Protocol 1: ULD, protocol 2: LD A, protocol 3: LD B, protocol 4: LD C, and protocol 5: CCT.

Table 3: Comparison of the number of nodules detected by all radiologists for every pair of protocols using McNemar's test.

Protocols	1/2	1/3	1/4	1/5	2/3	2/4	2/5	3/4	3/5	4/5
Nodules detected	244/255	244/247	244/255	244/319	255/247	255/255	255/319	247/255	247/319	255/319
p value	0.208	0.749	0.215	<0.001	0.302	1.000	<0.001	0.322	<0.001	<0.001

lower-attenuating nodules (CT HU < −600 HU) every radiologist presented at least one low-dose or ultralow-dose protocol in which the detection rate was significantly different when compared to CCT (protocol 5). For radiologist 1, protocol 4 was different from 5 ($p = 0.024$). For radiologist 2, protocols 1 and 3 were different from 5 ($p = 0.04$). For radiologist 3, all protocols were different from 5 ($p = 0.007$). For radiologist 4, protocols 1 and 4 were different from 5 ($p = 0.003$ and $p = 0.007$, resp.). There was no significant difference when comparing protocols for the detection rate of nodules with mean attenuation values from −600 to −500 HU ($p = 0.362$) and higher than −500 HU ($p = 0.406$).

κ-Values to evaluate interobserver agreement revealed that in all protocols there was at least moderate agreement (κ-value >0.41) between all radiologists, ranging from 0.522 to 1.000. When comparing the protocols (Table 4), the agreement between all ULD and LD was substantial (κ-values ranging from 0.617 to 0.766); however, their agreement levels when compared to CCT (protocol 5) were only fair or moderate (κ-values ranging from 0.398 to 0.502).

4. Discussion

Kim et al. [8] and Lee et al. [15] studied the same ULD protocol and reported effective doses of 0.31 and 0.29 mSv, respectively. As for the LD protocol, the mean effective dose in NLST was estimated in 1.5 mSv [16]. Depending on the values of kV and mA, literature shows different doses that range from 1.06 mSv to 2.7 mSv [8, 17]. Comparison between our results and others should be made carefully, due to different methodologies. Those studies report effective doses derived from DLP (dose-length product), a population dose metric that AAPM recommends not to be used to estimate dose or risk to an individual [11]. We decided to estimate dose using thermoluminescent dosimetry as an alternative that can be further reproduced by other authors.

Huber et al. [9] reported effective doses of 0.13 mSv using a ULD protocol, a value comparable to chest X-ray doses. The average effective dose for PA and lateral chest X-rays is approximately 0.16 mSv [18], what would make our protocol equivalent to about 3 X-rays. Again, this comparison is not

Table 4: Comparison of nodule detection rates between pairs of protocols (kappa values).

	Protocol 1	Protocol 2	Protocol 3	Protocol 4	Protocol 5
Protocol 1	—	0.617	0.766	0.605	0.398
Protocol 2	0.617	—	0.718	0.688	0.385
Protocol 3	0.766	0.718	—	0.694	0.494
Protocol 4	0.605	0.688	0.694	—	0.502
Protocol 5	0.398	0.385	0.494	0.502	—

entirely true due to different dosimetry approaches, but it still serves as an estimative of how CT can be performed with impressively low doses.

When trying to reduce patient exposure, ULDCT poses an interesting option, since it is possible to obtain considerably lower doses with similar nodule detection rate. When performing ULDCT is not an option, lowering kV and mA can reduce the equivalent dose without compromising image quality.

Literature shows conflicting results on the effects of dose reduction over lung nodules detection. Huber et al. [9] reported nodules detection rates of 93.3% in ULDCTs, compared to 95.5% in standard dose CTs (no significant difference). That study used a different anthropomorphic phantom, with different lung nodules sizes and attenuation values (−630 HU and 100 HU), which can partly explain the different results we obtained. Other studies show that low-dose images can reduce the detectability of peripheral lung nodules [19] and result in differences in nodules volumetry [20].

When evaluating interobserver agreement, it has been previously reported that even NLST participants presented substantial variability in false-positive rates [21]. Studies have shown that LDCT could result in poor accordance, with κ-values as low as 0.120 [22]. However, our degree of agreement is closer to the ones presented in more recent studies (kappa as high as 0.848 for 80 kV LDCT) [20]. The lowest κ-value for low-dose protocols in this study was 0.600, which still represents moderate agreement. The comparison of the performance of the radiologists between ULD and LD protocols revealed substantial agreement (kappa ranging from 0.605 to 0.766), indicating that although there was a small degree of heterogeneity, the final performance of the observers in different protocols was comparable, as shown in previous research [23].

Considering the effects of radiation dose over the detection of ground-glass nodules is also important. Literature shows that lepidic-growth adenocarcinomas tend to show CT attenuation values between −651 and −447 HU [24]. In this study, all 93 simulated lung nodules had attenuation values within this range. Although ULD and all three LD protocols had similar rates of detection for nodules with attenuation values lower than −600 HU, there was a significant difference when comparing the detection of those nodules with conventional dose CT (CCT). Funama et al. found that images obtained with lower milliampere settings (21 and 45 mA) can reduce the detection of simulated ground-glass lung nodules with attenuation coefficients of −650 HU in a phantom [25]. Our study reproduces this finding, showing that special attention should be given to lower-attenuating nodules, as scans performed with LD and ULD protocols can potentially miss small lepidic-growth adenocarcinomas.

Even though this study detected significant differences in lung nodules detection when comparing ULD and LDCT to conventional CT, the risk of radiation-induced cancer still has to be taken into account for all lung cancer screening programs. The dose reduction in LDCT can be responsible for reducing the risk of carcinogenesis from 8.6 to 0.35 per 100000 cases [26]. The "ALARA" (as low as reasonably achievable) principle of dose containment is still where the main efforts for lung cancer screening are driven [27].

This study has limitations: the main one being the use of a phantom instead of real patients. The methodology we chose for this study, in which five different protocols were repeated five times, would expose human participants to high levels of radiation, what would be ethically questionable. Our phantom simulates a 162 lb (73 kg) male, what limits the extrapolation of these results to different populations since different body types can have different qualities of images when scanned with the exact same protocols. There need to be further clinical studies in order to assure our results are reproductible in human patients and in different populations. Furthermore, all the analysis in this study were performed by radiologists, in contrast to many other similar ones that use computer aided detection software capable of reducing detection variability in lung nodules in different protocols [28]. Automatic tools have already proved to be efficient in detecting potentially malignant microcalcifications in digital mammograms [29] and are progressively being implemented for malignant nodules detection in CT scans [30], which can help to overcome human-analysis limitations potentially identifiable in this study.

In conclusion, it is possible to perform ULDCT exposing patients to less than a third of the equivalent dose seen in conventional LDCT and less than a tenth of conventional CT. There is no significant difference in lung nodules detection rates when comparing images obtained with ULDCT and LDCT. However, the detection rate for ULDCT and LDCT protocols differs from conventional CT, especially for lung nodules with lower density (CT Hounsfield units <−600 HU). These differences should be taken into account when selecting a protocol for the implementation of lung cancer screening programs.

References

[1] P. M. De Groot, C. C. Wu, B. W. Carter, and R. F. Munden, "The epidemiology of lung cancer," *Translational Lung Cancer Research*, vol. 7, no. 3, pp. 220–233, 2018.

[2] G. M. Strauss, R. E. Gleason, and D. J. Sugarbaker, "Chest X-ray screening improves outcome in lung cancer," *Chest*, vol. 107, no. 6, pp. 270S–279S, 1995.

[3] M. Kaneko, K. Eguchi, H. Ohmatsu et al., "Peripheral lung cancer: screening and detection with low-dose spiral CT versus radiography," *Radiology*, vol. 201, no. 3, pp. 798–802, 1996.

[4] The National Lung Screening Trial Team, "Reduced lung-cancer mortality with low-dose computed tomographic screening," *New England Journal of Medicine*, vol. 365, pp. 395–409, 2011.

[5] R. Wender, E. T. Fontham, E. Barrera Jr. et al., "American Cancer Society lung cancer screening guidelines," *CA: A Cancer Journal for Clinicians*, vol. 63, pp. 107–117, 2013.

[6] J. M. Albert, "Radiation risk from CT: implications for cancer screening," *American Journal of Roentgenology*, vol. 201, p. 1, 2013.

[7] C. Rampinelli, P. De Marco, D. Origgi et al., "Exposure to low dose computed tomography for lung cancer screening and risk of cancer: secondary analysis of trial data and risk-benefit analysis," *BMJ*, vol. 356, p. j347, 2017.

[8] Y. Kim, Y. K. Kim, B. E. Lee et al., "Ultra-low-dose CT of the thorax using iterative reconstruction: evaluation of image quality and radiation dose reduction," *American Journal of Roentgenology*, vol. 204, no. 6, pp. 1197–1202, 2015.

[9] A. Huber, J. Landau, L. Ebner et al., "Performance of ultralow-dose CT with iterative reconstruction in lung cancer screening: limiting radiation exposure to the equivalent of conventional chest X-ray imaging," *European Radiology*, vol. 26, no. 10, pp. 3643–3652, 2016.

[10] M. K. Gill, A. Vijayananthan, G. Kumar, K. Jayarani, K. H. Ng, and Z. Sun, "Use of 100 kV versus 120 kV in computed tomography pulmonary angiography in the detection of pulmonary embolism: effect on radiation dose and image quality," *Quantitative Imaging in Medicine and Surgery*, vol. 5, no. 4, pp. 524–533, 2015.

[11] American Association for Physicists in Medicine (AAPM), "AAPM lung cancer screening CT protocols version 5.1," 2019, https://www.aapm.org/pubs/CTProtocols/documents/LungCancerScreeningCT.pdf.

[12] C. H. McCollough and B. A. Schueler, "Calculation of effective dose," *Medical Physics*, vol. 27, no. 5, pp. 828–837, 2000.

[13] W. J. Conover, *Pratical Nonparametric Statistics*, John Wiley & Sons, Hoboken, NJ, USA, 3rd edition, 1999.

[14] F. Schoonjans, A. Zalata, C. E. Depuydt, and F. H. Comhaire, "MedCalc: a new computer program for medical statistics," *Computer Methods and Programs in Biomedicine*, vol. 48, no. 3, pp. 257–262, 1995.

[15] S. W. Lee, Y. Kim, S. S. Shim et al., "Image quality assessment of ultra low-dose chest CT using sinogram-affirmed iterative reconstruction," *European Radiology*, vol. 24, no. 4, pp. 817–826, 2014.

[16] National Lung Screening Trial Research Team, D. R. Aberle, C. D. Berg et al., "The national lung screening trial: overview and study design," *Radiology*, vol. 258, pp. 243–253, 2011.

[17] A. Neroladaki, D. Botsikas, S. Boudabbous, C. D. Becker, and X. Montet, "Computed tomography of the chest with model-based iterative reconstruction using a radiation exposure similar to chest X-ray examination: preliminary observations," *European Radiology*, vol. 23, no. 2, pp. 360–366, 2013.

[18] A. Lahham, A. Issa, and H. ALMasri, "Patient radiation dose from chest X-ray examinations in the West bank—Palestine," *Radiation Protection Dosimetry*, vol. 178, no. 3, pp. 298–303, 2018.

[19] H. Rusinek, D. P. Naidich, G. McGuinness et al., "Pulmonary nodule detection: low-dose versus conventional CT," *Radiology*, vol. 209, no. 1, pp. 243–249, 1998.

[20] S. Jin, B. Zhang, L. Zhang, S. Li, S. Li, and P. Li, "Lung nodules assessment in ultra-low-dose CT with iterative reconstruction compared to conventional dose CT," *Quantitative Imaging in Medicine and Surgery*, vol. 8, no. 5, pp. 480–490, 2018.

[21] P. F. Pinsky, D. S. Gierada, P. H. Nath, E. Kazerooni, and J. Amorosa, "National lung screening trial: variability in nodule detection rates in chest CT studies," *Radiology*, vol. 268, no. 3, pp. 865–873, 2013.

[22] J. K. Leader, T. E. Warfel, C. R. Fuhrman et al., "Pulmonary nodule detection with low-dose CT of the lung: agreement among radiologists," *American Journal of Roentgenology*, vol. 185, no. 4, pp. 973–978, 2005.

[23] X. Sui, F. G. Meinel, W. Song et al., "Detection and size measurements of pulmonary nodules in ultra-low-dose CT with iterative reconstruction compared to low dose CT," *European Journal of Radiology*, vol. 85, no. 3, pp. 564–570, 2016.

[24] H. Nomori, T. Ohtsuka, T. Naruke, and K. Suemasu, "Differentiating between atypical adenomatous hyperplasia and bronchioloalveolar carcinoma using the computed tomography number histogram," *The Annals of Thoracic Surgery*, vol. 76, no. 3, pp. 867–871, 2003.

[25] Y. Funama, K. Awai, D. Liu et al., "Detection of nodules showing ground-glass opacity in the lungs at low-dose multidetector computed tomography," *Journal of Computer Assisted Tomography*, vol. 33, no. 1, pp. 49–53, 2009.

[26] N. Staltybaeva, K. Martini, K. Frauenfelder et al., "Organ dose and attributable cancer risk in lung cancer screening with low-dose computed tomography," *PLoS One*, vol. 11, Article ID e0155722, 2016.

[27] M. Malscalchi and L. Sali, "Lung cancer screening with low dose CT and radiation harm—from prediction models to cancer incidence data," *Annals of Translational Medicine*, vol. 5, p. 360, 2017.

[28] P. Delogu, S. C. Cheran, I. De Mitri et al., "Preprocessing methods for nodule detection in lung CT," *International Congress Series*, vol. 1281, pp. 1099–1103, 2005.

[29] T. M. A. Basile, A. Fanizzi, L. Losurdo et al., "Microcalcification detection in full-field digital mammograms: a fully automated computer-aided system," *Physica Medica*, vol. 64, pp. 1–9, 2019.

[30] I. De Mitri and MAGIC-5 Collaboration, "The MAGIC-5 project: medical applications on a grid infrastructure connection," *Studies in Health Technology and Informatics*, vol. 112, pp. 157–166, 2005.

13

Correlation between Chest CT Severity Scores and the Clinical Parameters of Adult Patients with COVID-19 Pneumonia

Ghufran Aref Saeed,[1] **Waqar Gaba**,[2] **Asad Shah**,[1] **Abeer Ahmed Al Helali**,[1] **Emadullah Raidullah**,[2] **Ameirah Bader Al Ali**,[2] **Mohammed Elghazali**,[2] **Deena Yousef Ahmed**,[2] **Shaikha Ghanam Al Kaabi**,[2] **and Safaa Almazrouei**[1]

[1]*Department of Radiology, Sheikh Khalifa Medical City, Abu Dhabi, UAE*
[2]*Department of Internal Medicine, Sheikh Khalifa Medical City, Abu Dhabi, UAE*

Correspondence should be addressed to Ghufran Aref Saeed; gsaeed@seha.ae

Academic Editor: Daniele La Forgia

Purpose. Our aim is to correlate the clinical condition of patients with COVID-19 infection with the 25-point CT severity score by Chang et al. (devised for assessment of ARDS in patients with SARS in 2005). *Materials and Methods.* Data of consecutive symptomatic patients who were suspected to have COVID-19 infection and presented to our hospital were collected from March to April 2020. All patients underwent two consecutive RT-PCR tests and had a noncontrast HRCT scan done at presentation. From the original cohort of 1062 patients, 160 patients were excluded leaving a total number of 902 patients. *Results.* The mean age was 44.2 ± 11.9 years (85.3% males, 14.7% females). CT severity score was found to be positively correlated with lymphopenia, increased serum CRP, d-dimer, and ferritin levels ($p < 0.0001$). The oxygen requirements and length of hospital stay were increasing with the increase in scan severity. *Conclusion.* The 25-point CT severity score correlates well with the COVID-19 clinical severity. Our data suggest that chest CT scoring system can aid in predicting COVID-19 disease outcome and significantly correlates with lab tests and oxygen requirements.

1. Introduction

COVID-19 is an infection that has widely and rapidly spread all over the world and became a pandemic with significant impacts upon the sociopolitical milieu and healthcare delivery systems [1]. The clinical presentations vary from asymptomatic carriers to patients requiring assisted ventilatory support, and ICU admissions with increased mortality made it an unusual and unprecedented challenge [2, 3]. The nasopharyngeal swab RT-PCR test has been the diagnostic test used as the standard of reference for disease confirmation [4]. The test is a powerful tool; however, there is a small but significant proportion of false-negative results reported [5].

A noncontrast high-resolution CT chest imaging plays a pivotal and essential role in the early disease detection, particularly in patients with false-negative RT-PCR results, as well as in managing and monitoring the course of disease [6]. Moreover, the disease severity can be ascertained from the imaging findings, significantly supporting the clinicians in their clinical judgment and ensuring effective and timely management [7]. Prognosis can also be affected by the severity of the disease in the critically ill patients allowing appropriate selection of early involvement of the intensive care [8, 9].

Multiple studies have explored the pulmonary involvement on the chest CT images using both visual and software quantitative assessments [10, 11]. To our knowledge, ours is the first comprehensive study to describe the correlation of chest CT severity scores and the clinical picture of patients with COVID-19 disease in the Gulf and Arab region. Our study correlates the CT severity score with the clinical severity of the patients who were confirmed to have COVID-19 disease using the 25-point visual quantitative assessment.

2. Methods

2.1. Data Collection. Ethical approval was obtained from Institutional Review Board (IRB) and Department of Health (DOH), Abu Dhabi, United Arab Emirates (UAE). The informed consent was waved off as per the ethics committee. We collected clinical and laboratory data for analysis, derived from an electronic medical record system, from March to April 2020 of patients who were suspected to have COVID-19 infection and underwent a chest HRCT scan. The results for the chest HRCT images were collected and evaluated using the Picture Archiving and Communication Systems (PACS).

2.2. HRCT Inspection. All initial chest HRCT scans were performed on the day of patients' presentation using a VCT GE 64 scanner. Patients were placed in a supine position with single breath hold. Scanning parameters were as follows: scan direction (craniocaudally), tube voltage (120 kV), tube current (100–600 mA)-smart mA dose modulation, slice collimation (64 × 0.625 mm), width (0.625 × 0.625 mm), pitch [1], rotation time (0.5 s), and scan length (60.00–I300.00 s).

2.3. HRCT Image Analysis. Two radiologists with more than 8 years of experience evaluated the images to determine the disease severity score in each patient. The scans were first assessed whether negative or positive for typical findings of COVID-19 pneumonia (bilateral, multilobe, posterior peripheral ground-glass opacities) as defined by the *RSNA Consensus statement* [7, 12]. Severity then was assessed using the following scoring system which depends on the visual assessment of each lobe involved [13–15] (Figure 1) (see Tables 1 and 2).

2.4. Statistical Analysis. The analysis was performed using SPSS 21.0. Descriptive statistics of patients' demographics, clinical, and laboratory results were reported as numbers and relative frequencies. Frequencies of CT scores were calculated and compared with other clinical variables. The Pearson correlation coefficient test was used for correlations, and p value less than 0.05 was defined statistically significant.

3. Results

3.1. Baseline Information. Our population included 1,062 consecutive patients who were suspected to have COVID-19 infection. Infection with SARS-CoV-2 was confirmed from a nasopharyngeal swab using the U-TOP COVID-19 Detection Kit (Seasun Biomaterials Inc., Daejeon, Korea), which is a reverse transcriptase-polymerase chain reaction (RT-PCR) test that has received Emergency Use Authorization (EUA) from the US Food and Drug Administration (FDA). RT-PCR testing was performed using Clinical Laboratory Improvement Amendments (CLIAs) diagnostic standards according to current testing guidelines [16]. All patients underwent two consecutive RT-PCR tests and had a HRCT scan done.

160 patients were excluded from the study as per the following *exclusion criteria*: patients less than 18 years old, patients with negative RT-PCT results, discharge to another facility leading to lost follow-up, suboptimal HRCT scan due to significant motion artefacts, or CT with atypical findings for COVID-19 pneumonia.

Eventually, 902 patients were included with the following information been collected: age, gender, presence of comorbidities/risk factors, laboratory tests including lymphocyte count, CRP, d-dimer and ferritin levels, maximum O_2 requirement, need for intubation, ICU admission, length of hospital stay (LOS), and final clinical outcome (alive, expired, or still intubated at the time of study).

The mean age was 44.2 ± 11.9 years (range 19–87 years; 769 males (85.3%), 133 females (14.7%)). The age was further classified into 6 groups: <30, 30–39, 40–49, 50–56, 60–69, and >70 years.

The risk factors considered included hypertension, diabetes mellitus, asthma, COPD, coronary artery disease, and chronic kidney disease. Risk factors were found in 399/902 patients (44.2%) (one risk factor, $n = 206$ (22.8%); two risk factors, $n = 114$ (12.6%); and three or more risk factors, $n = 79$ (8.8%)).

Laboratory results showed lymphopenia (normal value $1.5–4 \times 10^9$/L) in 203 patients (22.5%), elevated CRP (50 mg/L) in 236 patients (40.3%), high d-dimer (>1 mcg/mL) in 147 (16.2%), and elevated ferritin level (>600 ng/mL) in 301 (33.3%).

Out of the 902 patients, 646 patients (71.6%) did not require any oxygen support. The remaining 256 patients required oxygen supplement as follows: 126 patients (14%) required nasal cannula, 32 patients (3.5%) required face mask, 15 patients (1.7%) required non-rebreather mask, 21 patients (2.3%) required a bilevel positive airway pressure (BiPAP) or a high-flow nasal cannula (HFNC), and 62 patients (6.9%) required intubation, out of which 32 patients (51.6%) were eventually extubated. ICU admission was required in 202 (22.4%) out of the 902 patients with a male predominance (182/202; 90.1%). The most common age group was that between 40 and 49 years old (53/202; 26.2%).

Regarding hospital stay, 631 patients (70%) stayed in the hospital for 5 days or less, 127 (14.1%) for 6–11 days, 50 (5.5%) for 11–15 days, and 94 (10.4%) for more than 16 days.

In terms of clinical outcome, 863 patients (95.7%) were found alive, 33 (3.7%) expired in hospital, and 6 (0.7%) were still intubated at the time of the study.

3.2. Correlation between CT Severity and Clinical Parameters

3.2.1. Age and Gender. Our results showed significant correlation ($p < 0.05$) between CT severity score and the male gender, raised inflammatory markers, maximum O_2 requirement, length of hospital stay (LOS), need for intubation, and clinical outcome.

The HRCT scans were negative in 203/202 (22.5%) of patients (75.9% males, 24.1% females). Mild disease was seen in 329/209 (36.5%) patients (84.5% males, 15.5% females), moderate in 309/902 (34.3%) (90.6 males, 9.4% females), and

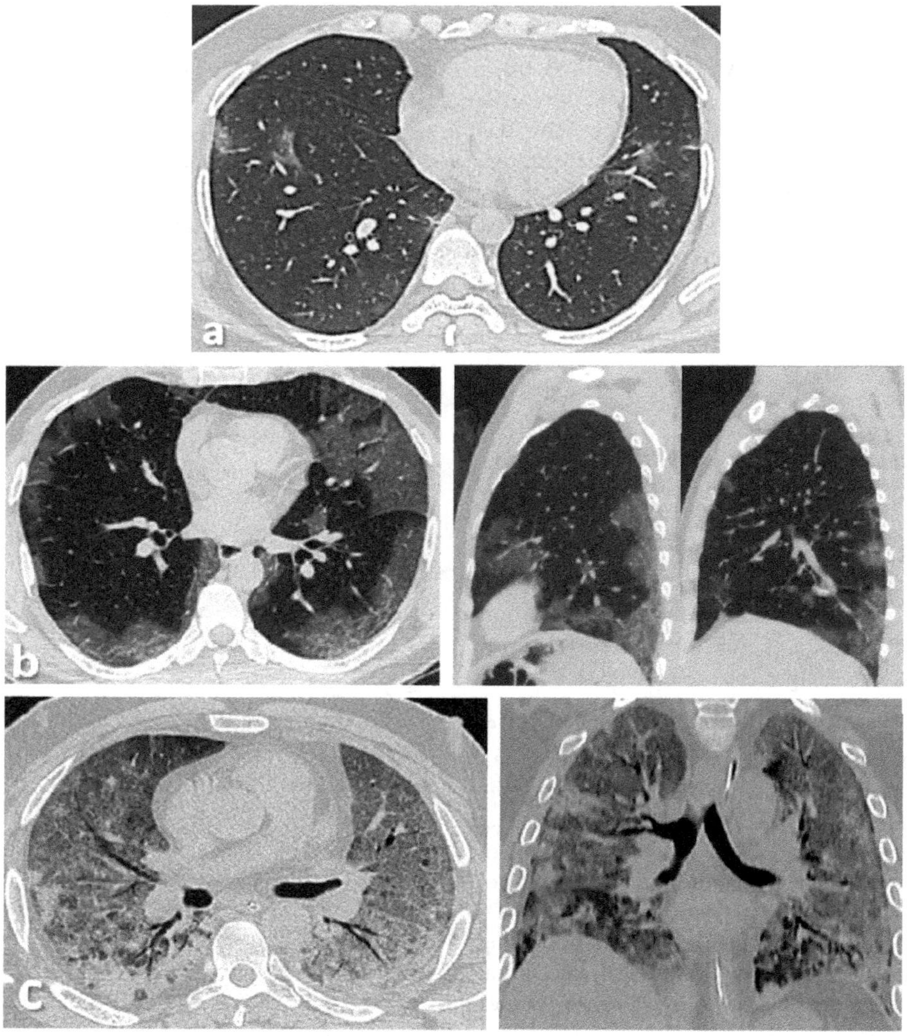

FIGURE 1: (a) Axial thin sections of unenhanced CT chest scan show mild GGO involving bilateral peripheral lower lobes. (b) Axial and sagittal sections show bilateral peripheral multilobe GGO of moderate disease severity. (c) Axial and coronal sections show diffuse crazy-paving pattern with areas of peripheral consolidations indicating severe disease.

severe in 61/209 (6.8%) patients (93.4% males, 6.6% females). A follow-up scan was done for 73/902 patients (8.1%).

The negative and mild scans were mainly seen in the 30- to 39-year age group, ($n = 62$, 30%) and ($n = 96$, 29.2%), respectively, and least in >70-year age group, ($n = 6$, 3%) and ($n = 4$, 1.2%), respectively. Moderate disease severity was mainly seen in the 40- to 49-year age group ($n = 98$, 31.7%) and least in >70 years old ($n = 4$, 1.3%). Severe disease was mainly seen in the 50- to 59-year age group ($n = 21$, 34.4%) and least in 18–29 years ($n = 0$, 0%) (Figure 2). The highest percentage of patients with 3 or more risk factors was seen in the severe group (11.5%).

3.2.2. Laboratory Results. Lymphopenia was detected in 17 patients (8.4%) of the negative group, 55 patients (13.7%) of the mild group, 110 patients (35.6%) of the moderate group, and 31 patients (50.8%) of the severe group. When compared with disease phase, lymphopenia was found to be more significant among patients with more severe scans ($p < 0.0001$).

CRP results were available for 897/902 patients. In patients with negative CT scan, CRP levels were <50 mg/L in 193 patients (96%) and in 308 patients (94.2%) with mild scan results. In patients with moderate CT scan, CRP levels were <50 mg/L in 151 patients (49%), 50–100 mg/L in 93 patients (30.2%), and >100 mg/L in 64 patients (20.8%). In patients with severe CT scan, CRP levels were <50 mg/L in 9 patients (14.8%), 50–100 mg/L in 13 patients (21.3%), and >100 mg/L in 39 patients (63.9%). These findings were found to have statistically significant correlation with the CT severity score ($p < 0.0001$, $r = 0.556$).

Moreover, the d-dimer level was assessed in 890/902 patients. Most patients with negative CT studies and mild CT severity scores had a normal d-dimer level: 182 patients (94.3%) and 304 patients (93%), respectively. In moderate category, the level was <1 mcg/mL in 239 patients (77.3%), 1–3 mcg/mL in 63 patients (20.4%), and >3 mcg/mL in 7 patients (2.3%). In the severe category, the level was <1 mcg/mL in 18 patients (29.5%), 1–3 mcg/mL in 28 patients (45.9%), and >3 mcg/mL in 15 patients (24.6%).

TABLE 1: Individual lobar scores based on percentage of involvement.

Lobar involvement	Score
5% or less	1
5%–25%	2
26%–49%	3
50%–75%	4
>75%	5

TABLE 2: Sum of the individual lobar scores indicates the overall severity of the five lobes.

Total score (numerical)	Severity (category)
7 or less	Mild
8–17	Moderate
18 or more	Severe

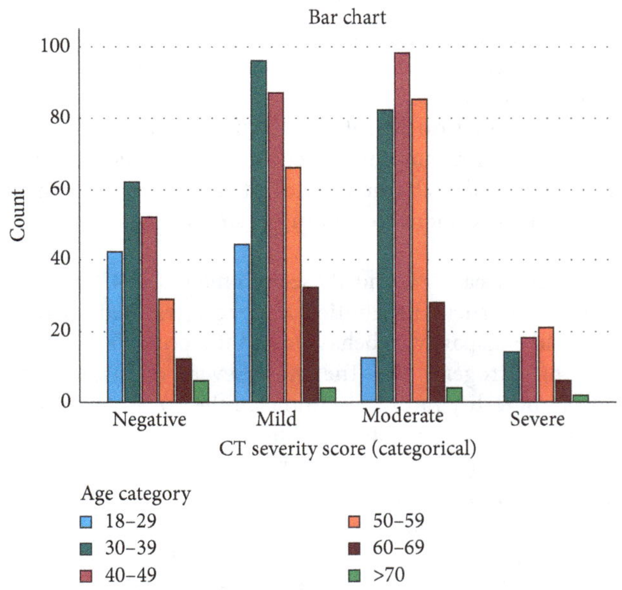

FIGURE 2: Prevalence of age categories for each CT severity score.

Ferritin level was assessed in 888/902 patients. In patients with negative and mild CT scan findings, ferritin level was <600 ng/mL in 176 patients (91.7%) and 267 patients (81.4%), respectively. In patients with moderate CT scans, ferritin level was <600 ng/mL in 131 patients (42.7%), 600–1200 ng/mL in 99 patients (32.2%), 1200–2400 ng/mL in 60 patients (19.5%), and >2400 ng/mL in 17 (5.5%). In patients with severe CT scan, ferritin level was <600 ng/mL in 13 patients (21.3%), 600–1200 ng/mL in 18 patients (29.5%), 1200–2400 ng/mL in 18 patients (29.5%), and >2400 ng/mL in 12 patients (19.7%).

3.2.3. Oxygen Requirement and Outcome. In relation to maximum oxygen requirement, 196/203 (96.6%) of patients with negative scan did not require any oxygen support, five patients (2.5%) required nasal cannula, one patient (0.5%) required BiPAP/HFNC, and one (0.5%) required intubation eventually. In the mild scan category, 293/329 (89.1%) patients did not require any oxygen support, 24 (7.3%) required nasal cannula, four (1.2%) required face mask, one (0.3%) required non-rebreather mask, one (0.3%) required BiPAP/HFNC, and six (1.8%) required intubation.

154/309 (49.8%) of patients with moderate scan findings did not require any oxygen support, 89 (28.8%) required nasal cannula, 20 (6.5%) required face mask, 9 (2.9%) required non-rebreather mask, 15 (4.9%) required BiPAP/HFNC, and 22 (7.1%) required intubation.

Only two patients (3.3%) with severe scan results did not require oxygen support, 8 (13.1%) required nasal cannula, 8 (13.1%) required face mask, 5 (8.2%) required non-rebreather mask, 4 (6.6%) required BiPAP/HFNC, and 34/61 (55.7%) required intubation (Table 3). The oxygen requirement and CT severity scores were found to have statistically significant correlation ($p < 0.0001$, $r = 0.529$).

In terms of length of hospital stay, 190/902 patients (21.1%) with negative scans, 276 patients (30.6%) with mild scans, 160 (17.7%) patients with moderate, and 5 patients (0.6%) with severe findings were either discharged the same day or required hospital admission for <5 days.

Six patients (0.7%) stayed in the hospital for 6–10 days from the negative group, 31 (3.4%) from mild, 79 (8.8%) from moderate, and 11 (1.2%) from severe groups.

Four patients (0.4%) stayed in the hospital for 11–15 days from the negative group, 8 (0.9%) from mild, 28 (3.1%) from moderate, and 10 (1.1%) from severe groups.

Three patients (0.3%) stayed in the hospital for >16 days from the negative group, 14 (1.6 %) from mild, 42 (4.7%) from moderate, and 35 (3.9%) from severe groups.

ICU admission was required in 202/902 (22.4%) patients. 23/902 (2.5%) patients with initial negative scan required ICU admission because of subsequent deterioration, 72 (8%) had mild CT scan findings, 69 (7.6%) had moderate, and 38 (4.2%) with severe CT findings (Figure 3).

Follow-up CT scans ($n = 73$) were done between 7 and 45 days from initial ones. 18 scans were done for patients who were in the ICU. Four scans (22.2%) showed improvement; 8 (44.4%) showed worsening of the findings, and the rest were relatively stable. 55 scans were done for patients who were not admitted to the ICU at that time. Sixteen scans (29.1%) showed improvement; 30 (54.5%) showed worsening, and the rest showed stable findings.

The best outcomes were associated with negative and milder CT findings, while death rate was increased among those with more severe scan results. Amongst the negative scan group, 201 patients (99%) are alive, 1 (0.5%) was expired, and 1 (0.5%) is still intubated. Among the mild ones, 325 (98.8%) patients are alive, 3 (0.9%) expired, and one (0.3%) is still intubated. In the moderate scan group, 292 (94.5%) patients are alive, 15 (4.9%) expired, and two (0.6%) are still intubated. In the severe scan group, 44 (72.1%) patients are alive, 14 (23%) expired, and 3 (4.9%) were still intubated at the time of study.

33 patients had in-hospital death, with ages ranging between 33 and 76 years (mean 55.2 years). 15/33 patients (45.5%) who expired were between 50 and 59 years, 30.3% between 60 and 69, 15.2 (40–49), 6 % (30–39), and 3% >70.

Table 3: Maximum oxygen requirement in each CT severity category.

			Maximum O_2 requirement						Total
			None	Nasal cannula	Face mask	Non-rebreather	HFNC/BIPAP	Intubation	
CT severity	Negative	Count	196	5	0	0	1	1	203
		% within category	96.6%	2.5%	0.0%	0.0%	0.5%	0.5%	100.0%
		% of total	21.7%	0.6%	0.0%	0.0%	0.1%	0.1%	22.5%
	Mild	Count	293	24	4	1	1	6	329
		% within category	89.1%	7.3%	1.2%	0.3%	0.3%	1.8%	100.0%
		% of total	32.5%	2.7%	0.4%	0.1%	0.1%	0.7%	36.5%
	Moderate	Count	154	89	20	9	15	22	309
		% category	49.8%	28.8%	6.5%	2.9%	4.9%	7.1%	100.0%
		% of total	17.1%	9.9%	2.2%	1.0%	1.7%	2.4%	34.3%
	Severe	Count	2	8	8	5	4	34	61
		% within category	3.3%	13.1%	13.1%	8.2%	6.6%	55.7%	100.0%
		% of total	0.2%	0.9%	0.9%	0.6%	0.4%	3.8%	6.8%
Total		Count	645	126	32	15	21	63	902
		% of total	71.5%	14.0%	3.5%	1.7%	2.3%	7.0%	100.0%

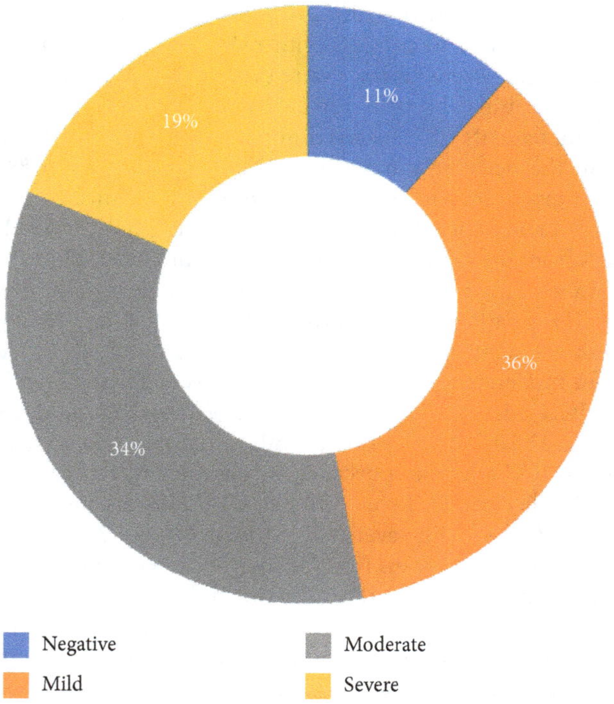

Figure 3: Percentage of patients admitted to the ICU in each CT severity category.

4. Discussion

The WHO advised the use of chest imaging as part of diagnostic workup of COVID-19 disease whenever RT-PCR testing is not available, in case of delayed test results or when there is a clinical suspicion of COVID-19 with initial negative RT-PCR testing. Clinicians should work hand in hand with the radiologists in order to make the proper choice of imaging modality [17].

CT scan can be a useful tool in evaluating the individual disease burden [18]. The quantitative severity can be assessed using a visual method (as in our study) or software that determines the percentage of affected lung volumes using the deep learning algorithms [10, 19, 20].

In our study, and due to unavailability of the software, we used the visual assessment of each of the 5 lung lobes. The severities were further classified based on the total cumulative severity score.

Our population revealed a relatively young age (mean 44.2 years) with male predilection. This can be explained by the particular characteristics of the population in the UAE, with prevalence of young male immigrant workers [21].

Severe disease was mostly seen in males (93.4%). Studies suggest that such distribution can be attributed to many factors like disparity in behavior and the possible protective effect of estrogen [22]. The most severe disease and the highest mortality rates were found in the 50- to 59-year age group. This can be affected by different factors like the stage of the pandemic when the study was carried, presence of patients' comorbidities, maturity and preparation of the healthcare system, and existence of elderly nursing homes services where disease can spread faster [23].

A number of existing literature suggested that the presence of risk factors, particularly hypertension, diabetes, lung, and coronary artery diseases, carries a poor prognosis, with even worse outcome when multiple risk factors are present [24,25]. Although in our study we did not find a statically significant correlation between the presence of risk factors and CT severity scores, there was however a significant correlation ($P < 0.0001$) between the ICU admission and presence of risk factors (Figure 4).

Lymphopenia correlated well with the increasing CT severity score. The presence of lymphopenia can be related to the inflammatory cytokine storm. Decreased T cell counts, particularly CD8+, has been observed in severe cases [26].

Furthermore, our results showed that the serum CRP level had significant correlation with CT severity. Studies have also suggested that early treatment at early disease stage can be considered using CRP as a predictive marker for likelihood of disease progression [27]. Similarly, serum ferritin is a vital mediator of immune dysregulation, and its level was closely linked to the severity of the disease [28]. D-dimer likewise can be used as a prognostic indicator, where higher levels are seen

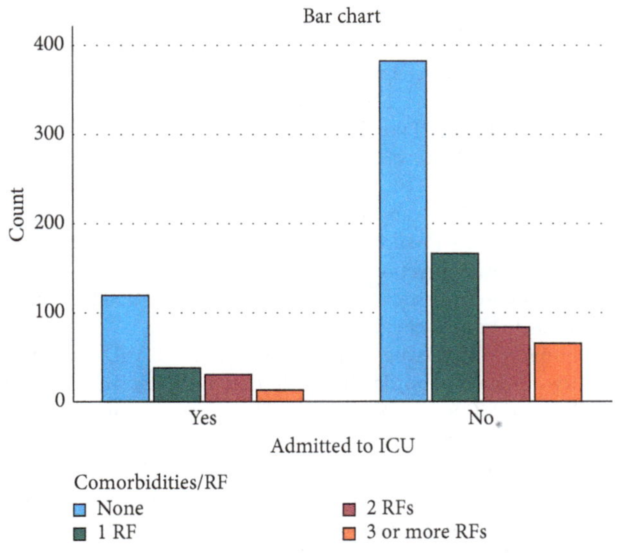

FIGURE 4: Number of patients admitted to ICU in relation to risk factors.

in more critical conditions. However, there is lack of evidence regarding the causal effect. It is not yet clear whether this increase is related to the direct effect of the virus or the systemic inflammatory response [29, 30].

As expected, and found in our data, oxygen requirements increase with the increasing CT severity. The progressive increase in oxygen requirement can be due to the direct damage of the lung by the virus causing inflammatory changes in alveolar wall that limit oxygen exchange, leading to acute respiratory distress, pulmonary fibrosis, and eventually death. Moreover, significant pulmonary thromboembolic effects were also found on autopsies from patients who died from COVID-19 disease [31–33].

Concerning the length of hospital stay for patients with COVID-19 disease, a systematic review done by Rees et al. has suggested that LOS varies depending on multiple factors such as admission and discharge criteria, bed demand and availability, and different timing within the pandemic [34]. Death rate in our cohort was significantly increased among patients with severe CT findings, as noted in other studies [35].

There are several limitations in this study: first, the need for a larger multicenter cohort to increase the accuracy of the findings and second, the fact that the assessment of disease severity on CT scans can be subjective. This was reduced by involving two experienced readers to reach a consensus. Finally, the other factors that might contribute to the disease outcome such as lifestyle and relying on self-reporting/underreporting of the comorbidities should be considered.

In conclusion, CT scans can have a pivotal role in assisting physicians in the management plan and work as an indicator for disease severity and possible outcome. CT severity score is positively correlated with inflammatory lab markers, length of hospital stays, and oxygen requirement in patients with COVID-19 infection. However, more research is needed to further clarify the value of chest CT for prognostication in COVID-19 disease, including correlation with patient outcome.

Abbreviations

COVID-19:	Coronavirus disease
CRP:	C-reactive protein
CT:	Computed tomography
GGO:	Ground-glass opacity
HRCT:	High-resolution computed tomography
PACS:	Picture archiving and communication systems
RT-PCR:	Reverse transcription polymerase chain reaction
WHO:	World Health Organization.

Acknowledgments

The authors would like to thank Mr. George Roy, Senior CT radiographer, for providing the technical information and Mrs. Maisoun Al Ali for assisting in the analysis. The authors would also like to acknowledge the radiological medical and technical team of the Radiology Department of Sheikh Khalifa Medical City, Abu Dhabi.

References

[1] http://www.who.int.https://www.who.int/emergencies/diseases/novel-coronavirus-2019?gclid=EAIaIQobChMImt2m3afS6wIVvSB7Ch3xdQDoEAAYASAAEgLb-_D_BwE Coronavirus Disease (COVID-19)—World Health Organization.

[2] Emedicine.medscape.com, *Coronavirus Disease 2019 (COVID-19) Clinical Presentation: History, Physical Examination, Complications*, https://emedicine.medscape.com/article/2500114-clinical.

[3] D. Thomas-Rüddel, J. Winning, P. Dickmann et al., ""Coronavirus disease 2019" (COVID-19): update für anästhesisten und intensivmediziner märz 2020," *Der Anaesthesist*, vol. 69, no. 4, p. 225, 2020.

[4] V. M. Corman, O. Landt, M. Kaiser et al., "Detection of 2019 novel coronavirus (2019-nCoV) by real-time RT-PCR," *Eurosurveillance*, vol. 25, no. 3, 2020.

[5] S. A. Bustin and T. Nolan, "Pitfalls of quantitative real-time reverse-transcription polymerase chain reaction," *Journal of Biomolecular Techniques: JBT*, vol. 15, no. 3, pp. 155–166, 2004, https://www.ncbi.nlm.nih.gov/pmc/articles/PMC2291693/.

[6] J. Liu, H. Yu, and S. Zhang, "The indispensable role of chest CT in the detection of coronavirus disease 2019 (COVID-19)," *European Journal of Nuclear Medicine and Molecular Imaging*, 2020, https://www.ncbi.nlm.nih.gov/pmc/articles/PMC7118704/#CR2, In press.

[7] A. Bernheim, X. Mei, M. Huang et al., "Chest CT findings in coronavirus disease-19 (COVID-19): relationship to duration of infection," *Radiology*, vol. 295, no. 3, p. 200463, 2020.

[8] A. Leonardi, R. Scipione, G. Alfieri et al., "Role of computed tomography in predicting critical disease in patients with covid-19 pneumonia: a retrospective study using a semiautomatic quantitative method," *European Journal of Radiology*, vol. 130, p. 109202, 2020.

[9] L. Meng, H. Qiu, L. Wan et al., "Intubation and ventilation amid the COVID-19 outbreak," *Anesthesiology*, vol. 132, no. 6, p. 1317, 2020.

[10] K. Li, Y. Fang, W. Li et al., "CT image visual quantitative evaluation and clinical classification of coronavirus disease (COVID-19)," *European Radiology*, vol. 30, no. 8, pp. 4407–4416, 2020.

[11] H.-t. Zhang, J.-s. Zhang, H.-h. Zhang et al., "Automated detection and quantification of COVID-19 pneumonia: CT imaging analysis by a deep learning-based software," *European Journal of Nuclear Medicine and Molecular Imaging* vol. 47, no. 11, p. 2525, 2020.

[12] S. Simpson, F. U. Kay, S. Abbara et al., "Radiological society of north America expert consensus document on reporting chest CT findings related to COVID-19: endorsed by the society of thoracic Radiology, the American college of Radiology, and RSNA," *Radiology: Cardiothoracic Imaging*, vol. 2, no. 2, p. e200152, Article ID e200152, 2020.

[13] Y.-C. Chang, C.-J. Yu, S.-C. Chang et al., "Pulmonary sequelae in convalescent patients after severe acute respiratory syndrome: evaluation with thin-section CT," *Radiology*, vol. 236, no. 3, pp. 1067–1075, 2005.

[14] Radiology Assistant, "The Radiology assistant: COVID-19 imaging findings," https://radiologyassistant.nl/chest/covid-19/covid19-imaging-findings.

[15] F. Pan, T. Ye, P. Sun et al., "Time course of lung changes at chest CT during recovery from coronavirus disease 2019 (COVID-19)," *Radiology*, vol. 295, no. 3, p. 715, 2020.

[16] World Health Organisation (WHO), "Use of laboratory methods for SARS diagnosis," 2020, https://who.int/csr/sars/labmethods/en/.

[17] http://www.who.int.. Use of Chest Imaging in COVID-19. https://www.who.int/publications/i/item/use-of-chest-imaging-in-covid-19.

[18] M. Francone, F. Iafrate, G. M. Masci et al., "Chest CT score in COVID-19 patients: correlation with disease severity and short-term prognosis," *European Radiology*, vol. 30, no. 12, p. 6808, 2020.

[19] L. Huang, R. Han, T. Ai et al., "Serial quantitative chest CT assessment of COVID-19: deep-learning approach," *Radiology: Cardiothoracic Imaging*, vol. 2, no. 2, p. e200075, 2020, https://pubs.rsna.org/doi/10.1148/ryct.2020200075.

[20] N. Lessmann, C. I. Sánchez, L. Beenen et al., "Automated assessment of CO-rads and chest CT severity scores in patients with suspected COVID-19 using artificial intelligence," *diology*, p. 202439, 2020, https://pubs.rsna.org/doi/10.1148/radiol.2020202439.

[21] Worldometers.info, *United Arab Emirates Population (2019)—Worldometers*, 2019, https://www.worldometers.info/world-population/united-arab-emirates-population/.*Ra-*

[22] A. Dangis, N. De Brucker, A. Heremans et al., "Impact of gender on extent of lung injury in COVID-19," *Clinical Radiology*, vol. 75, no. 7, pp. 554–556, 2020.

[23] S. Mallapaty, "The coronavirus is most deadly if you are older and male—new data reveal the risks," *Nature*, vol. 585, no. 7823, pp. 16-17, 2020.

[24] W.-j. Guan, W.-h. Liang, Y. Zhao et al., "Comorbidity and its impact on 1590 patients with covid-19 in China: a nationwide analysis," *European Respiratory Journal*, vol. 55, no. 5, p. 2000547, 2020.

[25] Japi. Clinico-radiological evaluation and correlation of CT chest images with progress of disease in COVID-19 patients. http://www.japi.org. https://www.japi.org/w2f4d464/clinico-radiological-evaluation-and-correlation-of-ct-chest-images-with-progress-of-disease-in-covid-19-patients.

[26] S. Tavakolpour, T. Rakhshandehroo, E. X. Wei, and M. Rashidian, "Lymphopenia during the COVID-19 infection: what it shows and what can be learned," *Immunology Letters*, vol. 225, pp. 31-32, 2020.

[27] Infectious Disease Advisor, *Elevated Level of C Reactive Protein May Predict Risk for Worsening COVID-19*, 2020, https://www.infectiousdiseaseadvisor.com/home/topics/covid19/high-crp-associated-with-increased-likelihood-of-progression-to-severe-covid-19/.

[28] http://www.paho.org. Ferritin levels and COVID-19. https://www.paho.org/journal/en/articles/ferritin-levels-and-covid-19.

[29] Y. Yao, J. Cao, Q. Wang et al., "D-dimer as a biomarker for disease severity and mortality in COVID-19 patients: a case control study," *Journal of Intensive Care*, vol. 8, no. 1, 2020.

[30] L. E. Gralinski and R. S. Baric, "Molecular pathology of emerging coronavirus infections," *The Journal of Pathology*, vol. 235, no. 2, pp. 185–195, 2015.

[31] J. B. Prudhomme and L. B. Ware, "Acute lung injury and acute respiratory distress syndrome: mechanisms and potential new therapies," *Drug Discovery Today: Disease Mechanisms*, vol. 1, no. 1, pp. 123–128, 2004.

[32] Europa.eu., *CORDIS*, European Commission, 2020, https://cordis.europa.eu/article/id/421597-how-covid-19-damages-the-lungs.

[33] M. Ackermann, S. E. Verleden, M. Kuehnel et al., "Pulmonary vascular endothelialitis, thrombosis, and angiogenesis in covid-19," *New England Journal of Medicine*, vol. 383, no. 2, p. 120, 2020.

[34] E. M. Rees, E. S. Nightingale, Y. Jafari et al., "COVID-19 length of hospital stay: a systematic review and data synthesis," 2020.

[35] Y. Li, Z. Yang, T. Ai, S. Wu, and L. Xia, "Association of "initial CT" findings with mortality in older patients with coronavirus disease 2019 (COVID-19)," *European Radiology*, vol. 30, no. 11, p. 6186, 2020.

14

Appendiceal Intraluminal Gas: A CT Marker for Gangrenous Appendicitis

Chantelle Ip,[1] Edward H. Wang,[2] Michael Croft,[1] and Wanyin Lim[1,3]

[1]*Royal Adelaide Hospital, Port Road, Adelaide 5000, Australia*
[2]*Flinders Medical Centre, Flinders Dr, Bedford Park 5042, Australia*
[3]*Dr Jones and Partners, 226 Greenhill Road, Eastwood 5065, Australia*

Correspondence should be addressed to Wanyin Lim; ynyn146@gmail.com

Academic Editor: Lorenzo Faggioni

Introduction. This manuscript aims to investigate the amount of intraluminal gas in acute, nonperforated appendicitis identified on computed tomography (CT) in diagnosing gangrenous appendicitis. *Methods.* This is a retrospective observational, case-control study with consecutive data collected at a tertiary institution over a two-year period, of patients with CT-diagnosed acute appendicitis who subsequently went on for surgery within 48 hours. Patients who were less than 16 years old, who had an interval between CT and surgery of more than 48 hours, or with CT evidence of appendiceal perforation were excluded. Images were independently assessed by 3 radiologists for intraluminal gas, and the results were then correlated with reference standards obtained from surgical and histopathology reports for the diagnosis of nongangrenous versus gangrenous appendicitis. The sensitivity, specificity, and predictive values of CT intraluminal gas in gangrenous appendicitis were calculated. *Results.* Our study identified 93 patients with nonperforated acute appendicitis who underwent surgery within the stated timeframe. Intraluminal gas in the appendix was identified in 26 patients (28%), of which 54% had macroscopic and/or microscopic evidence of gangrenous appendicitis. This is in contrast to the subgroup of patients who did not have intraluminal gas (72%), of which only 33% had gangrenous appendicitis. The specificity of intraluminal gas for gangrenous appendicitis is 79%, with a negative predictive value of 86% and likelihood ratio of 1.85. *Conclusion.* In cases of established acute appendicitis, the presence of intraluminal gas is a moderately specific sign for gangrenous complication. This is worth reporting as it can help prognosticate and triage patients accordingly, for a timelier surgical management and a better outcome.

1. Introduction

Acute appendicitis is an important cause of acute abdominal pain, with appendectomies being the most common emergency procedure performed in Australia [1]. Whilst acute appendicitis is a clinical diagnosis, CT scanning has become an important imaging tool to reduce the rate of negative or unnecessary surgeries by identifying other causes of abdominal pain which can mimic appendicitis. Appendicitis can have different clinical presentations, with overlapping clinical features between acute uncomplicated and complicated appendicitis such as perforation and abscess collection [2], and hence, imaging also plays an important role in differentiating between the simple and complicated cases [3]. These have important implications for patient management pathways, prognosis, and length of hospital stay.

There have been many studies focusing on CT signs differentiating perforated from nonperforated cases of appendicitis; however, few studies have focused on signs that differentiate simple phlegmonous appendicitis from gangrenous appendicitis in the nonperforated appendix [4]. This distinction is important as these two classifications of nonperforated appendicitis are associated with very different prognoses, with time-sensitive treatment pathways. Gangrenous appendicitis is estimated to occur in 17% of cases of acute appendicitis [5] and is associated with increased rates of complications such as intra-abdominal abscesses and appendiceal perforation [1] if surgical management is delayed.

The presence of intraluminal air within the appendix was traditionally thought to be a useful sign to exclude appendicitis, indicating that the appendix was patent, nonobstructed, and not inflamed [6]. However, there is increasing evidence that intraluminal gas on CT is common in appendicitis and may be seen in 19–27% of cases [7, 8]. One hypothesis is that there is an absence of intraluminal air in an acutely inflamed appendix due to gas displacement by intraluminal fluid and increased pressure. However, as the inflammation progresses towards gangrenous complication, intraluminal air develops in a similar pathophysiology as in the development of pneumatosis intestinalis.

This study aims to assess the presence of intraluminal air in the appendix on CT, an indicator for the gangrenous appendix in cases of acute nonperforated appendicitis.

2. Materials and Methods

Statement of Ethics. Ethical approval was granted for this project by the Institutional Human Research Ethics Committee (R20190408).

Data Collection. Data were collected from the picture archiving and communication system (PACS) of a tertiary hospital in South Australia using the keyword search "appendix, appendiceal inflammation, appendicitis." Consecutive patients over a two-year period (2018 and 2019) with CT prior to appendectomy for acute appendicitis were included in the study. Data extracted from existing databases included patient age, sex, time of CT, abdomen CT images, time of surgical intervention, operation report, and surgical histopathology report.

Exclusion Criteria. Exclusion criteria included the following patients with Ct-diagnosed appendicitis who did not proceed with surgery within 48 hours of CT scan, patients younger than 18 years of age, and patients with appendiceal perforation evident on CT at time of presentation.

Patients younger than 18 were excluded due to the small number of pediatric cases presenting to this adult institution and the increasing evidence that CT is not the recommended imaging modality in this cohort [4, 9].

Retrospective Image Review. The CT images, comprising volumetric CT scans with multiplanar reconstruction at 1 and 3 mm slices, were independently reviewed by three radiologists, including two registrars and one consultant radiologist with 4 years of experience, for the presence of appendiceal gas and perforation. Other signs of inflammation were noted to confirm diagnosis of appendicitis, and these included increased appendiceal diameter, wall thickness and enhancement, and associated appendicolith and periappendiceal fat stranding or collection [11].

Cases with CT-evident perforated appendicitis were then excluded. The CT findings indicative of perforation include a focal defect in the enhancing appendiceal wall, surrounding phlegmon or abscess, extraluminal air, and extraluminal appendicolith [10].

The reviewers were provided patient age and sex but were blinded to the original CT report and the subsequent surgical and histopathology reports. Any disagreements between the three reviewers were resolved by reviewing and discussing the images and correlating with the original CT report.

Reference Standards. Reference standards included the existing surgical records and histopathology reports. A definitive diagnosis of appendicitis was determined by the histopathologic documentation of transmural inflammation, ulceration, or thrombosis [12]. Gangrenous appendicitis was defined macroscopically as either a friable appendix with green, purple, or black colour changes or microscopically as the presence of transmural inflammation with necrosis. The presence of appendiceal perforation was determined by surgical documentation of visible perforation that was not caused by surgical handling or histopathologic documentation of appendiceal wall defect due to transmural necrosis.

Statistical Analysis. A readily available statistics calculator was used to calculate the sensitivity, specificity, positive and negative likelihood ratios, and positive and negative predictive values of CT intraluminal gas in nonperforated gangrenous appendicitis.

For sample size estimation, as gangrenous appendicitis is estimated to occur in 17% of cases of acute appendicitis [5], we had a minimum target of 100 total studies. This would result in an estimated 17 cases of gangrenous appendicitis and 83 cases of nongangrenous appendicitis. This sample size would be adequate to demonstrate a medium-to-large effect, with an estimated power of 0.8 and an alpha value of 0.05. An effect of this scale would be sufficient for our hypothesis.

3. Results

Demographic Information. The PACS database search yielded 305 patients. Of these, 135 patients had CT-diagnosed appendicitis prior to appendectomy within 48 hours of the CT scans. Of these, 3 patients younger than 18 years of age were excluded. 6 patients who underwent negative appendicectomies (four cases of histopathologically non-inflammed appendixes, one case of leukaemia with appendiceal involvement, and one case of appendiceal adenocarcinoma) were excluded. Finally, there were 31 cases of CT-evident perforated appendicitis which were also excluded.

The final study group comprised 93 patients with a mean (±SD) age of 49.0 ± 14.7 years (range, 19–95 years). There were 38 women (mean age, 52.6 ± 16.9 years; range, 20–95 years) and 55 men (mean age, 46.6 ± 12.3 years; range, 19–71 years).

Retrospective Review. There were 57 cases of surgically or pathologically confirmed simple (nongangrenous) acute appendicitis and 36 cases of nonperforated gangrenous appendicitis. The prevalence of gangrenous appendicitis in our study group was 39% (26/93).

Appendiceal intraluminal air on CT was present in 26 patients (26/93; 28%) and absent in 67 (67/93; 72%).

Of the 26 with appendiceal intraluminal air detected on CT, 14 patients (14/26; 54%) had histological/surgical evidence of gangrenous appendicitis and 12 patients (12/26; 46%) did not. Of the 67 without CT findings of appendiceal intraluminal air, 22 patients (22/67; 33%) had evidence of gangrenous appendicitis intraoperatively or surgically and 45 patients (45/67; 67%) did not (Table 1).

Figures 1–3 exhibit cases of CT-evident acute appendicitis with the presence of appendiceal intraluminal gas; gangrenous appendicitis was confirmed intraoperatively within 24 hours for all three patients and then histologically. Figure 4 exhibits a false-positive case; the appendix has low-grade surrounding fat stranding with appendiceal intraluminal gas; uncomplicated suppurative appendicitis was confirmed within 24 hours both surgically and histologically.

4. Statistical Analysis

As a marker for the gangrenous appendix in nonperforated appendicitis, intraluminal air on CT was found to have a specificity of 79% (95% CI, 66–89%), positive likelihood ratio of 1.85 (95% CI, 1.0–3.5), and negative predictive value of 86% (95% CI, 82–89%) (Table 2). The accuracy of correctly classifying the patient's appendicitis based on CT findings of intraluminal gas is 72%.

5. Discussion

Gangrenous appendicitis is associated with higher rates of complications such as perforation, abscess, and faeculent peritonitis. These have significant implications in patients, as they are associated with increased length of hospital stay, higher morbidity and mortality, and higher rates of open incision surgery and hospital readmission [1].

Due to the wide variation of clinical findings on examination in cases of acute appendicitis, CT has been a useful imaging modality to decrease the rate of negative appendicectomies and identify complicated cases such as perforation [13, 14]. There are many studies researching CT markers to differentiate perforated versus nonperforated appendicitis. However, when there is no CT evidence of perforation, there is scant data on whether there are CT markers which can differentiate between acute suppurative appendicitis and gangrenous appendicitis. It would be useful if radiologists could make this distinction, as accurately identifying patients with a higher risk for gangrenous complication would warrant more urgent appendicectomies which can, down the line, provide better service for the patients.

It is widely acknowledged that intraluminal gas in the appendix on CT is very commonly seen in the normal appendix [6, 7] as well as in a smaller percentage of patients with acute appendicitis [7, 8]. The diagnosis of acute appendicitis is often first made utilising a combination of other CT signs of appendiceal inflammation such as increased appendiceal diameter (6 mm), wall thickening and altered enhancement, and associated appendicolith and periappendiceal fat stranding or collection. In fact, it is much more common in cases of nonperforated acute appendicitis to have an absence of intraluminal air in the appendix (up to 66%) [7] as appendiceal inflammation from luminal obstruction leads to intraluminal fluid collection and displacement of prominent gas locules. Histologically, this is seen as transmural inflammation with infiltration of neutrophils. Further inflammation with gangrenous transformation, histologically seen as progression to focal necrosis, can then lead to the development of new gas locules from the gas-forming organisms, which can then be evident on CT.

Our study identified 93 consecutive patients with CT prior to appendectomy for nonperforated acute appendicitis between 2018 and 2019. Of these, 67 patients (67/93; 72%) demonstrated no gas in the appendix on CT. This is in keeping with other studies showing that intraluminal gas is more commonly absent in acute appendicitis. From this subgroup, only 33 percent (22/67) had macroscopic and/or microscopic evidence of gangrenous appendicitis. This is relatively less than the subgroup of patients with gangrenous appendicitis with intraluminal gas on CT, 54 percent (14/26).

From our results, intraluminal gas in nonperforated acute appendicitis on CT has a moderately high specificity of 79 percent, with a negative predictive value of 86 percent. This means that presence of gas is suggestive of suppurative appendicitis. As intraluminal gas may be present in either of these pathologies, it is within expectations that this marker has a lower sensitivity (39%) and positive predictive value (27%).

Even so, our data suggest that patients with acute appendicitis with intraluminal gas on CT are 1.85 times more likely to have gangrenous appendicitis and that the overall probability that an appendix is properly classified as gangrenous vs suppurative based on CT findings of intraluminal gas is 72% (62–81%).

Our study has focused on the intraluminal gas as a standalone finding in predicting gangrenous appendicitis. The specificity and likelihood ratio were externally validated and were similar to the recently published meta-analysis by HY Kim et al., using CT features to differentiate between complicated and uncomplicated appendicitis [11]. The group found that whilst being assessed in isolation, the sensitivity for intraluminal gas in complicated appendicitis is poor; however, if pooled with the other features of appendicitis that we know of, such as periappendiceal fat stranding and appendicolith, the presence of intraluminal gas is a useful feature in predicting complicated appendicitis.

The other limitations included the variability in reporting detail within database surgical and histopathological reports contributed to uncertainty when used as a reference standard. Only reports which stated the specific findings of either a friable appendix with green, purple, or black colour changes or the presence of transmural inflammation with necrosis were deemed positive results. This could have contributed to type II error and increased false-negative cases.

There may also be a discrepancy between the CT images and the surgical/histopathology reports due to

Table 1: Cases of appendicitis with or without CT-detected intraluminal gas, correlated with the final histopathological report of absence or presence of gangrenous appendicitis.

Intraluminal gas on CT	Gangrenous appendicitis	Nongangrenous appendicitis
Present	14	12
Absent	22	45

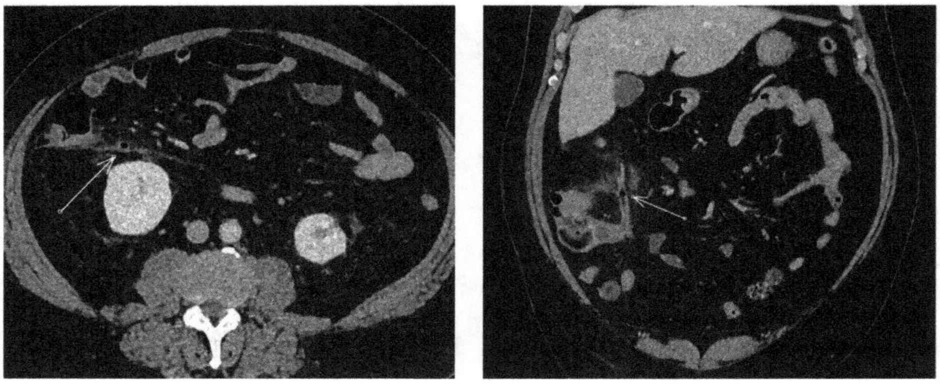

(a) (b)

Figure 1: A 64-year-old man with axial (a) and coronal (b) CT abdomen in the portal venous phase showing periappendiceal fat stranding and appendiceal wall hyperenhancement, confirming the clinical suspicion of acute appendicitis. There is a focus of intraluminal gas in the body of the appendix (arrow). Gangrenous appendicitis was confirmed intraoperatively and on subsequent histopathology.

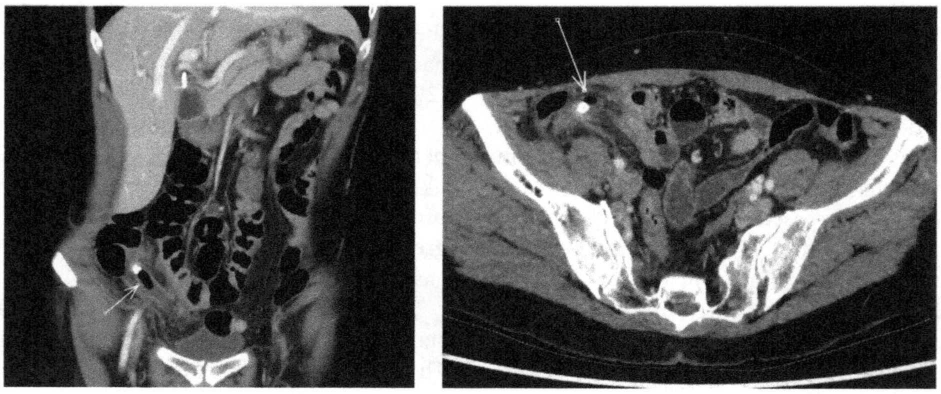

(a) (b)

Figure 2: A 58-year-old woman with clinical suspicion of acute appendicitis. Coronal (a) and axial (b) CT abdomen in the portal venous phase shows a distended appendix with periappendiceal fat stranding. There is intraluminal gas adjacent to the appendicolith towards the tip. Gangrenous appendicitis was confirmed on subsequent histopathology report and intraoperatively.

multifactorial extrinsic delays to surgery. The patient's clinical presentations which could influence management options, were not available to us. Furthermore, CT abdomen scans without contrast were not excluded, and this may have affected reporting accuracy with missed cases of CT perforation.

Ultimately, appendicitis remains a clinical diagnosis, and currently, CT is employed predominantly in atypical presentations to identify cases suspected to have complications or to exclude other differentials. This could be one of the reasons for our study population having a higher prevalence of gangrenous appendicitis (39%) when compared with other studies (17%).

Whilst the sample size is smaller than what we have initially hoped to achieve, it was calculated based on prevalence of 17%, for 17 cases of gangrenous appendicitis. Given the difference in prevalence of gangrenous appendicitis in our cohort, this study is still considered sufficiently powered.

Future studies in this area may include a large prospective multicentre cohort study, with collaboration between radiologists, surgeons, and pathologists to create a pro forma and standardised criteria for reporting appendicitis, and in particular for gangrenous change. This would provide external validation to our hypothesis. Future studies may also investigate gas patterns and exact location of the

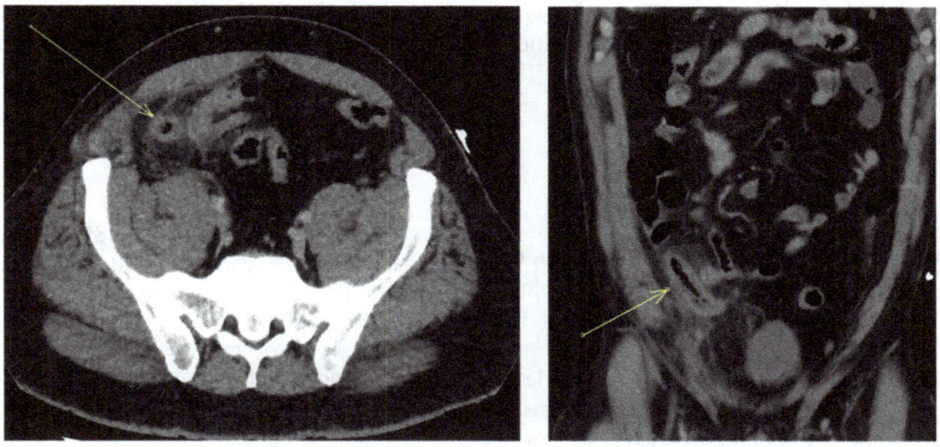

(a) (b)

Figure 3: A 45-year-old man with appendiceal intraluminal gas (arrow) on noncontrast CT in axial (a) and coronal (b) projections. Histological and surgical evidence of gangrenous appendicitis. Note the distended appendix with a thickened wall and surrounding fat stranding.

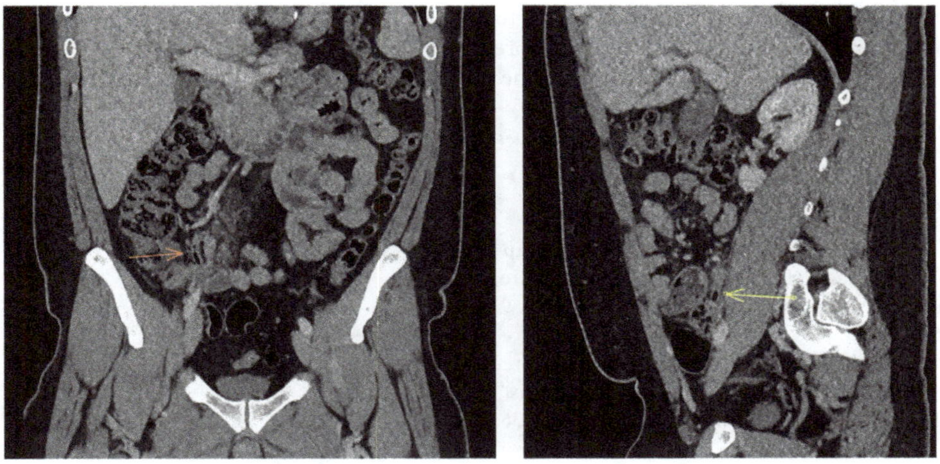

(a) (b)

Figure 4: A 33-year-old man with appendiceal intraluminal gas on CT (arrow). Coronal (a) and sagittal (b) CT abdomen in the portal venous phase. The appendix diameter is still within normal limits, but there is low-grade surrounding fat stranding. This is a false-positive case, with histological/surgical reports confirming uncomplicated suppurative acute appendicitis, without gangrenous complication.

Table 2: Statistical analysis of intraluminal gas in predicting gangrenous appendicitis.

Statistics	Value	95% confidence interval
Specificity	78.95%	66.1–88.6%
Sensitivity	38.89%	23.1–56.5%
Negative likelihood ratio	0.77	0.6–1.0
Positive likelihood ratio	1.85	1.0–3.5
Negative predictive value*	86.32%	82.5–89.4%
Positive predictive value*	27.45%	16.5–42.0%

*Disease prevalence = 17% [5] (Emil 2012).

appendiceal gas and the relationship of this CT marker with the development of complications (e.g., abscess, perforation, and peritonitis) depending on CT to surgery time. This would aim to provide further evidence for utilising this sign to triage patients for urgent appendicectomies.

6. Conclusion

This finding of intraluminal air as an indicator of gangrenous appendicitis is not well known amongst the radiology community, and the manuscript hopes to increase the awareness of this CT feature in the setting of acute appendicitis. Our study demonstrates a moderately high level of specificity (79%) but low sensitivity of intraluminal gas as a CT marker for gangrenous appendicitis in the setting of acute, nonperforated appendicitis. If there is intraluminal gas present, the appendix is 1.9 times more likely to be gangrenous, with moderate accuracy.

What is more important is that combined with other CT findings for acute appendicitis such as increased appendiceal diameter, wall enhancement, or adjacent fat stranding, intraluminal air is an important CT tool as it is a good predictor for gangrenous complication, before progression to perforated appendicitis [11]. Therefore, the presence of this sign in patients is an important feature for radiologists to note and convey to our surgical colleagues, to prompt a more timely surgical management and a better patient outcome.

References

[1] T. Arthur, R. Gartrell, B. Manoharan et al., "Emergency appendicectomy in Australia: findings from a multicentre, prospective study," *ANZ Journal of Surgery*, vol. 87, no. 9, pp. 656–660, 2017.

[2] O. O. Rasmussen and J. Hoffmann, "Assessment of the reliability of the symptoms and signs of acute appendicitis," *Journal of the Royal College of Surgeons of Edinburgh*, vol. 36, no. 6, pp. 372–377, 1991 Dec 1.

[3] Australian Commission on Safety and Quality in Health Care, *Australian Atlas of Heathcare Variation 2017: 4.5 Appendicectomy*, pp. 293–304, Sydney, NSW, 2017, https://www.safetyandquality.gov.au/sites/default/files/migrated/4.5-Appendicectomy.pdf.

[4] D. P. Ariza, E. M. Chamorro, J. C. Zornoza et al., *Intraluminal Gas in Non-perforated Acute Appendicitis: A CT Sign of Gangrenous Appendicitis*, European Congress of Radiology-ECR, 2012.

[5] S. Emil, F. Gaied, A. Lo et al., "Gangrenous appendicitis in children: a prospective evaluation of definition, bacteriology, histopathology, and outcomes," *Journal of Surgical Research*, vol. 177, no. 1, pp. 123–126, 2012.

[6] T. Rettenbacher, A. Hollerweger, P. Macheiner et al., "Presence or absence of gas in the appendix: additional criteria to rule out or confirm acute appendicitis-evaluation with US," *Radiology*, vol. 214, no. 1, pp. 183–187, 2000.

[7] M. Cabarrus, Y.-L. Sun, J. L. Courtier, J. W. Stengel, F. V. Coakley, and E. M. Webb, "The prevalence and patterns of intraluminal air in acute appendicitis at CT," *Emergency Radiology*, vol. 20, no. 1, pp. 51–56, 2013.

[8] H. C. Kim, D. M. Yang, S. W. Kim, and S. J. Park, "Reassessment of CT images to improve diagnostic accuracy in patients with suspected acute appendicitis and an equivocal preoperative CT interpretation," *European Radiology*, vol. 22, no. 6, pp. 1178–1185, 2012.

[9] R. R. Van Rijn, "Imaging pediatric appendicitis: time to put the discussion to bed?" *Radiology*, vol. 286, no. 3, pp. 1030–1032, 2018.

[10] M. M. Horrow, D. S. White, and J. C. Horrow, "Differentiation of perforated from nonperforated appendicitis at CT," *Radiology*, vol. 227, no. 1, pp. 46–51, 2003.

[11] H. Y. Kim, J. H. Park, Y. J. Lee, S. S. Lee, J.-J. Jeon, and K. H. Lee, "Systematic review and meta-analysis of CT features for differentiating complicated and uncomplicated appendicitis," *Radiology*, vol. 287, no. 1, pp. 104–115, 2018.

[12] A. Bhangu, K. Søreide, S. Di Saverio, J. H. Assarsson, and F. T. Drake, "Acute appendicitis: modern understanding of pathogenesis, diagnosis, and management," *The Lancet*, vol. 386, no. 10000, pp. 1278–1287, 2015.

[13] S. Akbulut, C. Koc, T. T. Sahin et al., "An investigation into the factors predicting acute appendicitis and perforated appendicitis," *Ulus Travma Acil Cerrahi Derg*, vol. 27, no. 3, pp. 315–324, 2021.

[14] A. S. Raja, C. Wright, A. D. Sodickson et al., "Negative appendectomy rate in the era of CT: an 18-year perspective," *Radiology*, vol. 256, no. 2, pp. 460–465, 2010.

15

Evaluation of Mental Foramen with Cone Beam Computed Tomography

Antoinette Pelé,[1,2] **Pierre-Alexandre Berry**,[1,2] **Charles Evanno**,[2,3] **and Fabienne Jordana**[1]

[1]*Oral and Maxillofacial Radiology, Dentistry Department, University Health Centre, University of Nantes, Orvault, France*
[2]*Private Practice, 34 Rue Jules Verne, 44700 Orvault, France*
[3]*Oral Implantology, Dentistry Department, University Health Centre, University of Nantes, Nantes, France*

Correspondence should be addressed to Fabienne Jordana; fabienne.jordana@univ-nantes.fr

Academic Editor: Lorenzo Faggioni

Purpose. The aim of this systematic review is to assess whether the anatomy of mental foramen is precisely evaluable with cone beam computed tomography (CBCT) before implantation in humans. *Methods*. A systematic review was carried out to evaluate the anatomy of mental foramen (size, position, symmetry, anterior loop, and accessory mental foramen or multiple mental foramina). According to Preferred Reporting Items for Systematic reviews and Meta-Analyses (PRISMA) guidelines, an electronic search of three databases (Medline, Web of Science, and Cochrane Library) was undertaken until June 2020 and was supplemented by manual searching. Two reviewers will independently perform the processes of study inclusion, data extraction, and quality assessment. Systematic reviews, studies about children, and case reports were excluded. Only studies using CBCT to do preoperative evaluation were selected. *Results*. From 728 potentially eligible articles, 72 were included in the qualitative analysis and quantitative synthesis. This systematic review provided an assessment of the anatomy of the mental foramen. The mental foramen was located mostly between the two premolars (between 50.4% and 61.95%) or apically to the second premolar (from 50.3% to 57.9%). The mean diameter of the mental foramen was bigger in males than in females; the difference between them could reach 0.62 mm. The anterior loop seemed to be longer in males (between 0.87 ± 1.81 and 7.25 ± 2.02 mm) than in females (between 0.81 ± 1.18 and 6.52 ± 1.63 mm) and with the presence of teeth (from 0.91 ± 1.18 to 2.55 ± 1.28 for dentate people and from 0.25 ± 0.61 to 2.40 ± 0.88 mm for edentate population). The anterior loop and the accessory mental foramina were detected more frequently with CBCT than panoramic X-ray: only between 0.0 and 48.6% AMFs detected with CBCT were also seen with panoramic images. *Clinical Significance*. The mental foramen (MF) is an important landmark for local anesthesia and surgical and implantology procedures. Its location, morphology, and anatomical variations need to be considered to avoid mental nerve injury. The aim of this review is to evaluate the mental foramen using CBCT through a systematic literature review to improve knowledge of this complex area for the clinician.

1. Introduction

The mental foramen (MF) is a strategically important landmark during implantology procedures. Its location, morphology, and anatomical variations need to be considered before surgery to avoid mental nerve injury [1].

Mental foramen is located on the mandible, a median and symmetric bone, which constitutes the low part of the face and the chin skeleton. The inferior alveolar nerve (IAN) progresses into the mandibular canal in the mandibular body on each side of the mandible. This canal opens posteriorly by the mandibular foramen and anteriorly by the mental foramen. Sometimes, small foramina in the surrounding area of the mental foramen are identified as accessory mental foramina (AMFs). This way, anteriorly, the IAN spreads into two branches: the mental nerve which goes out of the mandible through the mental foramen and enables the sensibility of the chin and the inferior lip while the incisive nerve stays into the mandible and enables the innervation of homolateral incisors and canine [2].

The mental nerve has different ways to reach the mental foramen. Solar et al. present a classification of intraosseous part of the mental nerve with three different types (Figure 1) [3].

The accessory mental foramina may present a continuity with the mandibular canal called "accessory branch of the mandibular canal" [5].

The area of the mental foramen shows complexity, with some anatomical particularities. The nerve can be hurt in different cases like during endodontic procedures and overfilling, teeth extractions, or surgical procedure like implantology; this could create temporary sensitive consequences for the patient similar to labiomental paresthesia [5, 6]. This is why a dentist has to take all the precautions to protect the mental nerve during surgeries.

CBCT, specifically developed for imaging of the teeth and jaws [7, 8], is a low-dose scanning system [9]. CBCT use backprojection reconstructed tomography to acquire data of the whole volume of interest through a rotation of the pyramidal or conical X-ray beam and reciprocal image detector. These data are then used to generate individual slice images or 3D reconstructions [7, 9–11]. The CBCT offers a three-dimensional reconstitution of buccal cavity and different slices (axial, transversal, and sagittal) of the studied area without superposition [12].

The aim of this review is to evaluate the mental foramen using CBCT through a systematic literature review to improve knowledge of this complex area for the clinician.

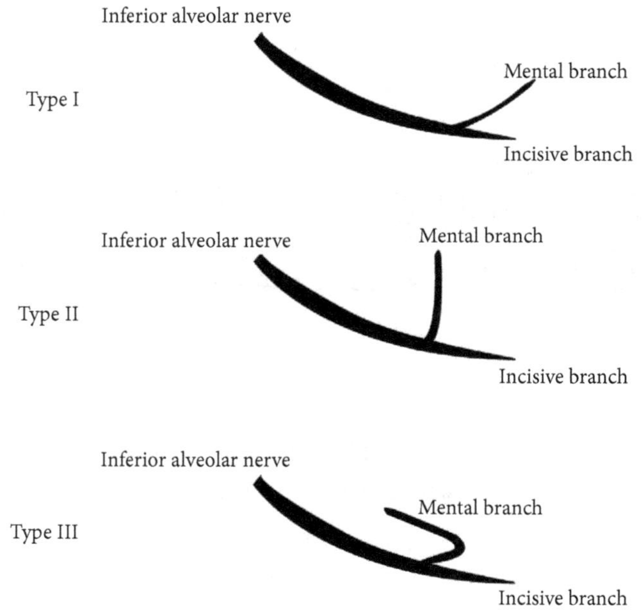

FIGURE 1: Solar et al. [3] classification of mental nerve paths. Type 1: no loop was found, and the anatomy was Y-shaped with the incisive branch usually as wide as the main branch. The mental branch leaves the inferior alveolar nerve posterior to the opening of the mental foramen [4]. Type 2: no loop was found, and the anatomy was T-shaped with the incisive branch usually as wide as the main branch. The mental branch leaves the inferior alveolar nerve perpendicular to the opening of the mental foramen [4]. Type 3: an anterior loop was found, and the anatomy was Y-shaped with the incisive branch usually as narrow as the main branch. The mental nerve branched from the inferior alveolar nerve anterior to the mental foramen [4].

2. Materials and Methods

The Preferred Reporting Items for Systematic Reviews and Meta-Analyses (PRISMA) system was adopted for this systematic review.

2.1. Study Protocol and Criteria. The protocol was designed to answer the following question: "do the CBCT studies evaluate the anatomic variations or individual parameters (sex, age, edentulism, and ethnic group) on the anatomy of mental foramen?"

It included studies reporting CBCT examination of the mental foramen and the surrounding area on patients before surgery or for routine examination or on cadavers. Some studies have also obtained results with panoramic radiography.

Inclusion criteria were as follows: only studies published in English in an international peer-reviewed journal were included. The observational studies had to describe the anatomy of mental foramen and the surrounding area using images obtained by CBCT.

Exclusion criteria were as follows: systematic reviews, studies about children, case reports, and studies using other types of computed tomography were excluded.

The following Population, Exposure to risk factor, Comparison, and Outcome (PECO) definitions were considered for systemic search:

(i) Population: studies had to include systemically cadavers or patients with CBCT examination
(ii) Exposure: no risk factor
(iii) Comparison: the specific comparisons investigated were anatomic variations or individual parameters (sex, age, edentulism, and ethnic group) on the evaluation of the anatomy of mental foramen
(iv) Outcome measures: characteristics of mental foramen (size, position, symmetry, accessory mental foramen, or multiple mental foramina)

2.2. Search Strategy. A literature search was performed in MEDLINE via the PubMed database of the US National Library of Medicine, Web of Science, and Cochrane Library databases as well as a hand search of other literature to identify articles of potential relevance. The search included articles accepted for publication from 2008 up to June 2020.

Previously published review articles on similar topics were also analyzed to assess potentially relevant publications.

The following keywords were used for this purpose:

Mental foramen OR mental foramina

AND CBCT OR Cone Beam Computed Tomography

2.3. Quality Assessment. Quality assurance was developed by independent screening by two reviewers (AP and PAB) according to Khan et al. [13]. When disagreement arose in the selection and eligibility, it was resolved by discussion between the two reviewers.

3. Results

The initial search of the literature up to June 2020 yielded 728 potentially suitable papers. Two independent reviewers (AP and PAB) analyzed titles and abstracts during the first stage of screening. Irrelevant articles and duplicates were discarded. Additional manual searching of reference lists in the papers selected as well as in a number of review articles was performed to source further relevant publications. Eighty-four full-text articles were assessed for eligibility. The full texts of the articles were read to determine whether the studies fulfilled the predetermined inclusion criteria. Seventy-two studies fulfilled the inclusion criteria and twelve were excluded (Figure 2). Following the exclusion of reviews, children studies, case reports, and studies using other types of computed tomography, 72 publications remained fully eligible for this review.

The κ value for interviewer agreement for study inclusion was 0.95 for titles and abstracts and 1.00 for full-text articles, indicating strong agreement.

Data was collated [4, 5, 12, 14–82] into tables (Tables 1–5 and Supplementary Tables 1–3) and grouped according to the anatomical characteristics studied. Data synthesis was performed based on the evidence tables alone, and the data was further interpreted.

3.1. The Mental Foramen

3.1.1. Localization. Mental foramina (MFs) were equidistant from the midline of the mandible [35–37]. The mean distance did not vary much from a study to another, from around 23 mm to 26 mm [35, 37]. The interforaminal distance seemed to correspond to the double of these values, about between 46.5 ± 5 mm and 51.4 ± 0.6 mm [35, 37]. Moreover, according to Parnia et al., the mental foramen was located around 5 mm away from the lingual border of the mandible, and according to von Arx et al., the shortest distance between MF and a tooth is around 5 mm [15, 36].

When looking vertically, the MF appeared to be approximately in the middle of the mandible regardless of the side with a longer distance between the MF and mandible borders in men. The mean distance between MF and inferior border of the mandible ranged from around 10 mm and 15 mm [16, 38]. This distance was longer in male. For example, according to Gungor et al., the mean distance was 13.35 ± 2.1 mm in men, whereas it was 12.0 ± 1.8 mm in women [39].

The mean distance between MF and superior border of the mandible ranged from 11.2 ± 1.99 to 14.3 mm [12, 22]. This distance was also longer in males than in females [12, 39, 40]. For example, Gungor et al. measured 14.03 ± 2.85 mm in males against 12.53 ± 2.54 mm in females [39].

3.2. No Significant Difference Was Found between Right and Left Sides.

The MF was located mostly between the two premolars (between 50.4% and 61.95%) or apically to the second premolar (PM2) (from 50.3% to 57.9%) [15, 16, 18–22, 25, 26]. Then, it was situated between the PM2 and the first molar (M1) (between 16.7% and 19.4%) or apically to the M1 (from 6.7% to 10.7%) and exceptionally before the PM1 or between M1 and second molar [12, 16, 19, 20, 22, 24]. Sex and side did not seem to have influence on the MF location in relation to the teeth. According to Chen et al., the presence of an anterior loop of the inferior alveolar nerve (AL) could have an influence on the position of MF to the teeth [16]. Indeed, at the majority position, without AL, the MF was found at 51.7% between PM1 and PM2, whereas when there was an AL, it was found at 73.3% apically to the PM2. On the contrary, in Krishnan et al.'s study [24], no significant difference was noticed (Table 1).

3.2.1. Shape. The majority of the shapes of MF in the general population were round (between 61.57% and 72.66%) or oval (between 60.7% and 73.1%) [18, 24, 41–44], and less frequently, it could be irregular (11.14%) [25]. None of the individual parameters studied seemed to have influence of the MF shape [18, 24, 41–44].

3.2.2. Diameter. The mean diameter of mental foramen ranged from 2.08 ± 0.53 mm to 4.44 ± 1.13 mm. Nevertheless, it was around 3 mm most of the time [21, 43]. The mean diameter was superior in males than in females in all the articles studied; the difference between them could reach 0.62 mm [12, 16, 25, 38–40, 45–47]. Moreover, when there was an accessory mental foramen (AMF) ipsilateral to the MF, its diameter was smaller (Supplementary Table 2) [18, 40, 48–50]. The diameter of AMF was smaller than mental foramen diameter, around 1.5 mm on average. It ranged from 0.87 ± 0.24 mm to 1.9 ± 0.6 mm [24, 40].

3.2.3. Area. The mean area of MF ranged from $9.41 \pm 4.58\ mm^2$ to $13.1 \pm 7.00\ mm^2$. MF area was larger than AMF area [51, 52]. According to Muinelo-Lorenzo et al. and Iwanaga et al., the MF ipsilateral to an AMF had a smaller area ($9.0 \pm 5{,}2$ and $12.9 \pm 8.0\ mm^2$) than the area measured in general (10.62 ± 5.00 and $13.1 \pm 7.0\ mm^2$) [18, 51]. On the contrary, MF was bigger on the contralateral side of an AMF or when a patient had no AMF than in general (11.36 ± 4.5 and $14.3 \pm 7.2\ mm^2$) [18, 51].

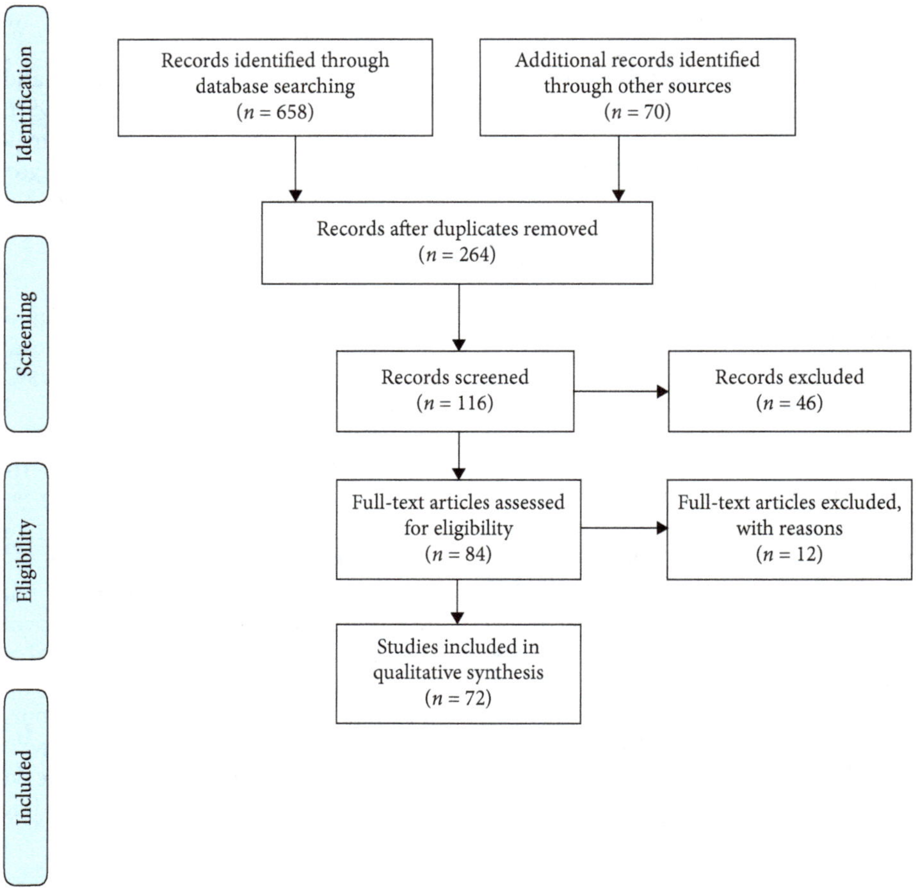

FIGURE 2: Preferred Reporting Items for Systematic Reviews and Meta-Analyses (PRISMA) flow diagram demonstrating the results of the systematic literature search.

TABLE 1: Location of the mental foramen (MF) in relation to adjacent teeth *n* MF (%).

Articles	Anterior to PM1	In line with PM1	Between PM1 and PM2	In line with PM2	Between PM2 and M1	In line with M1 (often to the mesial root)	Between M1 and M2	Total
[14]	0 (0.0)	18 (4.8)	231 (59.8)	120 (30.4)	16 (4.2)	1 (0.3)	0 (0.0)†	386 (100)
[15]	0 (0.0)	7 (4.2)	94 (56)	60 (35.7)	7 (4.2)	0 (0.0)	0 (0.0)	168 (100)
[16]	(0.0†) —	(3.33) (6.66†)‡	(51.67) (20)‡	(40.83) (73.33)‡	(4.17) 0‡	(0.0†) —	(0.0†) —	(100) (100)
[17]		57 (53.8)		1 (1)		48 (45.3)		106 (100)
[18]	0 (0.0)†	32 (5)	161 (25.3)	369 (57.9)	58 (9.1)	17 (2.7)	0 (0.0)†	637 (100)
[19]	0 (0.0)	1 (2.6)	9 (23.1)	22 (56.4)	7 (17.9)	0 (0.0)	0 (0.0)†	39 (100)
[20]	0 (0.0)†	0† (0.0†)	103 (33.0)	157 (50.3)	52 (16.7)	0 (0.0)†	0 (0.0)†	312 (100)
[21]	(0.0)†	(5.0)	(25.3)	(57.9)	(0.0)†	(2.7)	(9.1)	(100)
[22]	0 (0.0)†	62 (10.3)	179 (29.6)	319 (52.8)	36 (6)	8 (1.3)	0 (0.0)†	604 (100)
[23]	0 (0.0)†	(7.03)	(73.39†)	(17.74)	(1.83†)	(0.0†)	(0.0 †)	(100)
[12]	1 (0.6)	18 (10.7)	75 (44.4)	69 (40.8)	5 (3.0)	1 (0.6)	0 (0.0)†	169 (100)
[24]	0.0 —	(1.9) —	(43.5) (41.2)‡	(34.3) (37.3)‡	(19.4) —	(0.9) —	(0.0†) —	(100) (100)
[25]	0 (0.0)	5 (3.6)	70 (50.4)	57 (41.0)		7 (5.0)		139 (100)
[26]	2 (0.25)†	66 (8.26)†	495 (61.95)†	219 (27.41)†	11 (1.38)†	6 (0.75)†	—	799† (100)

PM1: first premolar, PM2: second premolar, M1: first molar, and M2: second molar. †Values calculated based on data from publications.‡In the presence of an anterior loop of the inferior alveolar nerve.

Table 2: Path of mandibular canal (MC) to the mental foramen *n* MC (%).

Articles	Straight	Perpendicular/vertical	Anterior loop
[27]	329 (33.30)†	442 (44.74)†	217 (21.96)†
[22]	279 (46.2)	233 (38.6)	92 (15.2)

†Values calculated based on data from publications.

Table 3: Distribution of mental nerve paths *n* (%) according Solar et al. [3] classification.

Articles	Type I (Y)	Type II (T)	Type III (AL + Y)	Others (AL)	Number of sites
[4]	48 (8.6)	178 (31.9)	332 (59.5)	—	558 (100)
[34]	15 (10.6)	39 (27.5)	50 (35.2)	38 (26.8)	142 (100)

AL: anterior loop.

Table 4: Comparison between cone beam computed tomography (CBCT) and panoramic radiograph (PAN) in measuring distances (mm).

Articles	Mean distance MF–midline of the mandible				Mean interforaminal distance		Mean length of the AL		Mean distance AL–inferior border of the mandible	
	Right side		Left side							
	CBCT	PAN	CBCT	PAN	CBCT	PAN	CBCT	PAN	CBCT	PAN
[35]	23 ± 2.8	21.3 ± 3.5	23 ± 2.4	21 ± 3.9	46.5 ± 5	41.9 ± 7.1	—	—	—	—
[31]	—	—	—	—	—	—	1.59 ± 0.93	2.82 ± 0.91	11.43 ± 1.81	11.64 ± 1.81
[32]	—	—	—	—	—	—	2.79 ± 0.82†	3.03 ± 0.92†	—	—

MF: mental foramen. AL: anterior loop.†Values calculated based on data from publications.

Table 5: Comparison between cone beam computed tomography (CBCT) and panoramic radiograph (PAN) for the visualization of anatomical structures.

Articles	Detection of accessory mental foramina (AMFs) *n* AMFs (%)		Visualization of the anterior loop (AL) *n* AL (%)	
	CBCT	PAN	CBCT	PAN
[28]	37 (100.00)	18 (48.60)	—	—
[29]	4 (100.00†)	0 (0†)	—	—
[30]	19 (100.00†)	3 (15.79†)	—	—
[31]	—	—	40 (48.80)/patient	30 (36.60)/patient
[18]	(100.00)	(45.83)	—	—
[32]	—	—	60[1] (30.30†)/side	41[1] (20.10†)/side
[33]	—	—	67 (37.20)/side	102 (56.75)/side

†Values calculated based on data from publications.

3.2.4. Opening Angle. The mean opening angle of MF ranged from 45.65 ± 10.8 and 55.84 ± 12.16 degrees [43, 45]. According to Çağlayan et al., there was a difference between sides (about 53.58 ± 11.39° on right sides and 58.09 ± 12.93° on left sides) [53]. Moreover, in the same study, the angle varied much more: 51.14 ± 8.90° and 54.66 ± 12.48° on right sides and 58.15 ± 13.40° and 58.07 ± 12.73° on left ones, respectively, in men and in women [53].

3.3. The Accessory Mental Foramen

3.3.1. Prevalence and Repartition. The prevalence of AMFs ranged from 2% to 26% among populations studied [26, 54]. For the sides, the maximum prevalence was 23.79%, which was quite the same than in the populations [26, 54, 55], more common in men [17, 21, 26, 29, 50, 51, 54, 56–59]. The AMF was seen more often on the right side of a patient; indeed, out of 10 studies, only three found more left sides with AMF than right ones [50, 51, 58]. Two studies found the same number of AMF on the right and left sides [26, 29, 54].

The AMF was more often found unilaterally in the studies, with a maximum of only 13 patients with AMFs on both sides in Aytugar et al.'s study [50]. Most of the time, the authors detected one to two AMFs per patient [5, 17, 24, 29, 40, 49].

3.3.2. Diameter. The mean diameter of AMF ranged from 0.87 ± 0.24 mm to 1.9 ± 0.6 mm, but it was around 1.5 mm most of the time [24, 40]. So, the AMF was smaller than the MF, about a half of it. For example, according to Gümüsok et al. [47], the mean horizontal and vertical diameters of MFs were, respectively, 2.80 ± 0.99 mm and 3.11 ± 0.89, whereas there were 1.27 ± 0.40 and 1.50 ± 0.63 mm for AMFs. No difference was found between the sex of the patient or sides on the AMF mean diameter (Supplementary Table 2).

3.3.3. Area. The mean area of AMF ranged from $1.20 \pm 1.10\,mm^2$ to $1.8 \pm 1.4\,mm^2$ [51, 52].

3.3.4. Localization. The AMF position the most seen was posteroinferior to the MF. Indeed, most of AMFs were found at this position in 8 studies out of 17 [18, 30, 40, 47, 50, 54, 57, 60]. However, it was not the first position in each study; for example, some authors did not find any AMF at this position [29]. The AMF was located from around 2.54 ± 1.09 mm to 8.7 ± 4.3 mm away from the MF, and AMF was situated in a radius of 1 cm around the MF [49, 51]. According to Sisman et al., eight AMF showed continuity with the mandibular canal out of 14 [54]. Among them, two were connected with the AL and six were directly connected to the mandibular canal posteriorly to the MF.

3.4. The Mandibular Canal. Two articles mentioned three paths of the MC to the mental foramen [22, 27]. First, there were "straight" type and "perpendicular" or "vertical" type and then less frequently the AL with 15.2% and 21.96% (Table 2) [22, 27].

According Solar et al.'s classification, the paths of the MC were in frequency order: type III (AL + Y), type II (T), and type I (Y) [3, 4, 34] (Table 3). Moreover, they had another type called "others," including other forms of AL seen at 26.8% [34].

3.5. The Anterior Loop of the Inferior Alveolar Nerve

3.5.1. Prevalence and Repartition. Within the different studies, the prevalence of the AL ranged from 10.4% to 94% and from 10% to 86% among sides observed [61–64]. The sex of the patient did not seem to have a significant influence on it. However, ALs were situated mostly on the right side of patient in six studies out of eight (that looked at this parameter) [4, 27, 32, 36, 65, 66]. The AL could be found unilaterally or bilaterally with no predominance of one or another.

3.5.2. Length. The mean AL length ranged from 0.89 ± 1.17 mm to 7.61 ± 1.81 mm [16, 38]. Among the extreme values, except for a minimal length of 0.0 mm meaning the absence of the AL, the smallest AL measured within the studies had a length of 0.15 mm, whereas the longest AL was equal to about 9.37 mm according to Yoon and al. [14, 52, 67]. The AL seemed to be longer in males (between 0.87 ± 1.81 and 7.25 ± 2.02 mm) than in female (between 0.81 ± 1.18 and 6.52 ± 1.63 mm); indeed, there were only two studies out of thirteen with a mean AL length bigger in females [16, 27]. The presence of teeth could be in favor of longer average length (from 0.91 ± 1.18 to 2.55 ± 1.28 for dentate people and from 0.25 ± 0.61 to 2.40 ± 0.88 mm with edentulous) [14, 67, 68]. Finally, the lengths measured on the left sides tended to be smaller except for Uchida et al. and Koivisto et al., who measured, respectively, 2.1 ± 1.9 mm and 3.5 mm on average against 1.7 ± 1.3 mm and 2.5 mm on the right sides (Supplementary Table 3) [62, 68].

3.5.3. Angle. Only one study measured the angle of the AL. Chen et al. found a mean angle of 19.13 ± 26.89° in the population [16]. This angle appeared to be bigger on the right sides than on left ones and in females (25.21 ± 28.89°) than in males (13.06 ± 23.43°).

3.6. Comparison between CBCT and PAN. Mean distances between MF and midline of the mandible and interforaminal mean distance measured with CBCT were greater than those measured with PAN. For example, Madrigal et al. [35] measured 46.5 ± 5 mm between the two MFs with CBCT, while they measured 41.9 ± 7.1 mm with PAN. It was the opposite for the AL mean length (Table 4) [31, 32, 35].

Moreover, AL and AMFs were detected more frequently with CBCT. For example, according to Vujanovik-Eskenazi et al., the AL was seen in 40 patients with CBCT against 30 with PAN [31]. Only 15.79% of AMFs detected with CBCT were also seen with PAN according to Neves et al. [30] (Table 5), and this could be explained by the small diameter of AMF (often inferior to 1 mm) and was spot with difficulty on panoramic radiograph [5].

4. Discussion

The mental foramen is a strategically important landmark during surgical procedures [1]. Its location, number of foramina, and possibility of anterior loop of the mental nerve or AMF being present need to be considered before surgery to avoid mental nerve injury. This article systematically reviews the literature with respect to the mental foramen to reduce unintentional damage to the mental nerve.

The damage to mental foramen or inferior alveolar nerve during oral surgery or implant placement is a serious complication [83]. The incidence of mental neurosensory disturbances resulting from orthodontic, periodontal, and surgical procedures cannot be determined [84]. Juodzbalys et al. reported the complication incidence, which varies from 0% to 40%, of implant related inferior alveolar nerve (IAN) injuries [83]. The IAN is the most commonly injured nerve (64.4%), followed by the lingual nerve (28.8%) [85]. The damages could be range from mild paresthesia or dysesthesia to complete anesthesia and/or pain [86]. Many functions (speech, eating, kissing, drinking, etc.) will be affected [87]. The damage can result from the traumatic local anaesthetic injections or during the dental implant site osteotomy or placement or direct injury with scalpel with extreme alveolar process resorption [83].

CBCT allows collecting extensive informations about the MF anatomy, its environment and anatomical variations that can exist when some clinical parameters vary as sex, side or dental status.

When comparing two- and three-dimensional imaging, some differences were noticed. The average distances between

MF and midline and between the mental foramina measured with cone beam were greater than those measured with PAN [35]. It was the contrary for AL lengths [31, 32]. CBCT overcomes certain limitations of two-dimensional imaging, such as distortion, magnification, and superimposition [88]. CBCT-reformatted panoramic images have been shown to be superior to PAN identifying the mandibular canal, because these images are free of magnification and superimposition [89]. So, according to Aminoshariae et al., CBCT is better in detecting anatomical particularities of each patient [90]. The authors supported the use of CBCT to evaluate the patient anatomy to avoid nerve injury before surgery [91].

To avoid nerve injury during surgery in the foraminal area, guidelines were developed based on the literature with respect to verifying the position of the mental foramen and validating the presence of an anterior loop of the mental nerve according to Greenstein and Tarnow [1]. The practitioner must be aware of the mental area anatomy and morphology before undertaking any treatment [84]. According to Juodzbalys et al. [83], the best way to prevent these damages is to have a clear three-dimensional vision of the jaw: proper presurgery planning, timely diagnosis, and treatment are the key to avoiding nerve sensory disturbances management. These guidelines included leaving a 2 mm safety zone between an implant and the coronal aspect of the nerve, three-dimensional radiographic evaluation, or surgical corroboration of the mental foramen's position [1].

Clinicians must also know the opening angle of the MF when operating on this area. For example, the diameter and length of an implant could be modified according to this angle. A smaller or thinner implant could be necessary when the opening angle of the MF increases since it means that the MF opens at a higher level than the mandibular canal one.

5. Conclusion

In dentistry, the acknowledgment of the anatomy of the oral cavity is necessary to treat patients correctly, especially for local anesthesia, in surgery or implantology consequently risking damage to critical structures, such as nerves and blood vessels. However, each person presents particularities, the anatomic variations, increasing the risks during our intervention. So, the clinician has to detect them during the preoperative phase to organize the patient treatment.

In the systematic review, the advantages of the CBCT technique were studied to analyze a surgical zone at anatomical risk within the mandible, that is, the mental foramen. The mental foramen was located mostly between the two premolars (between 50.4% and 61.95%) or apically to the second premolar (from 50.3% to 57.9%). The mean diameter of the mental foramen was bigger in males than in females, with a difference reaching 0.62 mm. The mean AL length ranged from 0.89 ± 1.17 mm to 7.61 ± 1.81 mm. The prevalence of the AL ranged from 10.4% to 94%, and from 10% to 86% among sides observed. The AMF, most seen in posteroinferior location to the MF, was situated from around 2.54 ± 1.09 mm to 8.7 ± 4.3 mm away from the MF.

References

[1] G. Greenstein and D. Tarnow, "The mental foramen and nerve: clinical and anatomical factors related to dental implant placement: a literature review," *Journal of Periodontology*, vol. 77, no. 12, pp. 1933–1943, 2006.

[2] T. Kawai, I. Sato, R. Asaumi, and T. Yosue, "Cone-beam computed tomography and anatomical observations of normal variants in the mandible: variant dentists should recognize," *Oral Radiology*, vol. 34, no. 3, pp. 189–198, 2018.

[3] P. Solar, C. Ulm, G. Frey, and M. Matejka, "A classification of the intraosseous paths of the mental nerve," *International Journal of Oral Maxillofacial Implants*, vol. 9, pp. 339–344, 1994.

[4] A. Demir, E. Izgi, and F. Pekiner, "Anterior loop of the mental foramen in a Turkish subpopulation with dentate patients: a cone beam computed tomography study," *Müsbed*, vol. 5, pp. 231–238, 2015.

[5] K. Katakami, A. Mishima, K. Shiozaki, S. Shimoda, Y. Hamada, and K. Kobayashi, "Characteristics of accessory mental foramina observed on limited cone-beam computed tomography images," *Journal of Endodontics*, vol. 34, no. 12, pp. 1441–1445, 2008.

[6] X. Wang, K. Chen, S. Wang, S. K. Tiwari, L. Ye, and L. Peng, "Relationship between the mental foramen, mandibular canal, and the surgical access line of the mandibular posterior teeth: a one-beam computed tomographic analysis," *Journal of Endodontics*, vol. 43, no. 8, pp. 1262–1266, 2017.

[7] Y. Arai, E. Tammisalo, K. Iwai, K. Hashimoto, and K. Shinoda, "Development of a compact computed tomographic apparatus for dental use," *Dentomaxillofacial Radiology*, vol. 28, no. 4, pp. 245–248, 1999.

[8] P. Mozzo, C. Procacci, A. Tacconi, P. T. Martini, and I. A. Andreis, "A new volumetric CT machine for dental imaging based on the cone-beam technique: preliminary results," *European Radiology*, vol. 8, pp. 1558–1564, 1999.

[9] A. Dawood, S. Patel, and J. Brown, "Cone beam CT in dental practice," *British Dental Journal*, vol. 207, pp. 23–28, 2009.

[10] P. Sukovic, "Cone beam computed tomography in craniofacial imaging," *Orthodontics & Craniofacial Research*, vol. 6, pp. 31–36, 2003.

[11] J. K. Mah, R. A. Danforth, A. Bumann, and D. Hatcher, "Radiation absorbed in maxillofacial imaging with a new dental computed tomography device," *Oral Surgery, Oral Medicine, Oral Pathology, Oral Radiology, and Endodontology*, vol. 96, no. 4, pp. 508–513, 2003.

[12] R. Dos Santos Oliveira, M. Rodrigues Coutinho, and F. Kühl Panzarella, "Morphometric analysis of the mental foramen using cone-beam computed tomography," *International Journal of Dentistry*, vol. 2018, Article ID 4571895, 7 pages, 2018.

[13] K. S. Khan, G. ter Riet, and J. Popay, "Stage II: conducting the review. Phase 5: study quality assessment," in *Undertaking Systematic Reviews of Research on Effectiveness*, K. S. Khan, G. ter Tiet, and J. Glanvill, Eds., pp. 1–20, University of York, York (UK), 2 edition, 2001.

[14] M. B. Rosa, B. S. Sotto-Maior, V. de Carvalho Machado, and C. E. Francischone, "Retrospective study of the anterior loop of the inferior alveolar nerve and the incisive canal using cone beam computed tomography," *The International Journal of Oral & Maxillofacial Implants*, vol. 28, no. 2, pp. 388–392, 2013.

[15] T. von Arx, M. Friedli, P. Sendi, S. Lozanoff, and M. M. Bornstein, "Location and dimensions of the mental foramen: a radiographic analysis by using cone-beam computed tomography," *Journal of Endodontics*, vol. 39, no. 12, pp. 1522–1528, 2013.

[16] Z. Chen, D. Chen, L. Tang, and F. Wang, "Relationship between the position of the mental foramen and the anterior loop of the inferior alveolar nerve as determined by cone beam computed tomography combined with mimics," *Journal of Computer Assisted Tomography*, vol. 39, no. 1, pp. 86–93, 2015.

[17] P. Carruth, J. He, B. W. Benson, and E. D. Schneiderman, "Analysis of the size and position of the mental foramen using the CS 9000 cone-beam computed tomographic unit," *Journal of Endodontics*, vol. 41, no. 7, pp. 1032–1036, 2015.

[18] J. Muinelo-Lorenzo, J. Suárez-Quintanilla, A. Fernández-Alonso, J. Varela-Mallou, and M. Suárez-Cunqueiro, "Anatomical characteristics and visibility of mental foramen and accessory mental foramen: panoramic radiography vs. cone beam CT," *Medicina Oral Patología Oral Y Cirugia Bucal*, vol. 20, pp. e707–e714, 2015.

[19] S.-S. Han, J. J. Hwang, and H.-G. Jeong, "Accessory mental foramina associated with neurovascular bundle in Korean population," *Surgical and Radiologic Anatomy*, vol. 38, no. 10, pp. 1169–1174, 2016.

[20] A. Safaee, S. Mirbeigi, F. Ezoddini, L. Khojastepour, and A. Navab-Azam, "Buccolingual course of the inferior alveolar canal in different mental foramen locations: a cone beam computed tomography study of an Iranian population," *International Journal of Applied and Basic Medical Research*, vol. 6, no. 4, pp. 262–266, 2016.

[21] J. Muinelo-Lorenzo, A. Fernández-Alonso, E. Smyth-Chamosa, J. A. Suárez-Quintanilla, J. Varela-Mallou, and M. M. Suárez-Cunqueiro, "Predictive factors of the dimensions and location of mental foramen using cone beam computed tomography," *PLoS ONE*, vol. 12, p. e0179704, 2017.

[22] H. Al-Mahalawy, H. Al-Aithan, B. Al-Kari, B. Al-Jandan, and S. Shujaat, "Determination of the position of mental foramen and frequency of anterior loop in Saudi population. A retrospective CBCT study," *The Saudi Dental Journal*, vol. 29, no. 1, pp. 29–35, 2017.

[23] M. Velasco-Torres, M. Padial-Molina, G. Avila-Ortiz, R. García-Delgado, A. Catena, and P. Galindo-Moreno, "Inferior alveolar nerve trajectory, mental foramen location and incidence of mental nerve anterior loop," *Medicina Oral Patologica Oral Y Cirugica Bucal*, vol. 22, pp. e630–e635, 2017.

[24] U. Krishnan, P. Monsour, K. Thaha, R. Lalloo, and A. Moule, "A limited field Cone-beam computed tomography-based evaluation of the mental foramen, accessory mental foramina, anterior loop, lateral lingual foramen, and lateral lingual canal," *Journal of Endodontics*, vol. 44, no. 6, pp. 946–951, 2018.

[25] F. Alsoleihat, F. A. Al-Omari, A. R. Al-Sayyed, A. A. Al-Asmar, and A. Khraisat, "The mental foramen: a cone beam CT study of the horizontal location, size and sexual dimorphism amongst living Jordanians," *Homo*, vol. 69, no. 6, pp. 335–339, 2018.

[26] Y. Y. Bosykh, A. Y. Turkina, R. P. A. V. Franco, A. Franco, and M. K. Makeeva, "Cone beam computed tomography study on the relation between mental foramen and roots of mandibular teeth, presence of anterior loop and satellite foramina," *Morphologie*, vol. 103, no. 341, pp. 65–71, 2019.

[27] H. Sahman and Y. Sisman, "Anterior loop of the inferior alveolar canal: a cone-beam computerized tomography study of 494 cases," *Journal of Oral Implantology*, vol. 42, no. 4, pp. 333–336, 2016.

[28] M. Naitoh, K. Yoshida, K. Nakahara, K. Gotoh, and E. Ariji, "Demonstration of the accessory mental foramen using rotational panoramic radiography compared with cone-beam computed tomography," *Clinical Oral Implants Research*, vol. 22, no. 12, pp. 1415–1419, 2011.

[29] T. S. N. Imada, L. M. P. d. S. R. Fernandes, B. S. Centurion, C. de Oliveira-Santos, H. M. Honório, and I. R. F. Rubira-Bullen, "Accessory mental foramina: prevalence, position and diameter assessed by cone-beam computed tomography and digital panoramic radiographs," *Clinical Oral Implants Research*, vol. 25, no. 2, pp. e94–e99, 2014.

[30] F. S. Neves, M. C. C. Nascimento, M. L. Oliveira, S. M. Almeida, and F. N. Bóscolo, "Comparative analysis of mandibular anatomical variations between panoramic radiography and cone beam computed tomography," *Oral and Maxillofacial Surgery*, vol. 18, no. 4, pp. 419–424, 2014.

[31] A. Vujanovic-Eskenazi, J. Valero-James, M. Sánchez-Garcés, and C. Gay-Escoda, "A retrospective radiographic evaluation of the anterior loop of the mental nerve: comparison between panoramic radiography and cone beam computerized tomography," *Medicina Oral Patología Oral Y Cirugia Bucal*, vol. 20, pp. e239–e245, 2015.

[32] S. Kumbargere Nagraj, E. Prashanti, H. H. Kyaw Soe, K. Salian, D. Chien, and C. Lin, "Radiographic evaluation of the anterior loop of the mental nerve: comparison between orthopantomograph and cone-beam CT-a pilot study," *Research Journal of Pharmaceutical, Biological and Chemical Sciences*, vol. 8, p. 2044, 2017.

[33] R. Kastala, C. David, and N. Jayapal, "Momentousness of the mental loop: a comparative study," *Contemporary Clinical Dentistry*, vol. 10, no. 1, pp. 86–92, 2019.

[34] B. Shaban, A. Khajavi, N. Khaki, Y. Mohiti, T. Mehri, and H. Kermani, "Assessment of the anterior loop of the inferior alveolar nerve via cone-beam computed tomography," *Journal of the Korean Association of Oral and Maxillofacial Surgeons*, vol. 43, no. 6, pp. 395–400, 2017.

[35] C. Madrigal, R. Ortega, C. Meniz, and J. López-Quiles, "Study of available bone for interforaminal implant treatment using cone-beam computed tomography," *Medicina Oral, Patologia Oral Y Cirugia Bucal*, vol. 13, no. 5, pp. E307–E312, 2008.

[36] F. Parnia, E. Moslehifard, A. Hafezeqoran, F. Mahboub, and H. Mojaver-Kahnamoui, "Characteristics of anatomical landmarks in the mandibular interforaminal region: a cone-beam computed tomography study," *Medicina Oral Patología Oral Y Cirugia Bucal*, vol. 17, pp. e420–e425, 2012.

[37] M. Sheikhi and M. K. Kheir, "CBCT Assessment of mental foramen position relative to anatomical landmarks," *International Journal of Dentistry*, vol. 2016, Article ID 5821048, , 2016.

[38] J. C.-H. Chen, L.-M. Lin, J. R. Geist, J.-Y. Chen, C.-H. Chen, and Y.-K. Chen, "A retrospective comparison of the location and diameter of the inferior alveolar canal at the mental foramen and length of the anterior loop between American and Taiwanese cohorts using CBCT," *Surgical and Radiologic Anatomy*, vol. 35, no. 1, pp. 11–18, 2013.

[39] E. Gungor, O. S. Aglarci, M. Unal, M. S. Dogan, and S. Guven, "Evaluation of mental foramen location in the 10-70 years age range using cone-beam computed tomography," *Nigerian Journal of Clinical Practice*, vol. 20, no. 1, pp. 88–92, 2017.

[40] M. Naitoh, Y. Hiraiwa, H. Aimiya, K. Gotoh, and E. Ariji, "Accessory mental foramen assessment using cone-beam computed tomography," *Oral Surgery, Oral Medicine, Oral Pathology, Oral Radiology, and Endodontology*, vol. 107, no. 2, pp. 289–294, 2009.

[41] M. Sheikhi, M. Karbasi Kheir, and E. Hekmatian, "Cone-beam computed tomography evaluation of mental foramen variations: a preliminary study," *Radiology Research and Practice*, vol. 2015, Article ID 124635, 5 pages, 2015.

[42] M. K. Alam, S. Alhabib, B. K. Alzarea et al., "3D CBCT morphometric assessment of mental foramen in Arabic population and global comparison: imperative for invasive and non-invasive procedures in mandible," *Acta Odontologica Scandinavica*, vol. 76, no. 2, pp. 98–104, 2018.

[43] S. Goyushov, M. D. Tözüm, and T. F. Tözüm, "Assessment of morphological and anatomical characteristics of mental foramen using cone beam computed tomography," *Surgical and Radiologic Anatomy*, vol. 40, no. 10, pp. 1133–1139, 2018.

[44] E. Zmysłowska, M. Radwański, S. Ledzion, M. Łęski, A. Zmyslowska, and M. Łukomska-Szymańska, "Evaluation of size and location of a mental foramen in the polish population using cone-beam computed tomography," *BioMed Research International*, vol. 2019, Article ID 1659476, 8 pages, 2019.

[45] A. Kalender, K. Orhan, and U. Aksoy, "Evaluation of the mental foramen and accessory mental foramen in Turkish patients using cone-beam computed tomography images reconstructed from a volumetric rendering program," *Clinical Anatomy*, vol. 25, no. 5, pp. 584–592, 2012.

[46] L. Ritter, J. Neugebauer, R. A. Mischkowski et al., "Evaluation of the course of the inferior alveolar nerve in the mental foramen by cone beam computed tomography," *International Journal of Oral Maxillofacial Implants*, vol. 27, pp. 1014–1021, 2012.

[47] M. Gümüşok, Z. Z. Akarslan, A. Başman, and Ö. Üçok, "Evaluation of accessory mental foramina morphology with cone-beam computed tomography," *Nigerian Journal of Clinical Practice*, vol. 20, no. 12, pp. 1550–1554, 2017.

[48] C. Oliveira-Santos, P. H. C. Souza, S. De Azambuja Berti-Couto et al., "Characterisation of additional mental foramina through cone beam computed tomography," *Journal of Oral Rehabilitation*, vol. 38, no. 8, pp. 595–600, 2011.

[49] M. Göregen, Ö. Miloğlu, I. Ersoy, I. Bayrakdar, and H. Akgül, "The assessment of accessory mental foramina using cone-beam computed tomography," *Turkish Journal of Medical Sciences*, vol. 43, pp. 479–483, 2013.

[50] E. Aytugar, C. Özeren, N. Lacin, I. Veli, and E. Çene, "Cone-beam computed tomographic evaluation of accessory mental foramen in a Turkish population," *Anatomical Science International*, vol. 94, no. 3, pp. 257–265, 2019.

[51] J. Iwanaga, K. Watanabe, T. Saga et al., "Accessory mental foramina and nerves: application to periodontal, periapical, and implant surgery," *Clinical Anatomy*, vol. 29, no. 4, pp. 493–501, 2016.

[52] T. Y. Yoon, A. G. Ahmadi, N. A. Saed, N. E. Estrin, D. E. Miller, and T. N. Dinh, "Prevalence and anatomical characteristics of the accessory mental foramen: a study using cone beam computed tomography," *General Dentistry*, vol. 67, pp. 62–67, 2019.

[53] F. Çağlayan, M. A. Sümbüllü, H. M. Akgül, and O. Altun, "Morphometric and morphologic evaluation of the mental foramen in relation to age and sex: an anatomic cone beam computed tomography study," *The Journal of Craniofacial Surgery*, vol. 25, no. 6, pp. 2227–2230, 2014.

[54] Y. Sisman, H. Sahman, A. Sekerci, T. T. Tokmak, Y. Aksu, and E. Mavili, "Detection and characterization of the mandibular accessory buccal foramen using CT," *Dentomaxillofacial Radiology*, vol. 41, no. 7, pp. 558–563, 2012.

[55] N. Raju, W. Zhang, A. Jadhav, A. Ioannou, S. Eswaran, and R. Weltman, "Cone-beam computed tomography analysis of the prevalence, length, and passage of the anterior loop of the mandibular canal," *Journal of Oral Implantology*, vol. 45, no. 6, pp. 463–468, 2019.

[56] L. Khojastepour, S. Mirbeigi, S. Mirhadi, and A. Safaee, "Location of mental foramen in a selected Iranian population: a CBCT assessment," *Iranian Endodontic Journal*, vol. 10, no. 2, pp. 117–121, 2015.

[57] Y. Li, X. Yang, B. Zhang, B. Wei, and Y. Gong, "Detection and characterization of the accessory mental foramen using cone-beam computed tomography," *Acta Odontologica Scandinavica*, vol. 76, no. 2, pp. 77–85, 2018.

[58] M. Lam, C. Koong, E. Kruger, and M. Tennant, "Prevalence of accessory mental foramina: a study of 4,000 CBCT scans," *Clinical Anatomy*, vol. 32, no. 8, pp. 1048–1052, 2019.

[59] X. Wei, P. Gu, Y. Hao, and J. Wang, "Detection and characterization of anterior loop, accessory mental foramen, and lateral lingual foramen by using cone beam computed tomography," *Journal of Prosthetic Dentistry*, vol. S22, pp. 30494–30499, 2019.

[60] D. Yovchev, H. Mihaylova, P. Stanimirov, A. Gusiyska, and M. Dimova, "Incidence, location and sizes of the accessory mental foramina in Bulgarian population assessed by cone-beam computed tomography," *Biomedical Research*, vol. 28, pp. 5122–5126, 2017.

[61] H. Eren, K. Orhan, N. Bagis, R. Nalcaci, M. Misirli, and E. Hincal, "Cone beam computed tomography evaluation of mandibular canal anterior loop morphology and volume in a group of Turkish patients," *Biotechnology & Biotechnological Equipment*, vol. 30, no. 2, pp. 346–353, 2016.

[62] T. Koivisto, D. Chiona, L. L. Milroy, S. B. McClanahan, M. Ahmad, and W. R. Bowles, "Mandibular canal location: cone-beam computed tomography examination," *Journal of Endodontics*, vol. 42, no. 7, pp. 1018–1021, 2016.

[63] P. Christopher, T. Marimuthu, C. Krithika, P. Devadoss, and S. M. Kumar, "Prevalence and measurement of anterior loop of the mandibular canal using CBCT: a cross sectional study," *Clinical Implant Dentistry and Related Research*, vol. 20, no. 4, pp. 531–534, 2018.

[64] S. K. Wong and P. G. Patil, "Measuring anterior loop length of the inferior alveolar nerve to estimate safe zone in implant planning: a CBCT study in a Malaysian population," *The Journal of Prosthetic Dentistry*, vol. 120, no. 2, pp. 210–213, 2018.

[65] Z. D. Kajan and A. Salari, "Presence and course of the mandibular incisive canal and presence of the anterior loop in cone beam computed tomography images of an Iranian population," *Oral Radiology*, vol. 28, no. 1, pp. 55–61, 2012.

[66] K. Filo, T. Schneider, M. C. Locher, A. L. Kruse, and H.-T. Lübbers, "The inferior alveolar nerve's loop at the mental foramen and its implications for surgery," *The Journal of the American Dental Association*, vol. 145, no. 3, pp. 260–269, 2014.

[67] D. Apostolakis and J. E. Brown, "The anterior loop of the inferior alveolar nerve: prevalence, measurement of its length and a recommendation for interforaminal implant installation based on cone beam CT imaging," *Clinical Oral Implants Research*, vol. 23, no. 9, pp. 1022–1030, 2012.

[68] Y. Uchida, N. Noguchi, M. Goto et al., "Measurement of anterior loop length for the mandibular canal and diameter of the mandibular incisive canal to avoid nerve damage when installing endosseous implants in the interforaminal region: a second attempt introducing cone beam computed tomography," *Journal of Oral and Maxillofacial Surgery*, vol. 67, no. 4, pp. 744–750, 2009.

[69] M. Naitoh, K. Nakahara, Y. Suenaga, K. Gotoh, S. Kondo, and E. Ariji, "Comparison between cone-beam and multislice computed tomography depicting mandibular neurovascular canal structures," *Oral Surgery, Oral Medicine, Oral Pathology, Oral Radiology, and Endodontology*, vol. 109, no. 1, pp. e25–e31, 2010.

[70] C.-I. Lu, J. Won, A. Al-Ardah, R. Santana, D. Rice, and J. Lozada, "Assessment of the anterior loop of the mental nerve using cone beam computerized tomography scan," *Journal of Oral Implantology*, vol. 41, no. 6, pp. 632–639, 2015.

[71] M. Panjnoush, Z. S. Rabiee, and Y. Kheirandish, "Assessment of location and anatomical characteristics of mental foramen, anterior loop and mandibular incisive canal using cone beam computed tomography," *Journal of Dentistry (Tehran)*, vol. 13, pp. 126–132, 2016.

[72] E. Zmysłowska-Polakowska, M. Radwański, M. Łęski, S. Ledzion, M. Łukomska-Szymańska, and M. Polguj, "The assessment of accessory mental foramen in a selected polish population: a CBCT study," *BMC Med Imaging*, vol. 17, p. 17, 2017.

[73] B. S. Chong, K. Gohil, R. Pawar, and J. Makdissi, "Anatomical relationship between mental foramen, mandibular teeth and risk of nerve injury with endodontic treatment," *Clinical Oral Investigations*, vol. 21, no. 1, pp. 381–387, 2017.

[74] X.-w. Yang, F.-f. Zhang, Y.-h. Li, B. Wei, and Y. Gong, "Characteristics of intrabony nerve canals in mandibular interforaminal region by using cone-beam computed tomography and a recommendation of safe zone for implant and bone harvesting," *Clinical Implant Dentistry and Related Research*, vol. 19, no. 3, pp. 530–538, 2017.

[75] L. Marieiro, D. Deluiz, D. Ferreira, and P. Tannure, "Measurement of distance between the mental foramina using cone beam computed tomography: a pilot study with a possible method for planning mandibular implants," *Pesquisa Brasileira em Odontopediatria e Clínica Integrada*, vol. 17, no. 1, pp. 1–6, 2017.

[76] M. R. Moghddam, Z. Davoudmanesh, N. Azizi, V. Rakhshan, and M. Shariati, "Prevalence and length of the anterior loop of the inferior alveolar nerve in Iranians," *Journal of Oral Implantology*, vol. 43, no. 5, pp. 333–336, 2017.

[77] G. Aoun, A. ElOuta, N. Kafrouny, and A. Berberi, "Assessment of the mental foramen location in a sample of fully dentate Lebanese adults using cone-beam computed tomography technology," *Acta Informatica Medica*, vol. 25, no. 4, pp. 259–262, 2017.

[78] M. Kheir and M. Sheikhi, "Assessment of the anterior loop of mental nerve in an Iranian population using cone beam computed tomography scan," *Dental Research Journal*, vol. 14, no. 6, pp. 418–422, 2017.

[79] M. do Carmo Oliveira, T. K. Tedesco, T. Gimenez, and S. Allegrini, "Analysis of the frequency of visualization of morphological variations in anatomical bone features in the mandibular interforaminal region through cone-beam computed tomography," *Surgical and Radiologic Anatomy*, vol. 40, no. 10, pp. 1119–1131, 2018.

[80] C. L. Vieira, S. d. A. R. Veloso, and F. F. Lopes, "Location of the course of the mandibular canal, anterior loop and accessory mental foramen through cone-beam computed tomography," *Surgical and Radiologic Anatomy*, vol. 40, no. 12, pp. 1411–1417, 2018.

[81] L. Xie, T. Li, J. Chen, D. Yin, W. Wang, and Z. Xie, "Cone-beam CT assessment of implant-related anatomy landmarks of the anterior mandible in a Chinese population," *Surgical and Radiologic Anatomy*, vol. 41, no. 8, pp. 927–934, 2019.

[82] S. Valdec, J. M. Borm, S. Casparis, G. Damerau, M. Locher, and B. Stadlinger, "Vestibular bone thickness of the mandible in relation to the mandibular canal-a retrospective CBCT-based study," *International Joural of Implant Dentistry*, vol. 5, p. 37, 2019.

[83] G. Juodzbalys, H.-L. Wang, and G. Sabalys, "Injury of the inferior alveolar nerve during implant placement: a literature review," *Journal of Oral and Maxillofacial Research*, vol. 2, no. 1, p. e1, 2011.

[84] W. Cheong Ngeow, "Is there a "safety zone" in the mandibular premolar region where damage to the mental nerve can be avoided if periapical extrusion occurs?" *Journal of Canadian Dental Association*, vol. 76, p. a61, 2010.

[85] A. B. G. Tay and J. R. Zuniga, "Clinical characteristics of trigeminal nerve injury referrals to a university centre," *International Journal of Oral and Maxillofacial Surgery*, vol. 36, no. 10, pp. 922–927, 2007.

[86] A. A. Alhassani and A. S. T. AlGhamdi, "Inferior alveolar nerve injury in implant dentistry: diagnosis, causes, prevention, and management," *Journal of Oral Implantology*, vol. 36, no. 5, pp. 401–407, 2010.

[87] V. B. Ziccardi and L. A. Assael, "Mechanisms of trigeminal nerve injuries," *Atlas of the Oral and Maxillofacial Surgery Clinics*, vol. 9, no. 2, pp. 1–11, 2001.

[88] R. Weiss and A. Read-Fuller, "Cone beam computed tomography in oral and maxillofacial surgery: an evidence-based review," *Dentistry Journal*, vol. 7, pp. 1–23, 2019.

[89] C. Angelopoulos, S. Thomas, S. Hechler, N. Parissis, and M. Hlavacek, "Comparison between digital panoramic radiography and cone-beam computed tomography for the identification of the mandibular canal as part of presurgical dental implant assessment," *Journal of Oral and Maxillofacial Surgery*, vol. 66, no. 10, pp. 2130–2135, 2008.

[90] A. Aminoshariae, A. Su, and J. C. Kulild, "Determination of the location of the mental foramen: a critical review," *Journal of Endodontics*, vol. 40, no. 4, pp. 471–475, 2014.

[91] Y. Uchida, Y. Yamashita, M. Goto, and T. Hanihara, "Measurement of anterior loop length for the mandibular canal and diameter of the mandibular incisive canal to avoid nerve damage when installing endosseous implants in the interforaminal region," *Journal of Oral and Maxillofacial Surgery*, vol. 65, no. 9, pp. 1772–1779, 2007.

16

Size of the Carotid Body in Patients with Cardiovascular and Respiratory Diseases Measured by Computed Tomography Angiography: A Case-Control Study

Sándor Csizmadia,[1] Gergely H. Fodor,[2] András Palkó,[3] and Erika Vörös[3]

[1]*Affidea Hungary Ltd. Budapest, 44-46 Bókay János Street, Budapest H-1083, Hungary*
[2]*Department of Medical Physics and Informatics, University of Szeged, Faculty of General Medicine, 9 Korányi Alley, Szeged H-6725, Hungary*
[3]*Department of Radiology, University of Szeged, Faculty of General Medicine, 6 Semmelweis Street, Szeged H-6725, Hungary*

Correspondence should be addressed to Sándor Csizmadia; csizmadia.sandor.89@gmail.com

Academic Editor: Lorenzo Faggioni

Objectives. Carotid bodies (CBs) play an important role in regulating sympathetic nervous system activity. Thus, they are likely to be enlarged in patients with certain cardiovascular and respiratory diseases. The aim of this case-control study was to verify this hypothesis using computed tomography angiography (CTA). *Methods.* We retrospectively analysed 141 CTAs including 16 controls, 96 patients with only hypertension (HT), 12 with HT and previous acute myocardial infarction (AMI), 9 with HT and heart failure (HF), and 8 with HT and chronic obstructive pulmonary disease (COPD). We assessed the data using analysis of variance, with $p < 0.05$ indicating significance. *Results.* CB average areas in the controls were 2.31 mm^2 (right side (RS)) vs. 2.34 mm^2 (left side (LS)). CB size was significantly enlarged in patients with HT: 3.07 mm^2 (RS) ($p = 0.019$) vs. 2.91 mm^2 (LS) ($p = 0.002$). If AMI (RS: 3.5 mm^2; LS: 3.44 mm^2) or HF (RS: 4.01 mm^2; LS: 4.55 mm^2) was associated with HT, the CB size was even more enlarged. COPD did not affect CB size (RS: 2.40 mm^2; LS: 2.29 mm^2). *Conclusions.* Our data showed that certain diseases with increased activity of the sympathetic nervous system were associated with significantly enlarged CBs.

1. Introduction

Carotid bodies (CBs) are small, paired organs that contain peripheral chemoreceptors and chromaffin cells. Richly supplied by blood vessels, CBs are located above the bifurcation of the common carotid artery. The amount of blood that flows through CBs is 20 times their weight per minute. Their main role is to sense the pressure of certain gases in the blood that passes through them, especially the partial pressure of O_2 and CO_2, as well as to monitor the pH level [1–4].

According to the literature, mitochondria in the glomus cells of CBs are sensitive to hypoxia. Therefore, if the arterial partial O_2 pressure decreases, the central nervous system is informed, resulting in the ventilation being stimulated. In addition to chemoreceptors, baroreceptors and thermoreceptors are also present, and some studies suggest that they play a role in glucose homeostasis as well. CBs are essential to regulating respiration and the blood circulation [5–8]. With their chromaffin cells, CBs take part in relevant processes of the sympathetic nervous system. By producing adrenaline and noradrenaline, they compensate the hypoxaemia-induced direct vasodilatation effect, promoting better adaptation [9, 10].

The hyperactivity of the chromaffin cells and their increased mass have been observed in patients with certain cardiovascular and respiratory diseases. Furthermore, the pathological processes of the liver and some metabolic or haematological states have an influence on the size of CBs' cells. Several articles have described the enlargement of CBs but did not compare the extent of the enlargement in the different diseases [11–21].

Previous studies with small groups of patients have shown that we can identify CBs reliably by computed tomography angiography (CTA) and can determine their exact size. We can identify CBs by searching for an avidly enhancing structure in its characteristic location, at the inferomedial aspect of the carotid bifurcation [22, 23].

The aim of this case-control study was to verify the enlargement of CBs with the help of CTA in a large number of patients with the following conditions: hypertension (HT); heart failure (HF) and HT; acute myocardial infarction (AMI) and HT; and chronic obstructive pulmonary disease (COPD) and HT. The second aim of the study was to determine the extent of the enlargement of CBs in the presence of the abovementioned conditions. Our purpose was to compare the measured data in order to better understand the operation of CBs and draw conclusions about their functions.

2. Materials and Methods

2.1. Study Group. The first phase of our study was to collect the records of neck carotid CTAs performed in the centre of Affidea Hungary Ltd., Szeged, during a one-year period. In total, 512 examinations were performed. Then, the conditions of the patients were investigated precisely with the help of the hospital informatics system Medsolution (International System House (ISH) Ltd., Budapest, Hungary). The International Statistical Classification of Diseases and Related Health Problems coding system provided significant help in this research. In all, 150 patients were found with sufficient information relevant to the study. Some diseases influence the size of CBs, including lesions of the liver (e.g., liver cirrhosis and hepatitis) and haematological or metabolic diseases (e.g., lactate acidosis and haemoglobinopathy). As only two patients suffered from liver cirrhosis, it was not enough for statistical analysis, so we excluded them from the study. Exclusionary haematological diseases or lactate acidosis could not be verified in any of the patients. In seven cases, we found more than two of the examined illnesses. Finally, 141 patients met the previously determined criteria and were classified according their conditions. There were 16 controls. HT alone was identified in 96 patients, HT associated with AMI in 12 patients, HF and HT in 9 patients, and COPD associated with HT in 8 patients.

All patients who suffered from HT had essential HT, and it was proven further by the criteria of blood pressure measurements. In all questionable cases, the patient underwent 24-hour ambulatory blood pressure monitoring (ABPM). In case the patient had an episode with typical ECG signs and the typical blood test, with elevated troponin level and creatine kinase level, AMI was proven in the anamnesis. In case of HF, the diagnosis was proven by echocardiography and the increased level of N-terminal pro-B-type natriuretic peptide (NT-proBNP) in the blood test. COPD was identified if spirometry proved the diagnosis by the decrease of forced expiratory volume during the first second (FEV1) and the decrease of the Tiffeneau-Pinelli index below 70%. Detailed information about the study groups is given in Table 1.

2.2. Measurement and Evaluation. The examinations were performed by using a 64-slice GE LightSpeed VCT XTe CT Scanner (General Electric, Fairfield, Connecticut, USA). The slices were obtained in the helical mode with 1.25 mm slice thickness. Patients were scanned from the aortic arch to the frontal sinus. The contrast agent (Omnipaque 350-General Electric, Fairfield, Connecticut, USA) was injected intravenously via an 18-gauge peripheral venous catheter. We used an antecubital vein if possible. When it was not feasible, the contrast material was injected into the dorsal venous network of the hand, with 50 ml of it used for each examination. We first administered 15 ml of contrast material at a rate of 2.5 ml/s and then 35 ml at a rate of 3.0 ml/s, followed by a 25 ml saline flush.

We managed the process with the SmartPrep technique. We began the examination when the contrast agent appeared in the region of interest which was in the aortic arch. The scans were uploaded to the Picture Archiving and Communication System database of GE. One of the authors, who was unaware of the clinical conditions of the patients, executed the identification and measurement of CBs twice at different times.

An axial scan was chosen for evaluation in each case because CBs could be best identified on axial scans. We used magnification if necessary. We measured the anteroposterior and the latero-lateral diameters of CBs on both sides on two occasions. The two measured areas were then averaged and used as final data. Figure 1 shows the identification processes. Figures 2 and 3 show examples from the examined groups.

2.3. Statistical Analysis. The analysis and evaluation of data were performed with SigmaPlot software package (version 13; SYSTAT Software Company Inc., San Jose, CA, USA). The Shapiro–Wilk test was used to test data for normality. The Kruskal–Wallis one-way analysis of variance on ranks test was executed to compare the results of all of the groups with each other, with $p < 0.05$ indicating significance. Dunn's multiple comparison procedure was applied to compare the groups. We also compared the measured data of the two measurement series (intraobserver variability) with the help of the Wilcoxon test.

3. Results

Successful identification of CBs was the primary criteria in the evaluation of the measured data. The identification was considered successful only if CBs were found on two separate occasions. The measured data were recorded and evaluated rigorously on both the right side (RS) and the left side (LS). On the RS, CBs were precisely detected in 129 of the 141 patients, with a success rate of 91%. Identification was even more successful on the LS, where they were clearly measured in 134 patients, with a 95% success rate.

We examined the two measurement series and compared them with each other to determine intraobserver variability. The average size ± standard deviation of the CB on the RS was $3.05 \pm 0.97\,mm^2$ for the first measurement

TABLE 1: Data for all patient groups.

Patient groups	Control	HT	AMI + HT	HF + HT	COPD + HT	Altogether
Number of patients	16	96	12	9	8	141
Female	7	47	3	5	4	66
Male	9	49	9	4	4	75
Average age (Min–Max in years)	48.63 (21–78)	65.79 (29–88)	63.58 (44–85)	65.78 (29–88)	65.38 (58–72)	61.83 (21–88)

HT, hypertension only; AMI + HT, previous acute myocardial infarction and hypertension; HF + HT, heart failure and hypertension; COPD + HT, chronic obstructive pulmonary disease and hypertension.

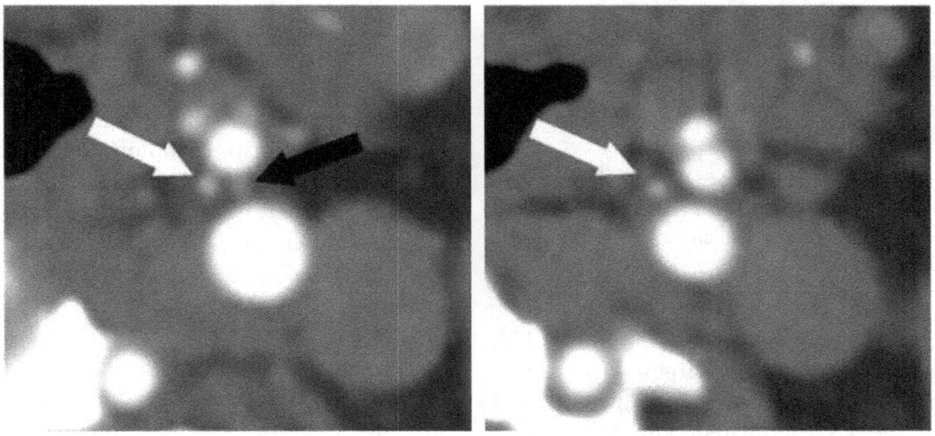

FIGURE 1: Images from a 53-year-old man in the control group (right: caudal image in which the small, avidly enhancing left carotid body (CB) (black arrow) is seen between the external carotid artery (smaller one on the ventral side) and the internal carotid artery (larger one on the dorsal side); left: a somewhat more cranial image in which the narrow branch of the external carotid artery (white arrows) is easily differentiated from the carotid body).

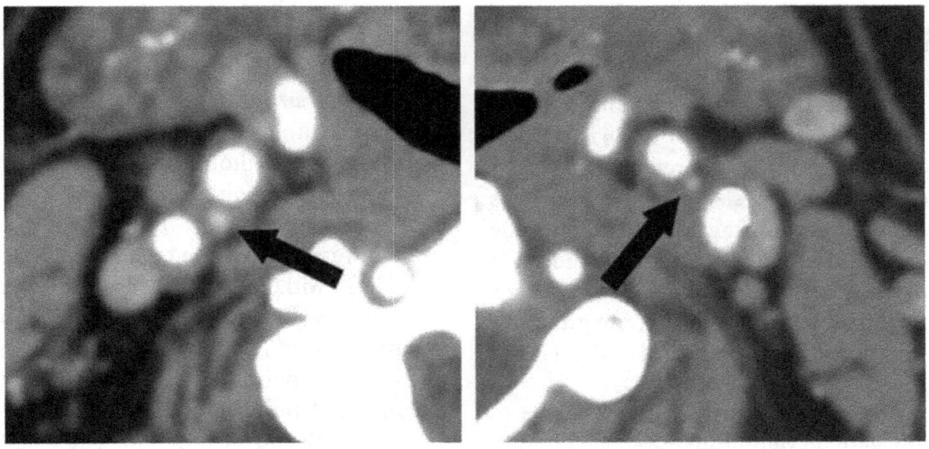

FIGURE 2: CTA shows moderately enlarged carotid bodies (arrow) on both sides in a 54-year-old woman who suffers from high blood pressure.

series and $3.04 \pm 0.89\,mm^2$ for the second one. On the LS, the average CB size was $2.94 \pm 0.88\,mm^2$ for the first measurement series and $2.95 \pm 0.87\,mm^2$ for the second series. No significant intraobserver variability was found for the cross-sectional areas ($p = 0.54$ for the RS and $p = 0.42$ for the LS).

In the control group, the average size of the CB was $2.31 \pm 0.82\,mm^2$ on the RS and $2.34 \pm 0.66\,mm^2$ on the LS. There was no significant difference between the two sides. The CB was larger in the HT-only patients ($3.07 \pm 0.81\,mm^2$ on the RS and $2.91 \pm 0.74\,mm^2$ on the LS) than in the control group. On the RS, there was a significant difference in its size between the HT-only patients and the control group ($p = 0.019$). On the LS, the difference was clear, but it was not quite at the level of significance ($p = 0.079$). In patients with AMI and HT, the average size of the CB was $3.5 \pm 0.74\,mm^2$ on the RS and $3.44 \pm 0.72\,mm^2$ on the LS. The measured data showed exactly the same tendency as in our previous assumptions: the CB was larger in patients with a prior heart attack and HT than in the HT-only patients or the controls. In the latter case, the difference was significant on both sides ($p = 0.002$ in both cases). Compared with patients with HT, the difference is detectable but not

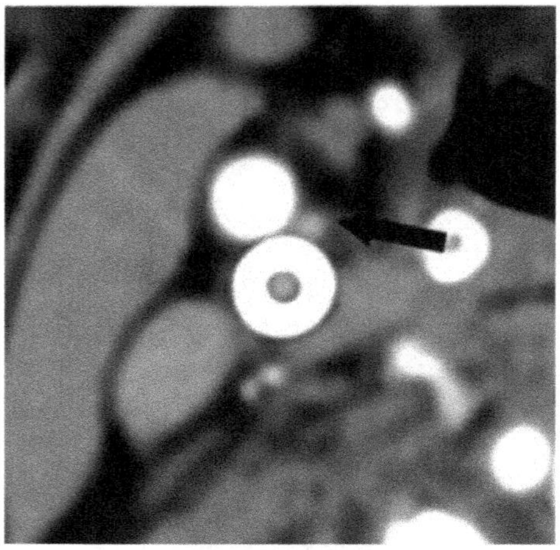

Figure 3: CTA axial slice from an 84-year-old man who had experienced a previous AMI and suffers from HT. The patient also had had a carotid stent implanted, but the enlarged CB (arrow) is still easily identified.

significant ($p = 0.583$ on the RS and $p = 0.180$ on the LS). Thus, patients with HF and HT had the largest CBs, with an average dimension of $4.01 \pm 1.39\,mm^2$ on the RS and $4.55 \pm 1.24\,mm^2$ on the LS. Compared with the control group, significance was obvious on both sides ($p = 0.003$ on the RS and $p < 0.001$ on the LS).

The average size of the CB in patients with COPD and HT was $2.40 \pm 0.54\,mm^2$ on the RS. It can be seen that the CB is smaller in these patients than in those who had HT alone. The size is almost the same as in the control group. No significant difference could be observed among the three groups. Statistically, the CB in patients who had COPD and HT was significantly smaller than that in patients with HT and HF and in those with HT and AMI ($p = 0.026$ in the first case and $p = 0.033$ in the second). Measurements on the LS showed the same results: the size of the CB was $2.29 \pm 0.27\,mm^2$. We found a significant difference with the HT and HF group ($p < 0.001$) and with the HT and AMI group ($p = 0.005$). We also compared the COPD and HT group with the control patients and the HT-only group on the LS. We could not identify a significant difference in either case.

The right and left sides were compared with each other in every examined group, with no significant differences found. The number of identified CBs, the success rate of identification, and the average size of CBs for the right side are shown in Table 2, and those for the left side are shown in Table 3. Figures 4 and 5 show the results and the significant pairs. The significant pairs and p values for every case are shown in Table 4.

4. Discussion

It is well known that CBs play an important role in regulating the respiratory and blood circulation systems. They are the most important chemosensors, baroreceptors, and thermoreceptors in the human body besides the brain. These sensors instigate the flow of information to the central nervous system about possible hypoxia. Their chromaffin cells participate in the activity of the sympathetic nervous system as well. As it is known, these cells are mostly located in the medulla of the adrenal gland. They produce noradrenaline and adrenaline, thereby playing a role in stimulating the sympathetic nervous system. It is important to compensate for the hypoxaemia-induced direct vasodilatation effect, thereby helping improve adaptation [3–10].

CBs enlarge significantly in the presence of cardiovascular diseases such as HT or HF. Moreover, it seems that respiratory diseases such as COPD and pathological processes of the liver as well as some metabolic or haematological states also influence the size and histologic structure of CBs. In these cases, the sympathetic nervous system might be overactivated, so the number of the chromaffin cells in this system could be increased. The role of CBs in the formation, progression, and maintenance of these diseases is still not fully clarified. The main problem is that some of the available data about CBs are derived from postmortem examinations, animal experiments, and studies with small groups of patients [7, 9, 12–14].

In patients with HT or HF or following AMI, the sympathetic tone could be intensified. In this study, we intended to evaluate the morphological signs related to this role of the CB based on alteration of its size. Hence, the carotid CTA examinations of 141 patients were reanalysed retrospectively. It was clearly proved that CBs could be reliably identified using this technique, with a success rate of >90%. Advanced calcification around the bifurcation or on a previously built-in metal stent makes measurement more difficult, as either situation deforms the normal anatomic conditions. As can be seen in Figure 3, there were some cases in which the size of the CB could be clearly measured despite the complicating conditions. Jie et al. [12] examined CBs by ultrasound. Even though they had studied a larger group, we could achieve a higher success rate of identification by our CTA study.

Our results confirmed that CBs are significantly enlarged in patients with HT. Previously, Habeck et al. [13] and Honig et al. [14] verified the enlargement of CBs in rats with high blood pressure. Presumably, because of the permanently increased activity of the sympathetic nervous system, the volume and number of chromaffin cells increase, thereby increasing the size of the CB. The significant enlargement proven by the measurements verified our assumptions and confirmed the results of previous studies. Sreejit et al. [23] proved that the volume of CBs also grows in patients with both HT and HF. Based on previous pathologic and pathophysiologic data, it is obvious that the simultaneous presence of the two diseases would further increase the sympathetic activity. Our CTA results verified this tendency of increase in vital situations. We measured significantly larger volumes on both sides in patients with both HT and HF versus the control group and the HT-only group. We also found that if the patients had not only HT but also a previous AMI, CBs had enlarged, although its size did not reach that in the HT and HF group. Perhaps the durations of the two diseases were responsible for the difference in the amount of enlargement.

TABLE 2: Success rate of identification and comparison of cross-sectional areas of the right CB.

Right side	Control	HT	AMI + HT	HF + HT	COPD + HT
Identified CBs	15	89	11	7	7
Success rate of identification (%)	93.75	92.7	91.67	77.78	87.5
Mean size of the CB (mm^2)	2.31	3.07	3.56	4.01	2.40
Standard deviation (±)	0.82	0.81	0.74	1.39	0.54

TABLE 3: Success rate of identification and comparison of cross-sectional areas of the left CB.

Left side	Control	HT	AMI + HT	HF + HT	COPD + HT
Identified CBs	16	91	12	7	8
Success rate of identification (%)	100	92.71	100	77.78	100
Mean size of the CB (mm^2)	2.34	2.91	3.44	4.55	2.29
Standard deviation (±)	0.66	0.74	0.72	1.24	0.27

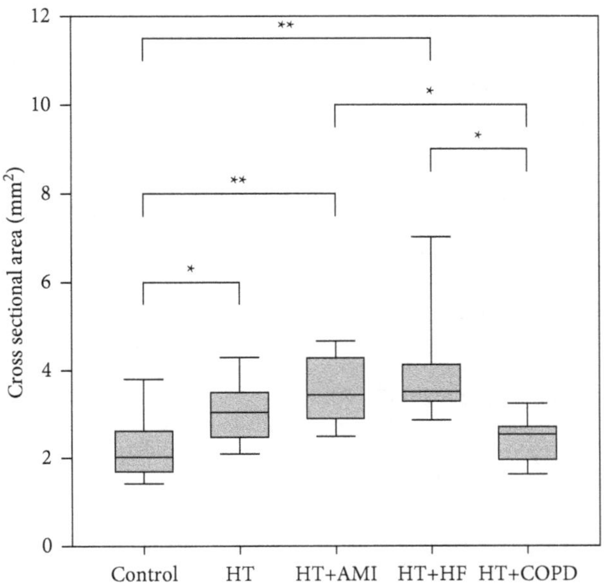

FIGURE 4: Our results and significant pairs ($^{*}p < 0.05$ and $^{**}p < 0.01$) for the right-side carotid bodies with the standard deviations. HT, hypertension; AMI, acute myocardial infarction; HF, heart failure; COPD, chronic obstructive pulmonary disease.

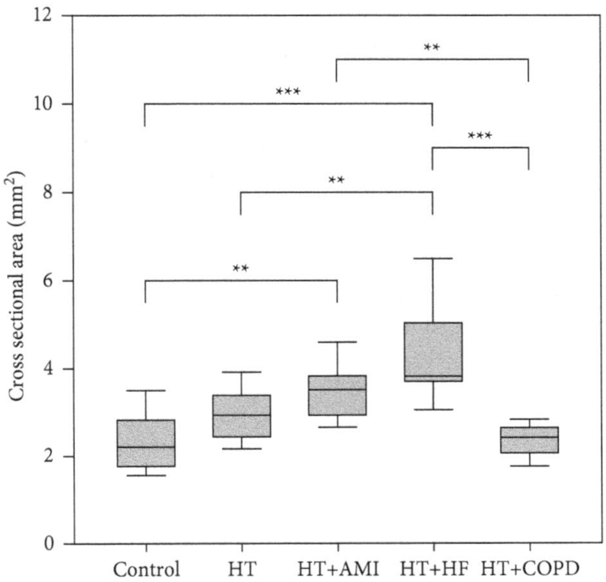

FIGURE 5: Significant differences ($^{*}p < 0.05$, $^{**}p < 0.01$, and $^{***}p < 0.001$) and the measured cross-sectional sizes of the left-side carotid bodies.

Based on previous studies, we assumed that the diameter of CBs enlarges in patients with COPD. Our measured data, however, did not corroborate that tendency. The recorded sizes on both sides were nearly the same as those in the control group with no significant difference. In a recent article, Vinhaes et al. [24] proved histologically that the construction of cells and their proportions change not only in COPD patients but also in those with acute respiratory distress syndrome. We thus assume that the increase in size is not the main determining change in COPD. Histologic remodelling is probably much more important in these diseases. Another reason we may not find larger areas is that COPD is an umbrella designation under which various illnesses reside. These different types of disease could affect CBs in different ways and to different degrees. Further analysis of the relations could be useful.

There are some limitations of our study, which we intend to solve in the future. First, it was not possible to measure catecholamine production by CBs directly, so we judged this function according to CB size. Second, although our study is based on a large group of patients, some of the subgroups were small. Thus, we have the data about medication of patients and the stage or grade of examined diseases; these could not submit accurate statistical analysis. It would be interesting to examine the nontreated or the not appropriately treated cases in separate groups. This evaluation could provide evidence to prove that the size of CBs correlate

TABLE 4: Significant pairs on the right and left sides using the p value.

Right side		p	Left side		p
Control	HT	0.019	Control	AMI + HT	0.002
Control	AMI + HT	0.002	Control	HF + HT	<0.001
Control	HF + HT	0.003	HT	HF + HT	0.005
COPD + HT	AMI + HT	0.033	COPD + HT	AMI + HT	0.005
COPD + HT	HF + HT	0.026	COPD + HT	HF + HT	<0.001

with the medical treatment and with the severity of the disease. It could be the subject of our following study.

The aims for the future are to widen the group of examined patients and to execute prospective measurements. These additions would provide more accurate information from the patients, and the abovementioned obstacles could be eliminated. Further improvement could be achieved if the resolution was enhanced and if the measurements were done on, for example, MRI scans as well or were compared with them [25–27].

5. Conclusion

We proved, using CTA, that CBs are indeed enlarged in patients with diseases that cause the sympathetic nervous system's operation to be intensified. Based on our measurements in patients with HT, the diameter of CBs is significantly larger than that of CBs in the average, healthy individuals. Its size further enlarges in patients who in addition to HT also have HF or AMI in the anamnesis. Taking our measurements into consideration allows the possibility of drawing conclusions about the physiologic and general state of the patient after analysing his or her anatomic structures on CTA. This protocol could provide us and clinicians additional information about the patient. In the future, it could be interesting to increase the number of patients and to analyse precisely the treatment used. It would allow the possibility of determining the efficacy of treatment of these diseases.

Abbreviations

ABPM:	Ambulatory blood pressure monitoring
AMI:	Acute myocardial infarction
CB:	Carotid body
COPD:	Chronic obstructive pulmonary disease
CTA:	Computed tomography angiography
FEV1:	Forced expiratory volume during the first second
HF:	Heart failure
HT:	Hypertension
LS:	Left side
RS:	Right side
NT-proBNP:	N-terminal pro-B-type natriuretic peptide.

Additional Points

Highlights.(1) The carotid body plays a role in sympathetic nervous system activity;(2) the size of the carotid body can be reliably measured by computed tomography angiography; and (3) the carotid body is enlarged in certain diseases with increased sympathetic activity.

Acknowledgments

The authors gratefully acknowledge the support of Affidea Hungary Ltd. The authors wish to thank Dr. Fanni Magdolna Márványkövi for English language editing and contributors of Department of Radiology, University of Szeged, for their technical assistance.

References

[1] D. Heath and P. Smith, "The nature of the carotid body," *Diseases of the Human Carotid Body*, Springer, London, UK, 1 edition, 1992.

[2] V. A. Safonov and N. N. Tarasova, "Structural and functional organization of the respiratory center," *Human Physiology*, vol. 32, no. 1, pp. 103–115, 2006.

[3] I. Rodrigo, "Translating carotid body function into clinical medicine," *Journal of Physiology*, vol. 596/15, pp. 3067–3077, 2018.

[4] J. Nanduri and N. R. Prabhakar, "Epigenetic regulation of carotid body oxygen sensing: clinical implications," *Advances in Experimental Medicine & Biology*, vol. 5/524, pp. 1–8, 2015.

[5] R. P. Nanduri, P. Ying-Jie, K. K. Ganesh, and N. Jayasri, "Peripheral chemoreception and arterial pressure responses to intermittent hypoxia," *Comprehensive Physiology*, vol. 5/2, pp. 561–577, 2015.

[6] I. Yuichi, "Oxygen sensing in the carotid body: inhibited hypoxic respiratory with muscle relaxant," *Journal of Anesthesia*, vol. 16, pp. 271-272, 2002.

[7] L. S. Gregg and R. P. Nanduri, "The role of hypoxia-inducible factors in carotid body (patho) physiology," *Journal of Physiology*, vol. 596/15, pp. 2977–2983, 2018.

[8] I. Rodrigo, C. A. David, and D. R. Rodrigo, "Enhanced carotid body chemosensory activity and the cardiovascular alterations induced by intermittent hypoxia," *Frontiers in Physiology*, vol. 5/468, pp. 1–9, 2014.

[9] J. K. Limberg, J. L. Taylor, M. T. Mozer et al., "Effect of bilateral carotid body resection on cardiac baroreflex control of blood pressure during hypoglycemia," *Hypertension*, vol. 65, no. 6, pp. 1365–1371, 2015.

[10] J. P. T. Ward, "Oxygen sensors in context," *Biochimica et Biophysica Acta (BBA) - Bioenergetics*, vol. 1777, no. 1, pp. 1–14, 2008.

[11] J.-O. Habeck, "Peripheral arterial chemoreceptors and hypertension," *Journal of the Autonomic Nervous System*, vol. 34, no. 1, pp. 1–7, 1991.

[12] T. Jie, X. Bo, Z. Yefeng, Y. Yuanqing, Q. Jun, and R. Shunkang, "Carotid body enlargement in hypertension and other comorbidities evaluated by ultrasonography," *Journal of Hypertension*, vol. 37/7, pp. 1455–1462, 2019.

[13] J. O. Habeck, C. Huckstorf, and A. Honig, "Influence of age on position, shape and size of the carotid bodies in spontaneously hypertensive (SHR) and normotensive (NCR) rats," *Anatomischer Anzeiger*, vol. 157, pp. 351–363, 1984.

[14] A. Honig, J. O. Habeck, C. Pfeiffer et al., "The carotid bodies of spontaneously hypertensive rats (SHR): a functional and morphologic study," *Acta Biologica et Medica Germanica*, vol. 40, pp. 1021–1030, 1981.

[15] P. Jaźwiec, P. Gać, M. Jurdziak et al., "Volume of carotid bodies and cardiac autonomic function in patients with essential hypertension," *Autonomic Neuroscience: Basic & Clinical*, vol. 190, pp. 26–32, 2015.

[16] H. D. Schultz and Y. L. Li, "Carotid body function in heart failure," *Respiratory Physiology & Neurobiology*, vol. 157, no. 1, pp. 171–185, 2007.

[17] D. S. Harold, J. M. Noah, and D. R. Rodrigo, "Role of the carotid body in the pathophysiology of heart failure," *Current Hypertension Reports*, vol. 15/4, pp. 356–362, 2013.

[18] J. M. Noah, D. R. Rodrigo, and D. S. Harold, "Central role of carotid body chemoreceptors in disordered breathing and cardiorenal dysfunction in chronic heart failure," *Frontiers in Physiology*, vol. 5/438, pp. 1–7, 2014.

[19] Y. Ding, Y. Li, K. G. Cornish, and H. D. Schultz, "Reduced blood flow in carotid arteries is a trigger contributing to peripheral chemoreflex hypersensitivity in chronic heart failure rabbits," *The FASEB Journal*, vol. 21/6, pp. 1268-1269, 2007.

[20] D. Heath and P. Smith, "The carotid bodies enlarge in some cases of cirrhosis of the liver," *Cardioscience*, vol. 5/1, pp. 37–41, 1994.

[21] C. Edwards, D. Heath, and P. Harris, "The carotid body in emphysema and left ventricular hypertrophy," *The Journal of Pathology*, vol. 104, no. 1, pp. 1–13, 1971.

[22] R. P. Nguyen, L. M. Shah, E. P. Quigley, H. R. Harnsberger, and R. H. Wiggins, "Carotid body detection on CT angiography," *American Journal of Neuroradiology*, vol. 32, no. 6, pp. 1096–1099, 2011.

[23] N. Sreejit, G. Ajay, F. Marat, R. Christopher, R. Vinay, and H. R. Sandra, "CT angiography in the detection of carotid body enlargement in patients with hypertension and heart failure," *Neuroradiology*, vol. 55, pp. 1319–1322, 2013.

[24] E. N. G. Vinhaes, M. Dolhnikoff, and P. H. N. Saldiva, "Morphological changes of carotid bodies in acute respiratory distress syndrome: a morphometric study in humans," *Brazilian Journal of Medical and Biological Research*, vol. 35, no. 10, pp. 1119–1125, 2002.

[25] J. F. R. Paton, P. A. Sobotka, M. Fudim et al., "The carotid body as a therapeutic target for the treatment of sympathetically mediated diseases," *Hypertension*, vol. 61, no. 1, pp. 5–13, 2013.

[26] S. F. Robert, "Carotid body: a new target for rescuing neural control of cardiorespiratory balance in disease," *Frontiers in Physiology*, vol. 5/304, pp. 1–4, 2014.

[27] D. R. Rodrigo, J. M. Noah, and D. S. Harold, "Carotid chemoreceptor ablation improves survival in heart failure: rescuing autonomic control of cardiorespiratory function," *Journal of the American College of Cardiology*, vol. 62/25, pp. 2422–2430, 2013.

17

A Study of a New Technique of the CT Scan View and Disease Classification Protocol Based on Level Challenges in Cases of Coronavirus Disease

Ahmed B. Salem Salamh,[1] **Abdulrauf A. Salamah**,[2] **and Halil Ibrahim Akyüz**[3]

[1]*Institute of Science, Material Science and Engineering, Kastamonu University, Kuzey Kent /P.O. Box, 37150, Kastamonu, Kastamonu, Turkey*
[2]*Tripoli Central Hospital, P.O. Box 15528, Tripoli, Libya*
[3]*Computer and Teaching Technologies Education, Kastamonu University, Kuzey Kent /P.O. Box, 37150, Kastamonu, Kastamonu, Turkey*

Correspondence should be addressed to Abdulrauf A. Salamah; abd.elr.salamah@gmail.com

Academic Editor: André Luiz Ferreira COSTA

The chest Computer Tomography (CT scan) is used in the diagnosis of coronavirus disease 2019 (COVID-19) and is an important complement to the Reverse Transcription Polymerase Chain Reaction (RT-PCR) test. The paper aims to improve the radiological diagnosis in the case of coronavirus disease COVID-19 pneumonia on forms of noninvasive approaches with conventional and high-resolution computer tomography (HRCT) scan images upon chest CT images of patients confirmed with mild to severe findings. The preliminary study is to compare the radiological findings of COVID-19 pneumonia in conventional chest CT images with images processed by a new tool and reviewed by expert radiologists. The researchers used a new filter called Golden Key Tool (GK-Tool) which has confirmed the improvement in the quality and diagnostic efficacy of images acquired using our modified images. Further, Convolution Neural Networks (CNNs) architecture called VGG face was used to classify chest CT images. The classification has been performed by using VGG face on various datasets which are considered as a protocol to diagnose COVID-19, Non-COVID-19 (other lung diseases), and normal cases (no findings on chest CT). Accordingly, the performance evaluation of the GK-Tool was fairly good as shown in the first set of results, where 80–95% of participants show a good to excellent assessment of the new images view in the case of COVID-19 patients. The results, in general, illustrate good recognition rates in the diagnosis and, therefore, would be significantly higher in normal cases with COVID-19. These results could reduce the radiologist's workload burden and play a major role in the decision-making process.

1. Introduction

In the first half of this year, on March 13, 2020, the World Health Organization (WHO) officially notified that the novel coronavirus disease (COVID-19) had become a global pandemic. COVID-19 is caused by severe acute respiratory syndrome coronavirus 2 (SARS-CoV-2) depicting a potentially fatal disease. [1]. Many previous studies have reported that the CT imaging features and correlation of chest computed tomography (CT) and reverse transcription polymerase chain reaction (RT-PCR) testing showed infections with SARS-CoV-2 [2–4]. The high false-negative rates and time-consuming RT-PCR affect the efficacy of this test [5, 6]. The asymptomatic cases of COVID-19 pneumonia CT scan images have definite characteristics and have important value in screening and detecting patients with COVID-19 pneumonia, especially in the highly suspicious cases with negative PCR testing. [7, 8]. Another diagnostic method to diagnosis and treatment guideline for COVID-19 pneumonia, issued by the National Health Commission of

The People's Republic of China is the CT, especially the high-resolution CT (HRCT) [9]. The CT examination of patients with COVID-19 pneumonia shows mixed and various patterns with both lung parenchyma and interstitial involvement. Represented with ground-glass opacity (GGO) with different manifestations which could be a solitary lesion at early-phase disease, the signs of aggravation and repair are seen in the advanced phase. Lesions presented with characteristic multifocal areas predominantly distributed in the middle and lower lung regions and in the posterior lung area. [10]. The most common chest findings of COVID-19 in CT images are multiple GGO, consolidation, crazy-paving, and interlobular septal thickening in both lungs, which are mostly distributed at subpleural locations in the lower lobes but the findings are nonspecific and can be found in other illness, including cancer [11]. There are significant correlations between the degree of pulmonary inflammation and the main clinical symptoms and laboratory results. In the emerging global health emergency, the computed tomography plays a major role in the diagnosis and evaluation [12, 13]. Usually, the chest CT abnormalities significantly increased in number up to 10 weeks (the peak at approximately 10 days). Subsequently, there were a short plateau phase and a gradual decrease in abnormalities with time [14]. There is obvious evidence that fatigue, particularly after long shift duty, is related to serious medical errors and can increase the risk of missing the image findings, especially during and pandemic time that complicates the situation and leads to more medical errors. [15, 16]. In general, it is divided into two main subtypes: the first one is physical and the second is mental fatigue. Especially in outbreak time, it is noted that physical fatigue comes first, which leads to deterioration in the muscle ability to create or sustain forces, which happens due to difficulties in controlling and coordinating muscles. Mental fatigue is a reduction in the ability to perform mental tasks and responses [17]. In general, newer techniques can potentially facilitate radiology department workflow, increase radiologist accuracy, improve detection of findings, reduce the possibility of medical error, and enhance patient health care [18]. Moreover, the outbreak likely persists for a foreseeable period as well with peaks. For immediate preparedness, the radiology in its ongoing battle against COVID-19 must reconsider and readjust the workflows and leverage new technologies and applications [19]. Recent modern trends show increased and rapid use of machine learning (ML) in the medical field, including computer-aided diagnosis (CAD), radio-mics, and radiology department [20]. In the last century, the first class of Neural Networks (NNs), called Convolutional Neural Network (CNN) was reported which showed enormous potential in machine vision (MV) related tasks [21]. The CNN designs are based on the architecture that performs traffic sign classification related tasks with a good recognition rate. This method uses a deep CNN which has been widely used for image classification and trained to classify faces using a VGG face (Deep Face) Figure 1 [8, 22]. The CNN "deep learning," in medical imaging is an explosively growing, promising field [23, 24].

2. Patients and Methods

2.1. Patients. Now we know that the COVID-19 chest CT view shows a pattern of ground-glass opacity in the lung leading to "consolidation" in advanced stages of the diseases. As seen in Figure 2. CT results become more widespread for a longer duration after the onset of symptoms, including consolidation, bilateral and peripheral disease, and overall lung involvement, linear opacities, "crazy-paving" pattern, and the "reverse halo" sign [25]. The data utility of CT views in the case of COVID-19 has been confirmed by a senior radiologist in Tongji Hospital, Wuhan, China, who had performed the diagnosis and treatment on a large number of COVID-19 patients during the outbreak of this disease between January and April [16, 26].

2.2. CT Images Acquisition and Preprocessing. The data of original CT images quality degradation during different utility and their negative impacts included Hounsfield unit (HU), any values lost, the number of bits per pixel, the resolutions reducing in comparison with original CT images, and putting into papers and about choosing only a few key slices to detect the diagnosis. The researchers consulted the aforementioned radiologist from China Tongji Hospital about these concerns. The problems posed in these considerations do not substantially affect the accuracy of diagnosis decision-making, according to the radiologist. They confirmed that any basic experienced radiologist will be able to make accurate diagnoses from low-quality CT images. The quality gap between CT images in papers and original CT images may not largely affect the accuracy of diagnosis. Moreover, one read of a single-slice of CT may provide enough clinical information for accurate decision-making. The information about the tomography type, brand, model, and fabrication companies are not available due to the characteristics of the retrospective study.

2.3. CT Image Square Root Equation. The main objective from design preprocessing filter to change lung CT image view from conventional view which means black and white to newer ones which can illustrate such improvement in the pattern with a new view. This can help in the major differentiation between the findings in COVID-19 cases. Square root equation (SRE) (1) operator's main idea is as follows: the first step is to convert lung CT image to gray-scale. The second step is taking pixel point (x_T, y_T) as the center point of 3–3 windows in an (m-n) image. The third step is applying the square root around the central point pixel value (x_T, y_T) as g_i, with the adjacent eight-pixel values being a_0-a_7, Figure 2.

Total summation of squaring adjacent eight-pixel values with the subtraction of 255 value with introducing the final feature point replaced by the central point pixel value as shown in the following equation:

$$SRE = 255 - \sum_{s=0}^{Z-1}\left(\sqrt[2]{(adjacent\ (g_s) * \sqrt[2]{p}}\right), \qquad (1)$$

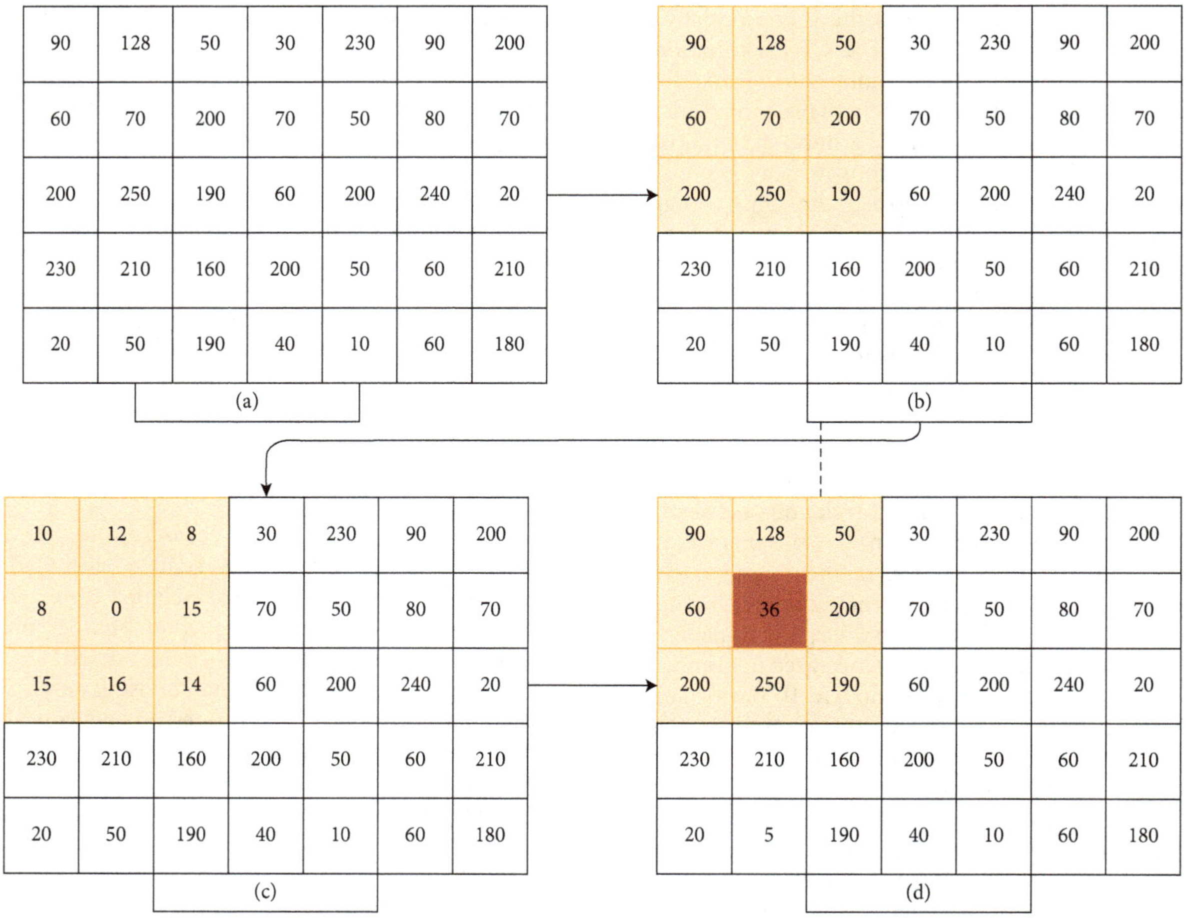

FIGURE 1: Demonstration of the steps to compute the square root value. The result would be varying based of P value and each value of square root must be rounded off. (a) Example of the original example of the image, (b) The determination of 3 neighbors, (c) The square root of 3 neighbors of center value, and (d) The final equation result value with $P = 5$.

where $z = 8$, $p = 1, 2, \ldots\ldots\ldots N : N \leq 16$ and g_s three neighbors of center value. The value of p is represented from 1 to 16 which introduce various differentiations. Based on this, each value of p must be selected to accommodate its applications. The pseudocode for the square root equation is as seen in Algorithm 1.

2.4. Deep Learning Model. In the case of image classification, Convolution Neural Network is the most important field in the sense of machine vision. CNN has obtained several achievements in the area of classification, segmentation, and recognition. The instant grayscale image is a 2D array and a color image is a combination of three 2D arrays. The CNNs are designed to operate on data that is in the form of multiple arrays [27].

The major field of CNN is in medical imaging, particularly for the diagnosis of cancer using image classification based on histopathological images. CNN recently is often used to diagnose images of breast cancer, and findings are contrasted with a network trained on a dataset containing local features descriptors [24, 28]. Figure 3 represents the VGG model of CNN used in this paper presenting in detail the CNN with its configuration in Table 1. The model used in this paper is based on the following steps:

(i) Pretrained model
(ii) Transfer learning
(iii) Fine-tune the model

2.5. Matrices Evaluation and Statistical Analysis. In order to evaluate and compare the performance of the CNNs, the indices were as follows:

(i) Accuracy (Acc):

$$ACC = \frac{TP + TN}{TP + TN + FP + FN}. \tag{2}$$

(ii) Error rate (ERR):

$$EER = 1 - ACC. \tag{3}$$

(iii) Sensitivity or true positive rate (TPR):

$$TPR = \frac{TP}{TP + FN}. \tag{4}$$

(iv) Specificity or true negative rate (TNR):

$$TNR = \frac{TP}{FP + TN}. \tag{5}$$

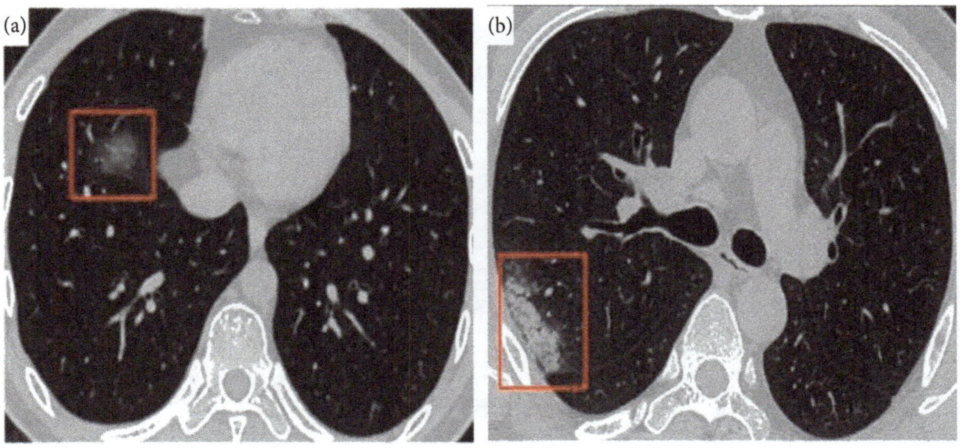

FIGURE 2: (a) Chest CT scan image shows a pure ground-glass opacity (GGO) in the right lower lobe (red frame). (b) Consolidation in the right lobe subpleural area (red frame).

(1) START
(2) INPUT CT_Scan_Image (Covid19)
(3) READ the value of **P**
(4) FOR each pixel in input image
(5) FOR each 3 ∗ 3 neighbors
(6) COMPUTE **SRE** new feature as SRE = $255 - \sum_{s=0}^{Z-1} (\sqrt[2]{(\text{adjacent}(g_s)} * \sqrt[2]{p})$.
(7) Replace the new value SRE with center pixel of 3 ∗ 3 with new image
(8) ENDFOR
(9) ENDFOR
(10) SHOW the new CT_Scan_Image (Covid19)
(11) End

ALGORITHM 1: Pseudocode for square root equation.

(v) Positive prediction value (PPV):

$$PPV = \frac{TP}{FP + TP}. \quad (6)$$

(vi) False positive rates (FPR):

$$FPR = 1 = TNR. \quad (7)$$

(vii) F-Measure or F1 score

$$\text{F1\_score} = \frac{2TP}{2TP + FP + FN}. \quad (8)$$

(viii) Matthews's correlation coefficient (MCC)

$$MCC = \frac{TP * TN - FP * FN}{\sqrt{(TP + FP)(TP + FN)(TN + FP)(TN + FN)}}. \quad (9)$$

3. Results and Discussions

The presentation images view in CT scan and the sensitivity in radiology diagnosis and detections can be improved. These improvements further have an effective potential in clinical applications, implementation, and structure. It also enhances the role of radiologists, who indirectly have a strong impact on radiology department outcomes especially during overload works. The diagnosis of COVID-19 by the use of imaging processes called GK-Tool with other conventional CT chest scans (COVID-19 pneumonia) is being compared and assessed by radiologists. In this study, the researchers have used CT images of patients already confirmed with COVID-19. The diagnosis has been made on patients belonging to both genders. The radiologists and experts in this field who reviewed the images have good experience in thoracic imaging for more than five years. All radiologists have reviewed the CT images of COVID-19 patients with defined regions of infections and reviewed the lung CT slices of different images with and without processing as seen in Figure 4. The performance reports were collected based on visual inspection of CT different images slices and views on a given scale from 1 to 5 points. The results illustrate that 80–95% of participants gave "good to excellent" assessment ratings on the images view improvement and the diagnosis sensitivity in the case of COVID-19 patients; refer to Tables 2 and 3. The researchers have considered engaging several radiologists from different hospitals and from different academic backgrounds to get an improved perspective and evaluation.

The critical and important issues for radiologists are to improve the sensitivity in the diagnosis and differentiating of

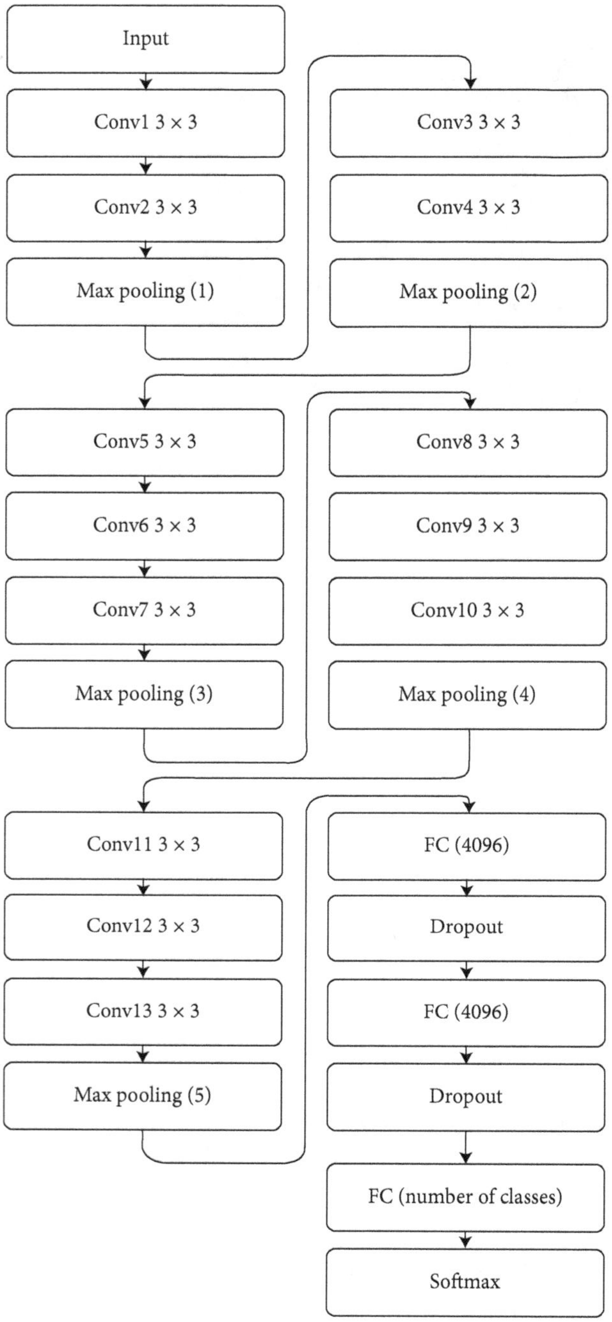

FIGURE 3: Deep learning VGG face architecture.

TABLE 1: Network configuration. Details of VGG face CNN configuration where N is the number of classes.

Layer name	Input size	Filters	Padding, stride, filter size
Conv1	224 × 224	64	1, 1, 3
Conv2	224 × 224	64	1, 1, 3
Max Pooling (1)	224 × 224	—	0, 2, —
Conv3	112 × 112	128	1, 1, 3
Conv4	112 × 112	128	1, 1, 3
Max Pooling (2)	112 × 112	—	0, 2, —
Conv5	56 × 56	256	1, 1, 3
Conv6	56 × 56	256	1, 1, 3
Conv7	56 × 56	256	1, 1, 3
Max Pooling (3)	56 × 56	—	0, 2, —
Conv8	28 × 28	512	1, 1, 3
Conv9	28 × 28	512	1, 1, 3
Conv10	28 × 28	512	1, 1, 3
Max Pooling (4)	28 × 28	—	0, 2, —
Conv11	14 × 14	512	1, 1, 3
Conv12	14 × 28	512	1, 1, 3
Conv13	14 × 14	512	1, 1, 3
Max Pooling (5)	28 × 28	—	0, 2, —
Output	7 × 7		
Fully connected	4096		
Dropout	0.5		
Fully connected	4096		
Dropout	0.5		
Fully connected	N classes		
Softmax	N classes		

COVID-19 from other typical diseases. The CNN's "deep learning" in medical imaging is rising exponentially thereby providing the detection of several diseases. The technology of using CNN VGG face can be very helpful to improve the performance in the radiology department. Further, it can give a rapid triaging of radiological findings detection and the technique that can potentially facilitate radiology department workflow. However, this paper is constrained to describe technical information and internal processing (data entry, implementation of CNNs, training, and result phases) about deep learning with CNNs by construction which contains different identities based on CT images' findings from our dataset. The four datasets taken as the protocol in order to assist the decision-making for any global pandemic are as mentioned below.

3.1. Dataset 1: COVID-19 and Normal Cases. Dataset 1 is a comparison between chest CT images of COVID-19 cases with normal cases. The researchers entered 349 CT images with different slices of confirmed cases of COVID-19 and 55 images of normal image cases. The dataset of COVID-19 cases included the early stage, presented with pure GGOs progressive stage; multiple GGOs, consolidations in lesions, crazy-paving pattern and the extensive stage, diffuse exudative lesions and white lung lesions [13, 29]. The evaluation performance of COVID-19 with normal cases achieved an accuracy of 100% for all matrices indicating that the system handles the problem perfectly. Refer to Figure 5.

3.2. Dataset 2: COVID-19 with Normal and Non-COVID-19 (20) Cases. Dataset 2 shows a comparison between chest CT images of COVID-19 cases with non-COVID-19 cases (other lung diseases that have similar findings in chest CT scan). The sample entered 349 chest CT images with different slices of confirmed cases of COVID-19, 55 images of normal image cases, and 20 images of non-COVID-19 cases. The evaluation matrices show fairly good accuracy 93.478% with an error of 6.5217% as seen in Figure 6. The precision showed the proportion of positive classes truly classified to the total number of positive predicted as 97.33%. F1 score gives the harmonic mean of precision and recalls with 87.5% indicating fairly good classification performance. Considering the other matrices evaluation in the figure, the system

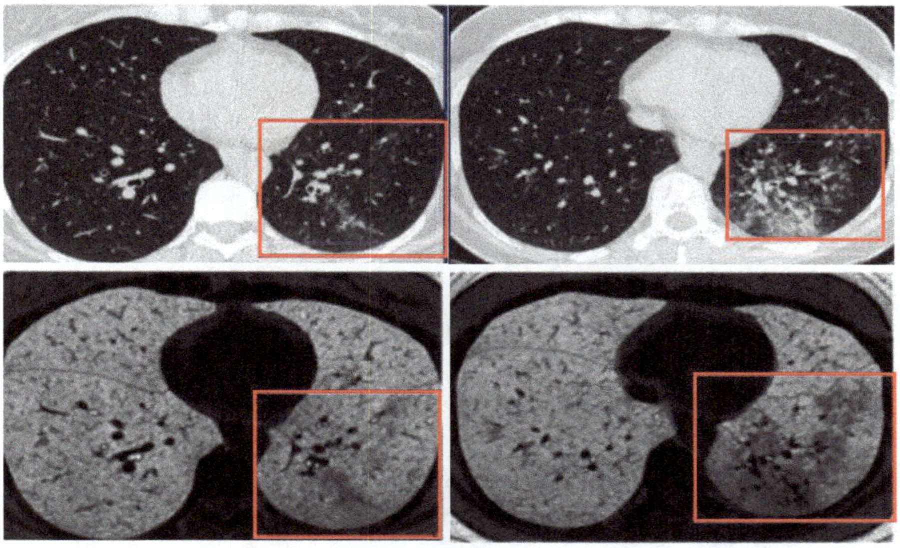

FIGURE 4: Lung CT images of COVID-19 findings before and after the process. The findings are in (red frame).

TABLE 2: The scale results illustrate a good assessment of the images view improvement by radiologists.

		Good			
		Frequency	Percent	Valid percent	Cumulative percent
Valid	4.00	15	78.9	100.0	100.0
Missing	System	4	21.1		
Total		19	100.0		

TABLE 3: The scale results illustrate an excellent assessment of the images view improvement by radiologists.

		Excellent			
		Frequency	Percent	Valid percent	Cumulative percent
Valid	5.00	18	94.7	100.0	100.0
Missing	System	1	5.3		
Total		19	100.0		

manages the challenges of COVID-19 and non-COVID-19 perfectly.

3.3. Dataset 3: COVID-19 and 20 of Non-COVID-19 Cases. Dataset 3 shows a comparison between chest CT images of COVID-19 cases with non-COVID-19 cases (other lung diseases that have similar findings in chest CT scan). The researchers entered 349 CT images with different slices of confirmed cases of COVID-19 along with 396 non-COVID-19 images cases. The most important challenge facing COVID-19 and Non-COVID-19 cases is disease similarity; for this reason, the differentiation is very hard to measure between two cases. The total accuracy of the system with COVID-19 and non-COVID-19 is 90.123% indicating good performance as seen in Figure 7. The misclassification rate is 9.87% and the precision is 90.6% for the percentage of positive classes to the total number of positive prediction. The false-positive rate is 8.6% seen as an indicator of the proportion of the negative classes that were falsely classified.

3.4. Dataset 4: COVID-19 and All Non-COVID-19 Cases. Dataset 4 is a comparison between chest CT images of COVID-19 cases with non-COVID-19 cases (other lung diseases that have related chest CT scan observations as stated earlier). The researchers entered 349 CT images with different slices of confirmed cases of COVID-19 and 396 images of non-COVID-19 cases. According to the original dataset, the challenges in this case have increased by using the total number of non-COVID-19. This means that in the cases of other COVID-19 diseases, and by considering this difficulty, the system has achieved total accuracy of 85.14%. The rate of misclassification was 14.86% which reflected the number of metrics misclassified cases of both positive and negative classes. By considering the challenges and problems of the datasets, the performance is fairly good for this case.

3.5. Performance Comparison of COVID-19 Datasets. The evaluation comparison of four datasets that represent different challenges of differentiation and similarity is consistent. This is evident from dataset 1 of COVID-19 with normal cases which achieved high performance with 100% accuracy as shown in Figure 8. In dataset 2, COVID-19 with a limited number of non-COVID-19 with normal cases achieved an accuracy of 93.48%, as the level of challenges index becomes higher, the accuracy decreases. In dataset 3, COVID-19 with non-COVID-19 (other diseases) showed accuracy at 90.123%, reflecting the difficulty of distinguishing the similarity between the two cases. The most difficult cases were observed in dataset 4 containing countless COVID-19 (other diseases) which achieved 85.14% accuracy.

The line of challenges for four datasets reflects the level of problems and this is clearly observed in the relationship between accuracy and level of challenges corresponding to

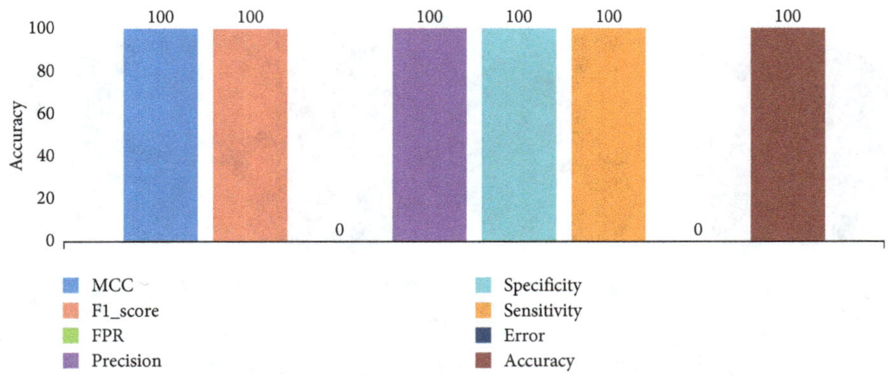

FIGURE 5: Overall, the values of COVID-19 with normal cases.

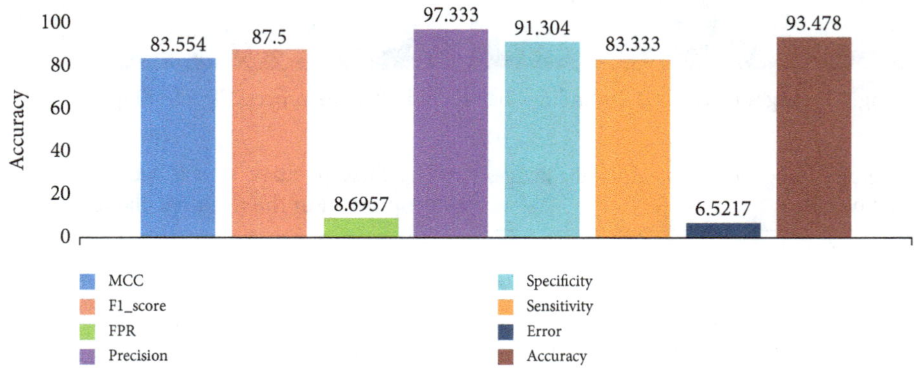

FIGURE 6: COVID-19 with normal and non-COVID-19 cases.

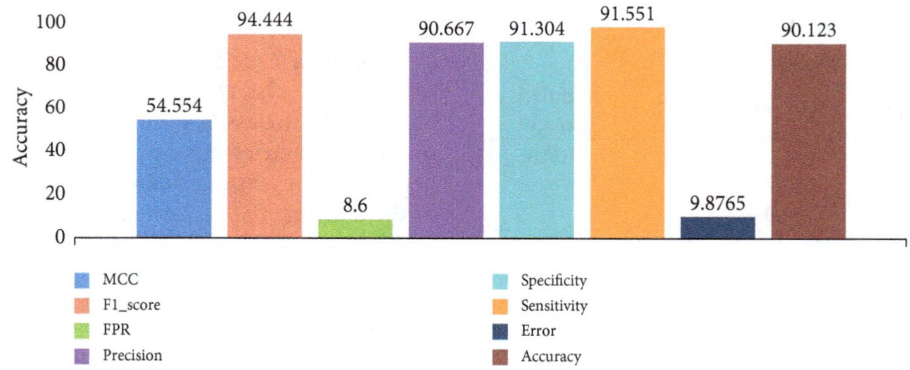

FIGURE 7: Overall values of COVID-19 with only 20 cases of Non-COVID-19 cases.

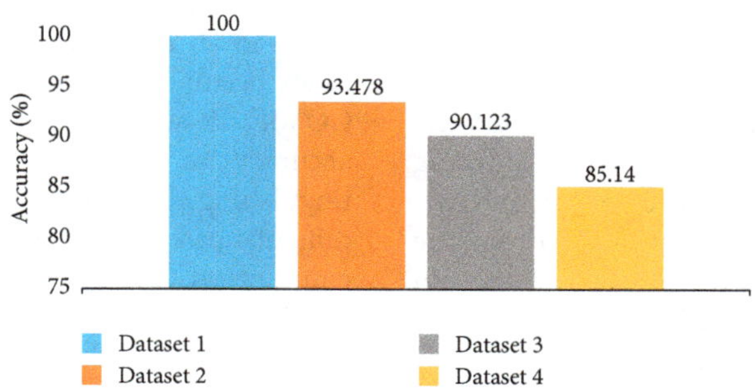

FIGURE 8: Total performance comparison of four datasets.

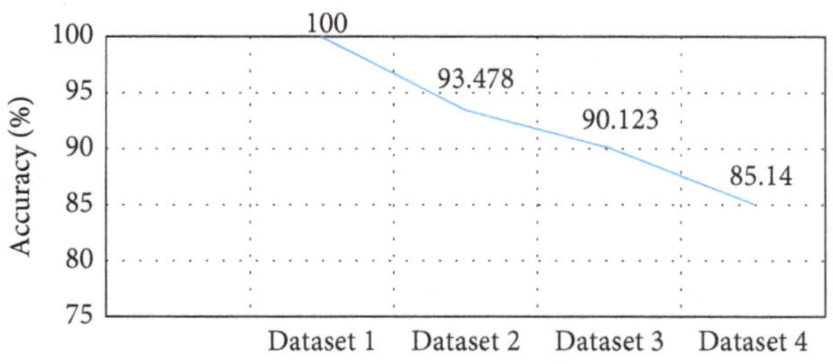

FIGURE 9: Datasets accuracy and challenges level representation.

the four datasets as seen in Figure 9. It can be stated that based on the result the accuracy will decrease as challenges increase in the datasets. This is considered the best protocol in order to diagnose the COVID-19 and help radiologists in their decision-making process.

The overall results achieved an excellent sensitivity of over 95%, at fewer than low evaluation in case of Golden Key Tool, and show an improvement of COVID-19 CT views. However, this facility can help respiratory specialists by giving a rapid triaging of radiological findings detection that increases the sensitivity of the diagnosis. The researcher's use of a Convolutional Neural Network on a chest CT case makes the recognition module more helpful when compared to other alternative approaches. A total of 800 images (349 COVID-19(+), 396 non-COVID-19 other diseases, and 55 normal which no-findings on chest CT) were used to develop the model. A fair result was obtained when the problems and the challenges of the dataset in this for binary and four groups were considered. The combination of individual systems with a new tool by new images view and by CNN classification process and detection illustrate a good impact on Radiology Order Entry Clinical Decision Support (CDS).

3.6. Challenges in the Datasets. The datasets were divided into four datasets that mean four protocols. The challenges in this paper present the protocol to help in the diagnoses of COVID-19 observed in CT findings in COVID-19 cases at different stages mainly related to pathogenesis. However, the consolidation superimposed on GGO as observed in the initial imaging presentation is found in a smaller number of cases, mainly among elderly people. With changes over time, very few cases have negative CT findings at the early stage. Advanced-phase disease is associated with a significantly increased frequency of CT pattern of COVID-19. There is much overlap of the CT-pattern of COVID-19 with other viral pneumonia and acute or chronic lung diseases. However, the advanced-phase disease makes the chest CT image more similar to non-COVID in some cases. Even though CNN is the best one to differentiate between image identities, there are small lines and time priority that can increase the false-negative rate, which may decrease the accuracy. In the case of vision evaluation, the quality difference between paper CT images and original CT images would not significantly harm the quality of the diagnosis as in the primary study but occurs in the case of CNN. If image enhancement is carried out before the convolution process to make the appearance of blurred or low resolution images better, the performance of a deep learning model can be enhanced. Missing data is a problem for deep learning networks because when large contiguous areas of images are missing, the network output deteriorates appreciably.

4. Conclusion

In the first study, the process is hardly new as a facility in the radiology department. But it continues to evolve in the face of newer technologies that can help and give more efficiency, improving the radiologist's performance and the accuracy in many cases as well as COVID-19 based on CT images. This tool provides impetus for early diagnosis and increases the sensitivity of the chest CT scan to distinguish the COVID-19 infection from other conditions. This study was assisted by specialists and experts who recommend that the appropriate test has the potential to make a difference in the field of radiology medicine. The second study focused on the diagnosis protocols by using different CNN classifications on chest CT cases of COVID-19 infection. These diagnosis protocols help the radiologists to make the right decisions. Moreover, the results can help respiratory specialists to study and observe the latest radiological findings which are based on patient management and may contribute to increasing diagnostic efficacy. Hence, this paper allows the usage of the new CT scan view and classification protocols based on challenges for other diseases.

Authors' Contributions

Ahmed Salamh and Abdulrauf Salamah contributed equally to this article. Ahmed Salamh and Halil Ibrahim Akyüz performed image classification of Convolutional Neural Networks (CNNs) processing and provided the results. Abdulrauf Salamah wrote the paper, provided the medical part, and developed the structures of the article. In this paper, the authors announce that they have complete access to all the data. There are no financial disclosures from the authors.

References

[1] W. C. Culp, "Coronavirus disease 2019," *A and A Practice*, vol. 14, no. 6, Article ID e01218, 2020.

[2] Q. Li, X. Guan, P. Wu et al., "Early transmission dynamics in Wuhan, China, of novel coronavirus-infected pneumonia," *New England Journal of Medicine*, vol. 382, no. 13, pp. 1199–1207, 2020.

[3] Z. Falaschi, P. S. C. Danna, R. Arioli et al., "Chest CT accuracy in diagnosing COVID-19 during the peak of the Italian epidemic: a retrospective correlation with RT-PCR testing and analysis of discordant cases," *European Journal of Radiology*, vol. 130, Article ID 109192, 2020.

[4] J.-L. He, L. Luo, Z.-D. Luo et al., "Diagnostic performance between CT and initial real-time RT-PCR for clinically sus-

pected 2019 coronavirus disease (COVID-19) patients outside Wuhan, China," *Respiratory Medicine*, vol. 168, Article ID 105980, 2020.
[5] X. Xie, Z. Zhong, W. Zhao, C. Zheng, F. Wang, and J. Liu, "Chest CT for typical coronavirus disease 2019 (COVID-19) pneumonia: relationship to negative RT-PCR testing," *Radiology*, vol. 296, no. 2, pp. E41–E45, 2020.
[6] T. Ai, Z. Yang, H. Hou et al., "Correlation of chest CT and RT-PCR testing for coronavirus disease 2019 (COVID-19) in China: a report of 1014 cases," *Radiology*, vol. 296, no. 2, pp. E32–E40, 2020.
[7] H. Meng, R. Xiong, R. He et al., "CT imaging and clinical course of asymptomatic cases with COVID-19 pneumonia at admission in Wuhan, China," *Journal of Infection*, vol. 81, no. 1, p. e33, 2020.
[8] M. Nakada, H. Wang, and D. Terzopoulos, "AcFR: active face recognition using convolutional neural networks," in *Proceedings of the 2017 IEEE Conference on Computer Vision and Pattern Recognition Workshops (CVPRW)*, pp. 35–40, Hawai, China, July 2017.
[9] National Health Commission, *National Health Commission of the People's Republic of China*, 2020, http://www.nhc.gov.cn/ (accessed Apr. 2020).
[10] S. Zhou, Y. Wang, T. Zhu, and L. Xia, "CT features of coronavirus disease 2019 (COVID-19) pneumonia in 62 patients in wuhan, China," *American Journal of Roentgenology*, vol. 214, no. 6, pp. 1287–1294, 2020.
[11] M. Parekh, A. Donuru, R. Balasubramanya, and S. Kapur, "Review of the chest CT differential diagnosis of ground-glass opacities in the COVID era," *Radiology*, vol. 297, Article ID 202504, 2020.
[12] J. Wu, X. Wu, W. Zeng et al., "Chest CT findings in patients with coronavirus disease 2019 and its relationship with clinical features," *Investigative Radiology*, vol. 55, no. 5, pp. 257–261, 2020.
[13] M. Carotti, F. Salaffi, P. Sarzi-Puttini et al., "Chest CT features of coronavirus disease 2019 (COVID-19) pneumonia: key points for radiologists," *La Radiologia Medica*, vol. 125, no. 7, pp. 636–646, 2020.
[14] F. Pan, T. Ye, P. Sun et al., "Time course of lung changes on chest CT during recovery from 2019 novel coronavirus (COVID-19) pneumonia," *Radiology*, vol. 295, Article ID 200370, 2020.
[15] S. Taylor-Phillips and C. Stinton, "Fatigue in radiology: a fertile area for future research," *The British Journal of Radiology*, vol. 92, no. 1099, p. 20190043, 2019.
[16] Z. Zhu, S. Xu, H. Wang et al., "COVID-19 in Wuhan: sociodemographic characteristics and hospital support measures associated with the immediate psychological impact on healthcare workers," *EClinicalMedicine*, vol. 24, p. 100443, 2020.
[17] R. Xu, C. Zhang, F. He et al., "How physical activities affect mental fatigue based on EEG energy, connectivity, and complexity," *Frontiers in Neurology*, vol. 9, no. Oct, 2018.
[18] G. Choy, M. Michalski, S. Do et al., "Current applications and future impact of machine learning in radiology," *Radiology*, vol. 288, no. 2, pp. 318–328, 2018.
[19] B. P. Tan, K. C. Lim, Y. G. Goh et al., "Radiology preparedness in the ongoing battle against COVID-19: experiences from large to small public hospitals in Singapore," *Radiology: Cardiothoracic Imaging*, vol. 2, no. 2, Article ID e200140, 2020.
[20] M. K. Santos, J. R. Ferreira Júnior, D. T. Wada, A. P. M. Tenório, M. H. N. Barbosa, and P. M. d. A. Marques, "Artificial intelligence, machine learning, computer-aided diagnosis, and radiomics: advances in imaging towards to precision medicine," *Radiologia Brasileira*, vol. 52, no. 6, pp. 387–396, 2019.
[21] Y. B. Yann LeCun, P. Haffner, L. Bottou, *Object Recognition With Gradient Based Learning*, Springer, New York, NY, USA, Lecture Notes in Computer Science, 1989.
[22] M. A. Wani, F. A. Bhat, S. Afzal, and A. I. Khan, "Advances in deep learning," *Studies in Big Data*, vol. 57, 2020.
[23] K. Yasaka, H. Akai, A. Kunimatsu, S. Kiryu, and O. Abe, "Deep learning with convolutional neural network in radiology," *Japanese Journal of Radiology*, vol. 36, no. 4, pp. 257–272, 2018.
[24] G. Murtaza, L. Shuib, A. W. Abdul Wahab et al., "Deep learning-based breast cancer classification through medical imaging modalities: state of the art and research challenges," *Artificial Intelligence Review*, vol. 53, no. 3, pp. 1655–1720, 2020.
[25] A. Bernheim, X. Mei, M. Huang et al., "Chest CT findings in coronavirus disease-19 (COVID-19): relationship to duration of infection," *Radiology*, vol. 295, no. 3, Article ID 200463.
[26] D. Liu, P. Cui, S. Zeng et al., "Risk factors for developing into critical COVID-19 patients in Wuhan, China: a multicenter, retrospective, cohort study," *EClinicalMedicine*, vol. 25, Article ID 100471, 2020.
[27] R. Jiang, C.-T. Li, D. Crookes, W. Meng, and C. Rosenberger, *Deep Biometrics, Unsupervised and Semi-Supervised Learning*, 1st ed. Cham, Switzerland, Springer International Publishing, 2020.
[28] D. Bardou, K. Zhang, and S. M. Ahmad, "Classification of breast cancer based on histology images using convolutional neural networks," *IEEE Access*, vol. 6, pp. 24680–24693, 2018.
[29] W.-c. Dai, H.-w. Zhang, J. Yu et al., "CT imaging and differential diagnosis of COVID-19," *Canadian Association of Radiologists Journal*, vol. 71, no. 2, pp. 195–200, 2020.

18

Accuracy of Pelvic Ultrasound in Diagnosing Adnexal Torsion

Labib Ghulmiyyah,[1] Anwar Nassar,[1] Dib Sassine,[1] Sally Khoury,[1] Joseph Nassif,[1] Hadi Ramadan,[1] Elie Najem,[2] and Ghina Berjawi[2]

[1]*Department of Obstetrics and Gynecology, American University of Beirut Medical Center, Lebanon*
[2]*Department of Diagnostic Radiology, American University of Beirut Medical Center, Lebanon*

Correspondence should be addressed to Ghina Berjawi; gb02@aub.edu.lb

Academic Editor: Paul Sijens

Ovarian/adnexal torsion is a rather frequent occurrence in women of reproductive age group worldwide. Etiologies are quite diverse with ovarian lesions and corpus luteal cysts being the most two common. Pelvic or intravaginal ultrasound remains the first-line imaging modality used for diagnosis and evaluation of suspected ovarian/adnexal torsion. In this study, we have adopted a case-based statistical analysis to identify important sonographic markers and further evaluated their contribution in identifying ovarian torsion. Our study successfully determined the important sonographic markers. Our observation and analysis suggest that ovarian enlargement is the most sensitive marker. Ovarian edema was found to be the most specific marker to identify the ovarian torsion with higher level of accuracy and confidence. This pioneer study will provide valuable information and direction to the medical practitioners and radiologists for better diagnosis. Further studies with large sample size will help in establishing our findings universally.

1. Introduction

Adnexal torsion accounts for almost 3% of surgical emergencies [1]. It involves twisting of the ovary and/or fallopian tube leading to either a necrotic ovary or an undamaged ovary with impaired vascularization. This incidence is most common in women aged between 14 and 45 years. To prevent the loss of the ovary or adnexa and severe conditions such as thrombophlebitis or peritonitis, delay in the diagnosis should be avoided [2]. The presence of an ovarian mass of at least 5 cm is the primary risk factor that can cause torsion [3, 4].

Diagnosis of an ovarian torsion is challenging due to lack of sensitivity and specificity of its clinical signs [5]. Mostly, patients with ovarian torsion show abdominal pain as the major clinical symptom [6, 7]. To the present, the diagnosis of ovarian torsion has been based on clinical findings.

Reports from existing evidence suggest that sonography along with ovarian vasculature Doppler flow studies help in the correct diagnosis of only 66% of surgical cases [1]. The ultrasonography based diagnostic technique is known to be operator-dependent and, thus, may involve human error.

Our study aims to identify the sonographic marker(s) that are most helpful in making an accurate diagnosis of adnexal torsion. We also aim to assess the accuracy and predictive value of such identified sonographic markers to aid the early intervention.

2. Materials and Methods

This study was approved by the Institutional Review Board at the American University of Beirut. The study subjects were retrieved from the Department of Diagnostic Radiology of the American University of Beirut Medical Center (AUBMC) database. All women aged between 14 and 45 years presenting to AUBMC Emergency Department between July 2009 and February 2015 with acute lower abdominal pain suggestive of ovarian/adnexal were identified. Among the selected subjects, only those with positive ultrasound findings suggestive of ovarian/adnexal torsion and underwent laparoscopic surgery were included in this study.

The ultrasound machine used for the acquisition of sonographic images is a PHILIPS EPIQ 5G. A curvilinear probe C5-1 was used with a 5 MHz frequency. Both axial and sagittal cuts were obtained.

Relevant information including patient demographics, past medical and surgical history, and operative and pathology notes were collected from the electronic medical records. All retrieved data were then tabulated into an excel sheet. To avoid bias, a second sheet containing only the patients' study number, demographics, and clinical history was sent to a specialized women imaging Diagnostic Radiologist at the Diagnostic Radiology department at AUBMC for reevaluation of the ultrasound images. Ultrasound findings and the sonographic markers—ovarian edema, ovarian enlargement, ovarian location, and presence/absence of an ovarian cyst/mass, ovarian blood flow, fluid in the pouch of Douglas, fluid around the ovary, distention of fallopian tubes, and bleeding within ovaries— were then added to the excel sheet and sent for statistical analysis.

Initial data tabulation was done in a Microsoft Excel sheet and later loaded into the Statistical Package for Social Sciences (SPSS) package version 22 for analyses. Descriptive statistical analysis was carried out by reporting the number and percentage of the categorical variables whereas continuous variables were summarized by mean and standard deviation. Fisher's Exact test was used to compare the presence of sonographic signs between the samples with and without laparoscopic evidence of torsion. To assess the statistical outcome, the sensitivity, specificity, positive predictive value (PPV), and negative predictive value (NPV) were calculated. During these analyses, 95% confidence intervals (CI) were considered for each statistical measure.

3. Results

Table 1 summarizes the characteristics of the 37 patients who met the inclusion criteria. The baseline characteristics were found to be similar in the torsion and no torsion groups (Table 2).

Table 3 represents the frequency of various sonographic markers associated with ovarian torsion in women with and without evidence of ovarian torsion determined by laparoscopy. In patients with ovarian torsion, the most frequent sonographic markers observed were relative enlargement of the affected ovary, ovarian edema, and the presence of an ovarian mass/cyst. Ovarian edema and ovarian enlargement were both found to be statistically significant markers ($p = 0.03$).

Three out of 10 ovarian torsion cases had abnormal ovarian location noted on ultrasound ($p = 0.02$).

Interestingly, none of the 10 torsion cases had abnormal ovarian blood flow using Doppler ultrasound.

Table 4 summarizes the sensitivity, specificity, PPV, and NPV of the various sonographic markers. Ovarian enlargement was found to be the most sensitive marker (80%) with a specificity of 63%. On the other hand, ovarian edema was found to be the most specific marker (100%) and a CI of 0.8-1. In this study, abnormal ovarian blood flow was not found to be sensitive as the calculated sensitivity was 0%.

TABLE 1: Patient characteristics.

	N=37
Age*	27.16 ± 6.58
Gravidity*	1.05 ± 1.54
Parity*	0.84 ± 1.32
Smoking**	
No	36 (97.3)
Yes	1 (2.7)
Past Surgical History**	
None	17 (45.9)
Abdomino-Pelvic	12 (32.4)
Other	8 (21.6)
Body Mass Index*	24.01 ± 4.10
History of PCOS**	
Yes	3 (8.1)
No	34 (91.9)
Pain location**	
Left	13 (35.1)
Right	20 (54.1)
Mid	4 (10.8)

*Mean ± SD; **n (%); PCOS=polycystic ovary syndrome.

Table 5 shows the frequency of the combination of sonographic markers found during the scan in patients suspected to have ovarian torsion. It was found that 11 had only 1 marker, whereas 15 had 3 or more markers.

It was observed that when only a single marker was detected on ultrasound, the sensitivity approached 90% whereas the presence of 3 combined markers increased the specificity to 96% (Table 6). Therefore, we calculated the Youden score which simultaneously reflects the sensitivity and the specificity for a combination of markers. It was observed that a combination of 2 markers detected on ultrasound had the highest Youden score of 0.4.

4. Discussion

At present, there is no reliable method to confirm the diagnosis of adnexal torsion preoperatively. To prevent the loss of the ovarian function and its potential association with fertility problems, an early diagnosis of an adnexal torsion is needed [8]. Moreover, delay in diagnosis and treatment or mistake in diagnosis may lead to potentially fatal thrombophlebitis or peritonitis [8, 9].

This study demonstrates the importance of combining both clinical and ultrasonographic findings together to diagnose ovarian torsion with better accuracy and reliability.

The existing literature suggests that torsion occurs in the right side in most of the cases accounting for almost 67-71% [10, 11]. This is since the right uteroovarian ligament is physiologically longer than its left counterpart. The presence of the sigmoid colon on the left side reduces the space needed and may aid in the occurrence of torsion. Our study showed that 60% of the adnexal torsion occurred in the left side.

TABLE 2: Patient characteristics in the two patient groups.

Variables	Negative† (N=27)	Positive†† (N=10)	P-Value
Age*	27.15 ± 6.91	27.20 ± 5.94	1
Gravidity*	1.11 ± 1.58	0.90 ± 1.52	0.67
Parity*	0.89 ± 1.34	0.70 ± 1.34	0.72
Smoking**			
No	26 (96.3)	10 (100.0)	1
Yes	1 (3.7)	0 (0.0)	
Past Surgical History**			
None	11 (40.7)	6 (60.0)	0.51
Abdomino-Pelvic	9 (33.3)	3 (30.0)	
Other	7 (25.9)	1 (10.0)	
Body Mass Index*	23.95 ± 4.31	24.16 ± 3.66	0.65
History of PCOS**			
Yes	3 (11.1)	0 (0.0)	0.55
No	24 (88.9)	10 (100.0)	
Pain location**			
Left	7 (25.9)	6 (60.0)	0.16
Right	16 (59.3)	4 (40.0)	
Mid	4 (14.8)	0 (0.0)	

Negative† refers to patients with no proven ovarian torsion determined by laparoscopy.
Positive†† refers to patients with proven ovarian torsion determined by laparoscopy.
*Mean ± SD; **n (%); PCOS=polycystic ovary syndrome.

TABLE 3: Presence of the various sonographic markers in the torsion and no torsion groups.

Variables	Negative† (N=27)	Positive†† (N=10)	P-Value
Ovarian edema	0 (0.0)	4 (40.0)	0.003
Ovarian enlargement	10 (37.0)	8 (80.0)	0.03
Ovarian cyst or mass	11 (40.7)	6 (60.0)	0.3
Abnormal ovarian location	0 (0.0)	3 (30.0)	0.002
Abnormal ovarian blood flow	0 (0.0)	0 (0.0)	NA
Free fluid in pouch of Douglas	6 (22.2)	2 (20.0)	1
Fluid around the ovary	0 (0.0)	0 (0.0)	NA
Distended fallopian tube	0 (0.0)	0 (0.0)	NA
Sites of bleeding within the affected ovary	0 (0.0)	0 (0.0)	NA

Negative† refers to patients with no proven ovarian torsion determined by laparoscopy.
Positive†† refers to patients with proven ovarian torsion determined by laparoscopy.
Data presented as n (%).

Our findings will help in future diagnosis and early detection of ovarian torsion and will guide the medical practitioners or radiologists in handling such cases.

We observed that ovarian enlargement was the most sensitive marker in our series in diagnosing ovarian torsion. The sensitivity found was 80% and specificity of 63% was achieved for this specific marker. Similar outcome was also shown in another case series of 63 ovarian torsion cases by Mashiach et al., where ovarian enlargement was the most sensitive sonographic finding with a sensitivity of 85% and specificity of 18.8% [1].

Comparison of the enlarged ovarian size with the unaffected ovarian size in normal subjects is of major importance. However, normal looking ovaries do not necessarily rule out the possibility of ovarian torsion [12].

According to Pena et al. [10], 60% of the cases of torsion are missed by Doppler, while its positive predictive value was 100.

Abnormal flow detected by Doppler sonography can be highly predictive of adnexal torsion and is therefore useful in the diagnosis of ovarian torsion. In fact, several studies have previously concluded that completely normal venous

TABLE 4: The observed outcome of sensitivity, specificity, PPV, and NPV.

Signs	Sensitivity (95% CI)	Specificity (95% CI)	PPV (95% CI)	NPV (95% CI)
Ovarian edema	0.40 (0.14 - 0.73)	1.00 (0.84 - 1.00)	1.00 (0.40 - 1.00)	0.82 (0.64 - 0.92)
Ovarian enlargement	0.80 (0.44 - 0.96)	0.63 (0.42 - 0.80)	0.44 (0.22 - 0.69)	0.89 (0.65 - 0.98)
Ovarian cyst or mass	0.60 (0.27 - 0.86)	0.59 (0.39 - 0.77)	0.35 (0.15 - 0.61)	0.80 (0.56 - 0.93)
Abnormal ovarian location	0.30 (0.08 - 0.65)	1.00 (0.84 - 1.00)	1.00 (0.40 - 1.00)	0.79 (0.61 - 0.91)
Abnormal ovarian blood flow	0.00 (0.00 - 0.34)	1.00 (0.84 - 1.00)	NA	0.73 (0.56 - 0.86)
Free fluid in the pouch of Douglas	0.20 (0.03 - 0.56)	0.78 (0.57 - 0.91)	0.25 (0.04 - 0.64)	0.72 (0.52 - 0.86)
Presence of fluid around the ovary	0.00 (0.00 - 0.34)	1.00 (0.84 - 1.00)	NA	0.73 (0.56 - 0.86)
Distended fallopian tube	0.00 (0.00 - 0.34)	1.00 (0.84 - 1.00)	NA	0.73 (0.56 - 0.86)
Sites of bleeding within the affected ovary	0.00 (0.00 - 0.34)	1.00 (0.84 - 1.00)	NA	0.73 (0.56 - 0.86)

TABLE 5: Frequency of the number of sonographic markers observed.

Number of markers	Frequency (N=37)	Percent	Cumulative Percent
0	2	5.4	5.4
1	11	29.7	35.1
2	9	24.3	59.5
3	10	27.0	86.5
4	4	10.8	97.3
5	1	2.7	100.0

waveforms are very unlikely in cases of ovarian torsion [13, 14]. However, when normal flow is detected, it does not necessarily exclude an ovarian torsion; in fact, torsion can be missed in 60% of cases [10]. In addition, Murat et al. (xxxx) also reported velocity loss in Doppler sonography in 46.4% of the patients.

Unlike the literature, in our case series, no abnormal arterial or venous Doppler flow was noted in any of the 10 ovarian torsion cases, not enabling us to calculate the positive predictive value (PPV) in this case.

Therefore, relying on normal Doppler sonography could have resulted in missing all cases of torsion. Normal Doppler studies should not delay surgical intervention in the presence of a high clinical index of suspicion.

Our study suggests that using multiple sonographic markers can be helpful to confirm the presence of torsion and initiate surgical intervention in a timely fashion. Marker combination was able to increase the specificity value of the test. Using two sonographic markers increased the specificity up to 70% compared with 44% specificity with the use of a single marker.

Interestingly, incorporating more than two of such markers would eventually reduce the overall sensitivity. Our results also showed that a single torsion marker achieved a sensitivity of 90% whereas considering three markers reduced the sensitivity up to 40%. Similar findings were observed by Reuven et al., where the combination of sonographic markers displayed higher specificity and lower sensitivity values [1].

For better evaluation and optimal outcome and to understand the impact of the combination of the markers with best possible specificity and sensitivity, we considered Youden score.

The highest observed Youden score was 0.4, suggesting that combination of any two sonographic markers related to the ovarian torsion could provide the best possible sensitivity and specificity for the accounted dataset.

Our study has several limitations the most important of which is the small sample size. Despite this, we believe that our study is a pioneer study in Lebanon and in the Middle East region in this direction. Utmost care was taken to extract the best possible results through extensive and reliable statistical measures such as Youden scoring and blinded evaluation of the sonographic images by the radiologist.

With time, along with the increment of complications such as PCOD and other, the number of cases of ovarian

TABLE 6: Sensitivity, specificity, and Youden score for combined markers.

Number of markers	Sensitivity	Specificity	Youden
1	0.9	0.44	0.34
2	0.7	0.7	0.4
3	0.4	0.96	0.36
4	0.1	1	0.1

torsion is increasing. Reports are available from all geographical regions in this context. Ultrasonography is the most commonly used and cost-effective method of diagnosis so far. Early and accurate diagnosis remains a challenge for ovarian torsion. Early detection of ovarian torsion also helps in the further treatment decision which may have less complication. Reports suggest that MRI and CT scan have been attempted as an alternative protocol towards better diagnosis [15–17]. But ultrasound remains the most cost-effective, easily accessible diagnostic measure for adnexal torsion all over the world.

Studies have reported that ultrasound-based methods are quite reliable in diagnosing torsions where significant signs such as abnormal blood flow [18], positive whirlpool sign [19], and other markers could serve as best predictors and confirm the presence of adnexal torsion. Therefore, our study will help in considering specific markers which could be the best possible markers in terms of their sensitivity and specificity while doing such diagnosis.

5. Conclusion

The increment in the number of cases of adnexal torsion demands specific, quick, and accurate diagnostic measure. Ultrasound has been the most successful technique in this scenario. Yet, considering the consequences and probable loss of the patient due to delayed diagnosis or misdiagnosis, better detection accuracy is required.

The common symptoms are unspecific in nature in most of the cases of adnexal torsion and sometimes Doppler method may not be able to detect the abnormalities as well. At present, the accurate diagnosis of ovarian torsion can only be achieved and treated by surgery. Therefore, increased sensitivity and specificity in diagnosis through ultrasound is an urgent need.

Along with the clinical suspicion and estimations, this study will provide ample valuable information towards understanding the impact of the sonographic markers during the diagnosis of ovarian torsion accurately.

Authors' Contributions

Labib Ghulmiyyah and Anwar Nassar equally contributed to this work.

References

[1] R. Mashiach, N. Melamed, N. Gilad, G. Ben-Shitrit, and I. Meizner, "Sonographic diagnosis of ovarian torsion," *Journal of Ultrasound in Medicine*, vol. 30, no. 9, pp. 1205–1210, 2011.

[2] D. H. Nichols and P. J. Julian, "Torsion of the Adnexa," *Clinical Obstetrics and Gynecology*, vol. 28, no. 2, pp. 375–380, 1985.

[3] M. Varras, A. Tsikini, D. Polyzos et al., "Uterine adnexal torsion: pathologic and gray-scale ultrasonographic findings," *Clinical and Experimental Obstetrics and Gynecology*, pp. 31–34, 2004.

[4] S. C. Oltmann, A. Fischer, R. Barber, R. Huang, B. Hicks, and N. Garcia, "Cannot exclude torsion—a 15-year review," *Journal of Pediatric Surgery*, vol. 44, no. 6, pp. 1212–1217, 2009.

[5] M. White and J. Stella, "Ovarian torsion: 10-year perspective," *Emergency Medicine Australasia*, vol. 17, no. 3, pp. 231–237, 2005.

[6] E. R. Kokoska, M. S. Keller, and T. R. Weber, "Acute ovarian torsion in children," *The American Journal of Surgery*, vol. 180, no. 6, pp. 462–465, 2000.

[7] C. Lee, S. Raman, and V. Sivanesaratnam, "Torsion of ovarian tumors: A clinicopathological study," *International Journal of Gynecology & Obstetrics*, vol. 28, no. 1, pp. 21–25, 1989.

[8] C. Huchon and A. Fauconnier, "Adnexal torsion: a literature review," *European Journal of Obstetrics & Gynecology and Reproductive Biology*, vol. 150, pp. 8–12, 2010.

[9] L. T. Hibbard, "Adnexal torsion," *American Journal of Obstetrics & Gynecology*, vol. 152, no. 4, pp. 456–461, 1985.

[10] J. E. Peña, D. Ufberg, N. Cooney, and A. L. Denis, "Usefulness of Doppler sonography in the diagnosis of ovarian torsion," *Fertility and Sterility*, vol. 73, no. 5, pp. 1047–1050, 2000.

[11] M. A. Warner, A. C. Fleischer, S. L. Edell et al., "Uterine adnexal torsion: sonographic findings.," *Radiology*, vol. 154, no. 3, pp. 773–775, 1985.

[12] L. L. Shadinger, R. F. Andreotti, and R. L. Kurian, "Preoperative sonographic and clinical characteristics as predictors of ovarian torsion," *Journal of Ultrasound in Medicine*, vol. 27, no. 1, pp. 7–13, 2008.

[13] M. Ben-Ami, Y. Perlitz, and S. Haddad, "The effectiveness of spectral and color Doppler in predicting ovarian torsion," *European Journal of Obstetrics & Gynecology and Reproductive Biology*, vol. 104, no. 1, pp. 64–66, 2002.

[14] F. Albayram and U. M. Hamper, "Ovarian and adnexal torsion: spectrum of sonographic findings with pathologic correlation.," *Journal of Ultrasound in Medicine*, vol. 20, no. 10, pp. 1083–1089, 2001.

[15] I. Petkovska, E. Duke, D. R. Martin et al., "MRI of ovarian torsion: Correlation of imaging features with the presence of perifollicular hemorrhage and ovarian viability," *European Journal of Radiology*, vol. 85, no. 11, pp. 2064–2071, 2016.

[16] C. Moore, A. B. Meyers, J. Capotasto, and J. Bokhari, "Prevalence of abnormal CT findings in patients with proven ovarian

torsion and a proposed triage schema," *Emergency Radiology*, vol. 16, no. 2, pp. 115–120, 2009.

[17] M. S. Lee, M. H. Moon, H. Woo et al., "CT findings of adnexal torsion: A matched case-control study," *PLoS ONE*, vol. 13, no. 7, Article ID e0200190, 2018.

[18] A. Rostamzadeh, S. Mirfendereski, M. J. Rezaie, and S. Rezaei, "Diagnostic efficacy of sonography for diagnosis of ovarian torsion," *Pakistan Journal of Medical Sciences*, vol. 30, no. 2, pp. 413–416, 1969.

[19] S. B. Vijayaraghavan, "Sonographic whirlpool sign in ovarian torsion," *Journal of Ultrasound in Medicine*, vol. 23, no. 12, pp. 1643–1649, 2004.

19

Advanced Ultrasound Screening for Temporomandibular Joint (TMJ) Internal Derangement

Saul N. Friedman[1] **Miriam Grushka,**[2] **Hussam K. Beituni,**[3] **Madhu Rehman,**[3] **Hart B. Bressler**[4] **and Lawrence Friedman**[3]

[1]*Division of Nuclear Medicine, Mallinckrodt Institute of Radiology, Washington University School of Medicine, Saint Louis, MO 63110, USA*
[2]*974 Eglington Avenue West, Toronto, Ontario M6C 2C5, Canada*
[3]*Department of Medical Imaging, North York General, 4001 Leslie Street, Toronto, Ontario M2K 1E1, Canada*
[4]*Department of Family and Community Medicine, University of Toronto, Mount Sinai Hospital, 600 University Ave, Toronto, Ontario M5G 1X5, Canada*

Correspondence should be addressed to Saul N. Friedman; saul.friedman@gmail.com

Academic Editor: Henrique M. Lederman

Purpose. To present an advanced ultrasound (US) technique and propose its use as a screening diagnostic tool for temporomandibular joint (TMJ) internal derangement. *Materials and Methods.* The technique is based on maintaining the US probe parallel to the articular disc, rather than traditional axial and coronal views, with the position described relative to a clock face. Validation was achieved by direct comparison with magnetic resonance imaging (MRI). A total of 61 patients, with age ranging from 13 to 67 years, were prescreened for TMJ pain and internal derangement, underwent US imaging for screening, and MRI evaluation for final diagnosis. *Results.* 29 of the 61 patients had disc pathology on MRI. US screening produced no false positive results and only 6 false negative results, corresponding to a sensitivity of 79% and specificity of 100%. Half of the false negative cases involved disc pathology with a medial component to the disc displacement. *Conclusion.* US is both a sensitive and a specific screening tool for TMJ dysfunction when used by an appropriately trained operator, with the exception of medially displaced discs. If TMJ assessment is found to be abnormal, the patient should be referred for MRI, and any patient scheduled for surgery must have the diagnosis confirmed by MRI. If a component of medial disc displacement is suspected, MRI should be performed despite a normal screening US.

1. Introduction

In the past, internal derangement of the temporomandibular joint (TMJ) has been assessed with plain film radiographs as the initial investigation [1] followed by arthrography [2] and computed tomography (CT) [3]. More recently, magnetic resonance imaging (MRI) [4–7] has provided a noninvasive accurate method of assessing the TMJ without associated radiation risks. Its advantages over previous methods include its ability to directly visualize the disc and accurately determine the position of the disc with respect to the condyle of the mandible and eminence of the temporal bone. The examination, however, takes 20 to 45 minutes on average to perform depending on the scanner and protocol, and patients have difficulty keeping still and having their mouths open for extended periods of time, especially if they are experiencing pain. In addition, the examination is costly and access is still limited in many centres. Many patients also experience claustrophobia and are unable to complete or even undergo the examination.

Ultrasound is relatively inexpensive, is readily accessible, and can be performed in most outpatient facilities; studies take only an average of 10 to 15 minutes in total, and it is without any known risks. In addition, US provides the opportunity to converse with patients and identify the exact locations of pain, while the probe can be used as a palpable tool for real-time identification of crepitus, clicking, motion, and snapping sensations. The disadvantages of US remain the long learning curve and the fact that the test is operator dependent. There is also the question of ultrasound being effectively used as a diagnostic tool [8–13], given the many constraints that will be discussed. In particular, Katzberg [12] questioned its validity stating that ultrasound images do not appear to be anatomically correct, that tissues indicated to be discs were not convincing, and that interpretation was not blinded. He also believed that given the bone blockade barrier and inability of the ultrasound beam to bend around curved narrow structures, ultrasound does not allow for adequate diagnosis. However, more recently, Katzberg and colleagues have proposed the use of sagittal transoral US to evaluate the TMJ [14].

Additional and more recent works by numerous investigators provide strong support for the use of conventional US techniques. For example, Li et al. [13] in 2012 calculated a sensitivity and specificity of 76% and 82% for disc displacement with reduction, respectively, and 79% and 91% without disc reduction, respectively. They also stated that ultrasound is acceptable as a rapid initial method to exclude some potential patients but recommended MRI if treatment is necessary. In addition, they noted that the ability to diagnose lateral and posterior displacements by ultrasound is not clear. More recently, Su et al. published a meta-analysis in 2018 noting an overall sensitivity and specificity of 75–81% and 73–80%, respectively, for disc displacement in the closed-mouth position and 65–74% and 86–91%, respectively, for disc displacement in the open-mouth position [15].

Katzberg [12] attempted to quantify the distribution of disc displacements in a prospective study of 76 volunteers and 102 patients studied with MRI. He noted 52% of abnormal joints had anterior displacement, 27% of abnormal joints had anteromedial displacement, 12% of abnormal joints had medial displacement, 34% of abnormal joints had anterolateral displacement, and 4% of abnormal joints had lateral displacement. He also stated that anteromedially and medially displaced discs, totalling 39%, would not be visualized by ultrasound.

1.1. Goal. Using knowledge of the normal US appearance and dynamic motion of the articular disc, we present a new technique for visualization and assessment of the TMJ using ultrasound, where the probe is positioned parallel to the disc throughout movement; this technique differs from traditional vertical and horizontal probe positioning, where the focus has been on obtaining true axial and coronal plains of imaging. MRI of the TMJ is used as the gold standard for technique validation.

2. Materials and Methods

Institutional review board approval from North York General Ethics Committee was obtained, and verbal consent was obtained from all patients and subjects prior to inclusion in the study.

2.1. Ultrasound Technique Details. The patient can be in a sitting position or lying down on a stretcher. We prefer the patients lying supine with the jaw tilted away from the side to be examined, as this position not only offers more stability for probe positioning but also allows for further patient comfort. The joint is then palpated while we have the patient open and close their mouth. Once the joint is located, the probe is placed over the joint using a liberal amount of warm gel.

Traditional ultrasound techniques have included positioning of the probe on the skin surface in the axial (Figure 1(a)) and coronal (Figure 1(b)) planes [12, 13]. We employ a method whereby the position of the probe can be compared to that of a clock face in a clockwise rotation. The probe is angled appropriately parallel to the right disc in the sagittal plane initially at an angle 50–60° down from the horizontal as measured from the anterior side of the probe or 5 o'clock in the closed-mouth position on the right (Figure 1(c)), followed by 0° angulation or 3 o'clock in the semiopen position (Figure 1(d)), and finally an anterior angle of 50–60° up from the horizontal as measured from the anterior side of the probe or 1 o'clock in the fully open-mouth position on the right (Figure 1(e)). In a similar manner, these angles would correspond to 7 o'clock, 9 o'clock, and 11 o'clock positions, respectively, when investigating the left TMJ. Dynamic video clips of movement can be obtained by swivelling the probe or by keeping the probe just off the horizontal, which varies from patient to patient.

The disc was considered normal in the static closed-mouth position if the intermediate zone or centre of the hypoechoic disc was located between the anterosuperior aspect of the condyle and the posteroinferior aspect of the articular eminence. During movement, the disc was considered normal if the intermediate zone or centre of the disc maintained its central location to the condyle from the closed-mouth to fully open-mouth positions. All other disc locations were considered to exhibit either anterior or posterior displacement.

2.2. Imaging Equipment. Ultrasound images were obtained using a 15–7 MHz L15-7io hockey stick transducer (Philips iU22 Ultrasound System, Netherlands). The total US image acquisition time was approximately 10 minutes per patient.

MRI was performed using T1 coronal and sagittal images in both open- and closed-mouth positions as well as gradient kinetic dynamic sagittal images (GE Signa HDxt 1.5T, Milwaukee, USA) with the following parameters: coronal T1-weighted images with repetition time (TR) = 405 ms and echo time (TE) = 10 ms, sagittal proton-density-weighted images with TR = 2025 ms and TE = 30 ms, and sagittal T2*-weighted kinematic dynamic images with TR = 100 ms and TE = 10 ms. The total acquisition time was approximately 30 minutes per patient.

2.3. Validation with Normal Volunteers. Normal anatomy was first reviewed through the evaluation of both TMJs in 10 normal volunteers between the ages of 20 and 30 years.

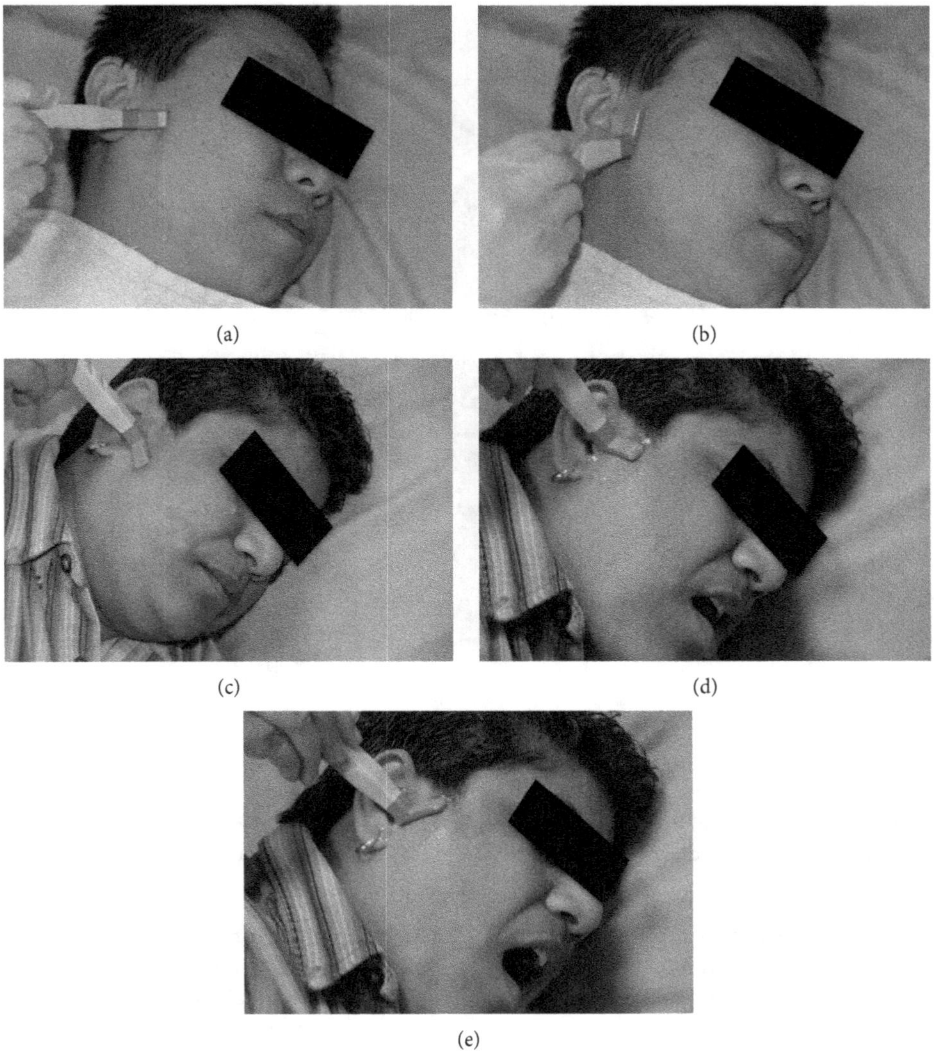

FIGURE 1: Position of the probe on the skin surface for traditional (a) transverse and (b) coronal scans. The probe position during routine interrogation of the TMJ is (c) angled parallel to the disc in the sagittal plane at 50–60° below the horizontal as measured from the anterior side of the probe or 5 o'clock position in the closed-mouth position on the right, (d) angled parallel to the disc or 3 o'clock position in the half-open-mouth position on the right, and (e) angled 50–60° above the horizontal as measured from the anterior side of the probe in the fully open-mouth or 1 o'clock position on the right. In a similar manner, these angles represent 7 o'clock, 9 o'clock, and 11 o'clock positions when investigating the TMJ on the left.

2.4. Assessment of Patient Pathology. Patients were prescreened for TMJ pain and internal derangement based on the history and clinical exam by our TMJ pathology specialist (author MG) or our pain specialist with particular experience in TMJ pathology (author HBB). Recommendations on the physical exam technique have been described in detail elsewhere [16]. A total of 61 symptomatic patients were recruited, of which 43 were male and 18 female with a mean age of 40 years and age range of 13 to 67 years. MR and US imaging was obtained using the same equipment and protocol as above. All US images were acquired by the senior radiologist (author LF), who had over 20 years of specialized US MSK experience. Contrast was not used for either MR or US imaging. MRI interpretations were performed by 4 radiologists, each with a minimum of 5 years of experience working in a practice, and typically completed first to avoid delay in patient care. The same senior MSK radiologist with over 20 years of specialized US MSK training performed all US interpretations. To avoid recall bias, the US reader remained blinded to all MRI results performed by other readers. In addition, in the situation where the US reader also interpreted the MRI first, a period of 3-4 weeks was waited after the MRI interpretation before interpreting the associated US.

The US screen was considered positive if displacement was observed, regardless of the direction (anterior, posterior, medial, or lateral) and regardless of whether it reduced or remained fixed. In cases where displacement was observed in multiple directions (e.g., anteromedial), the displacement was labelled by the predominant direction of displacement. Pathology was then further subdivided into fixed displacement and recapture subgroups. Osteoarthritic changes and

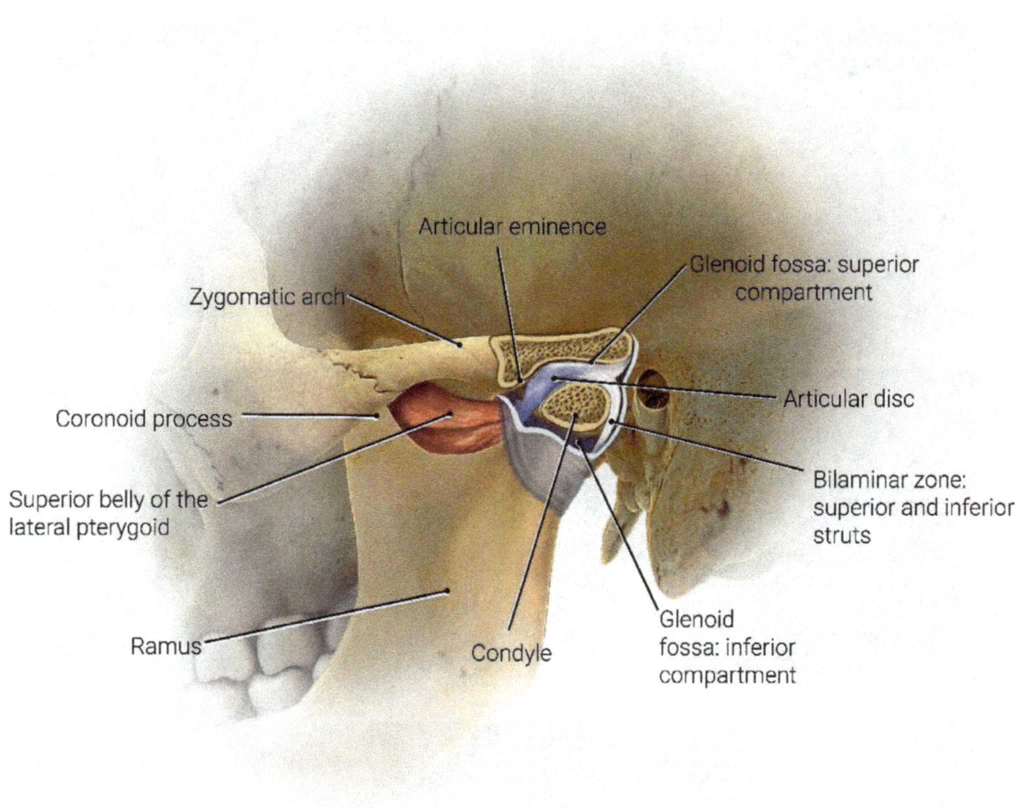

FIGURE 2: Normal anatomy illustrating the condyle of the mandible, superior and inferior belly of the lateral pterygoid muscle, articular disc, articular eminence of the temporal bone, and articular fossa (glenoid fossa) of the temporal bone.

evidence of inflammation as determined through increased blood flow were also evaluated but could only be performed on US as MRI postcontrast imaging was not performed.

3. Results

3.1. Normal TMJ. A diagram of basic anatomy is presented in Figure 2 as a visual aid. The articular disc in the normal TMJ is a fibrous structure composed of a superficial band, a slightly more thickened deep band, and a very thin intermediate zone that is attached posteriorly to the temporal bone through the bilaminar zone and anteriorly to the lateral pterygoid muscle superior belly. A lower synovial-lined joint space separates it from the head of the condyle, and a noncommunicating upper joint separates it from the bony glenoid fossa and the articular eminence of the temporal bone.

On MRI, the disc has a bowtie or saddle appearance. On sonography, a normal disc usually appears as an inverted more hypoechoic c-shaped structure that straddles the hyperechoic cortex of the condyle, as seen in Figure 3. However, the disc can also appear isoechoic to hyperechoic especially as it becomes less hydrated and more calcified with disease.

During normal movement and disc translation, the disc maintains a constant relationship between the condyle head of the mandible and the eminence of the temporal bone. From the closed-mouth to the fully-open-mouth position, the thin intermediate zone should be between the closely applied cortical surface of the condyle and the eminence. Close attention to this relationship is critical in separating a normal from an abnormal disc on both MRI and ultrasound interrogation. For a right-sided TMJ in the closed-mouth position in the sagittal plane, the anterior angle of the normal disc is 50–60° down from the horizontal. When midway between open- and closed-mouth positions, the anterior angle is 0° to the horizontal, and in the fully-open-mouth position, it is 50–60° up from the horizontal. The mirror image configuration is present in the left-sided TMJ.

3.2. Abnormal TMJ. Pathology for the 61 patients included in the study as determined by MRI is summarized in Table 1. The 29 patients positive for TMJ pathology correspond to a prevalence of 47.5%. Fixed posterior displacement was not observed. Of the 14 patients with fixed anterior displacement, 3 were noted to have a medial component to the displacement. Lateral disc displacement was not observed.

Ultrasound screening identified 23 of the 29 patients with pathology, corresponding to 6 false negatives. No false positive results were obtained. This corresponds to a sensitivity of 79% and specificity of 100%; results are summarized in Table 2. The 6 false negative cases all corresponded to fixed anterior displacement and included all 3 cases that were noted to contain a medial component of displacement. Based on the calculated prevalence of 47.5%,

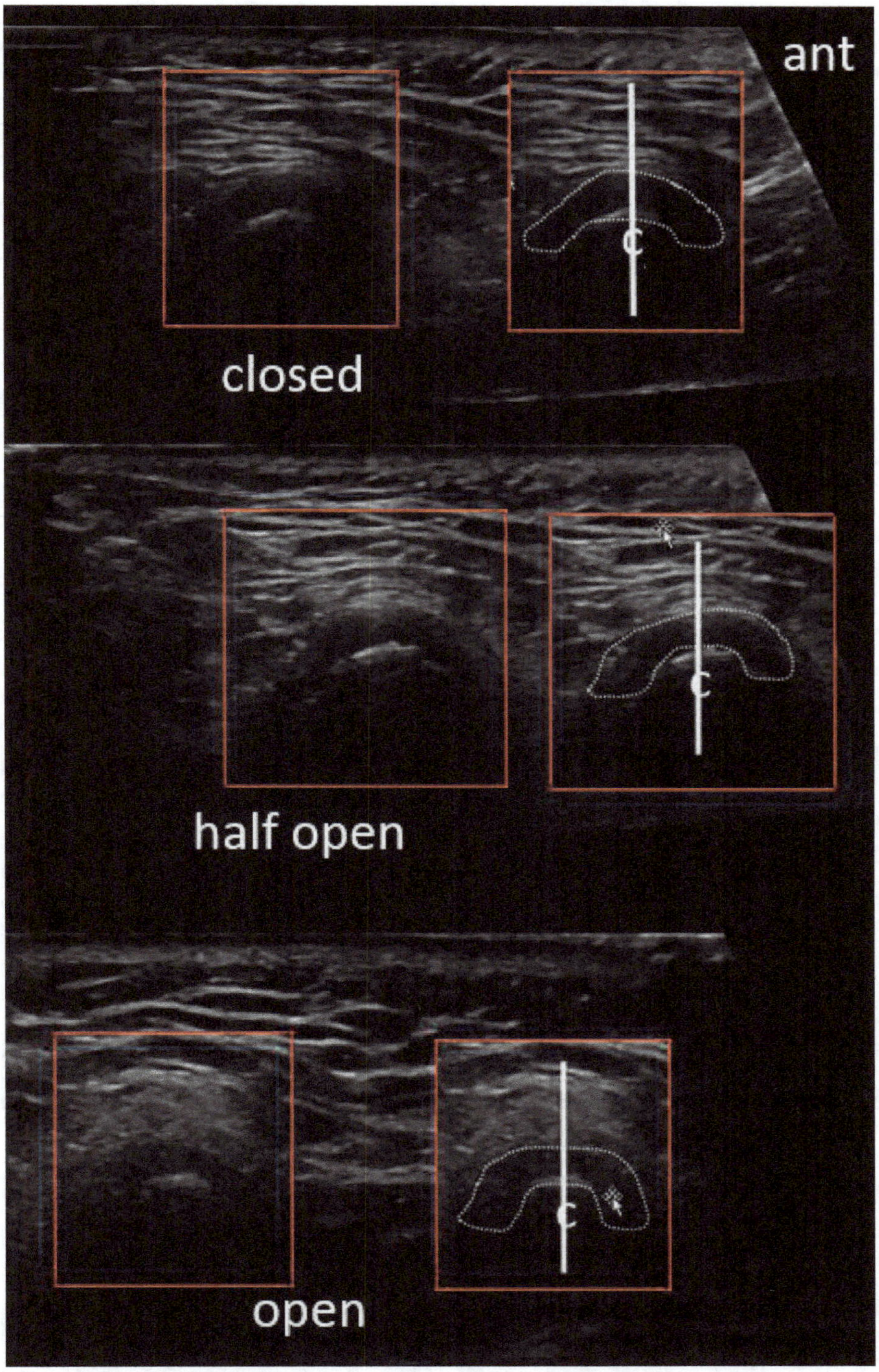

FIGURE 3: Normal ultrasound appearance of the articular disc in the sagittal plane, seen as an inverted hypoechoic c-shaped structure. Note that the disc maintains a constant central appearance with respect to the centre of the condyle, "c," outlined by a central vertical line during the closed-mouth, half-open-mouth, and fully-open-mouth views. The anterior ("ant") band and posterior band of the articular disc appear symmetrical in size with respect to the centre of the condyle. A focal annotated view was provided to aid visualization with the articular disc outlined with a dotted contour.

the calculated positive predictive value is 100% and the negative predictive value is 84%.

US and MRI of anterior disc displacement with recapture of the disc in the open-mouth position are demonstrated in Figure 4. Note the normal MRI bowtie appearance in Figure 4(b). Corresponding pathology without recapture, labelled as fixed anterior dislocation, is demonstrated in Figure 5. While the morphology of the disc usually remains normal with an anteriorly displaced disc that recaptures, it more often appears morphologically abnormal with fixed anterior dislocation, as noted in Figure 5. Posterior displacement is demonstrated in Figure 6. Bony deformity and bony

Table 1: A total of 29 of the 61 patients experiencing temporomandibular symptoms had pathology visible on magnetic resonance imaging (MRI), corresponding to a disease prevalence of 47.5%. Pathology is subdivided into anterior, posterior, and medial displacements and summarized here, with the number demonstrating the presence of recapture, osteoarthritic changes, and presence of inflammation (as determined from ultrasound imaging) noted.

Pathological disc displacement	Fixed	Recapture present	Total
Anterior	14*	14	28
Posterior	0	1	1
Medial	0	0	0
Lateral	0	0	0
Total	14	15	29

*3 cases were further noted to have a medially displaced component.

Table 2: Summary of results of the 61 patients prescreened for temporomandibular symptoms using ultrasound (US) and compared to the gold standard of magnetic resonance imaging (MRI). US results are split into true positive and true negative (concordant with MRI), and false positive and false negative (discordant with MRI), corresponding to a sensitivity of 79% and specificity of 100%.

	MRI screened positive	MRI screened negative
US screened positive	23	0
US screened negative	6	32

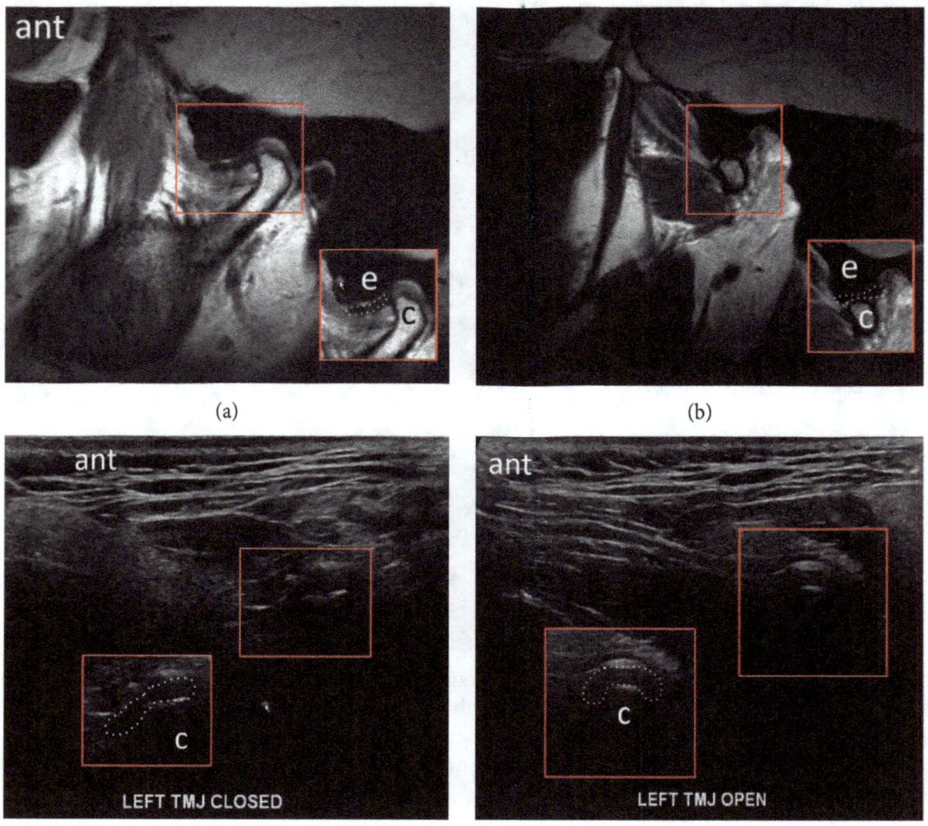

(a) (b)

(c) (d)

Figure 4: Images demonstrating anterior displacement of the disc in the sagittal plane in the (a) closed-mouth position with MR, (b) disc recapture in the open-mouth position with MR, (c) closed-mouth position with US, and (d) recapture in the open-mouth position with US. The disc retains normal morphology. A focal annotated view was provided to aid visualization with the articular disc outlined with a dotted contour; condyle = "c"; eminence = "e"; anterior = "ant."

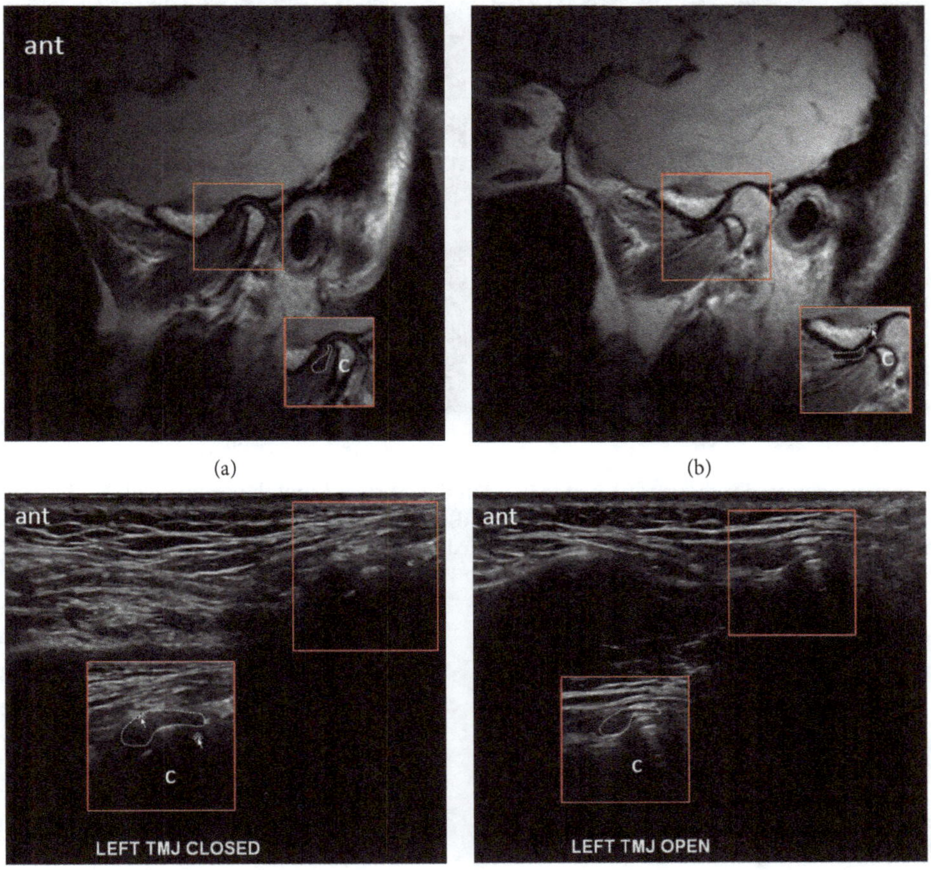

(a) (b)

(c) (d)

FIGURE 5: Images demonstrating a deformed disc with fixed anterior dislocation in the sagittal plane in the (a) closed-mouth position with MRI, (b) open-mouth position with MRI, (c) closed-mouth position with US, and (d) open-mouth position with US. A focal annotated view was provided to aid visualization with the articular disc outlined with a dotted contour; condyle = "c"; anterior = "ant"; left = "LT."

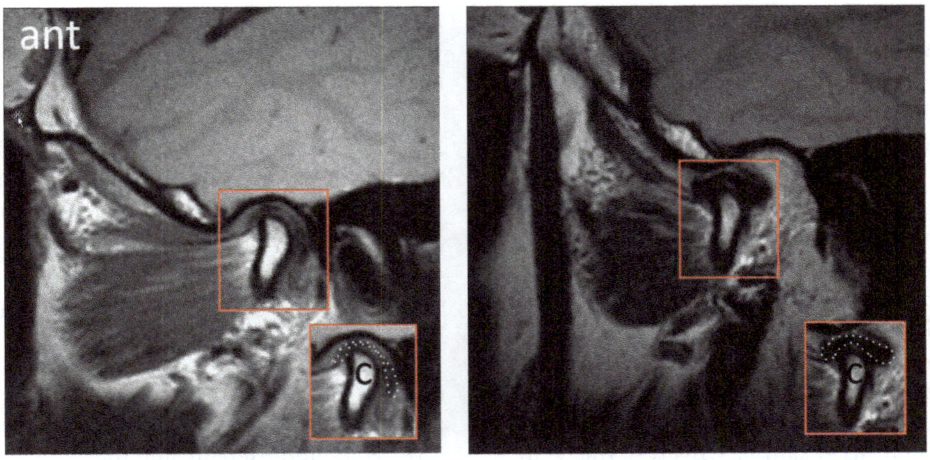

(a) (b)

FIGURE 6: Continued.

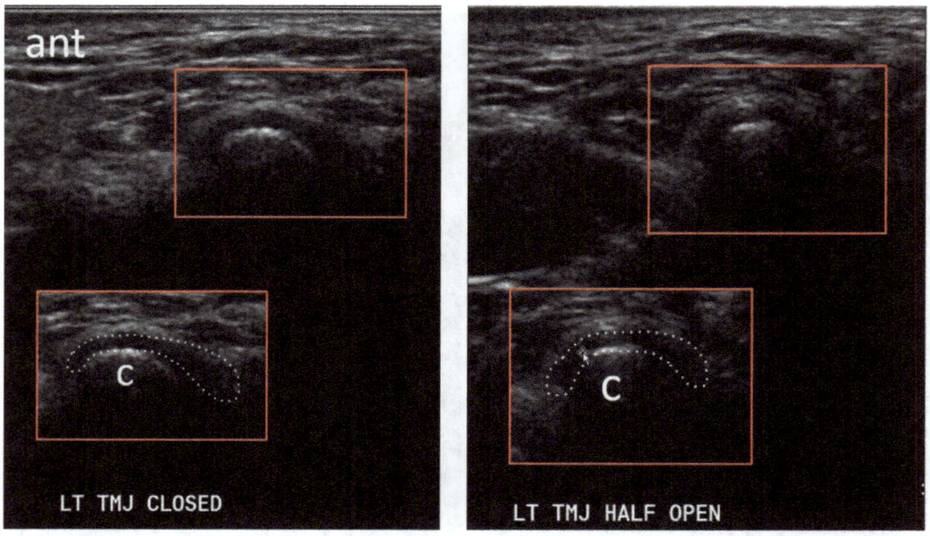

(c) (d)

FIGURE 6: Images demonstrating posterior displacement of the disc in the (a) closed-mouth position with MRI, (b) recapture in the open-mouth position with MRI, (c) closed-mouth position with US, and (d) recapture in the open-mouth position with US. A focal annotated view was provided to aid visualization with the articular disc outlined with a dotted contour; anterior = "ant"; condyle = "c"; left = "LT."

osteophyte formation in osteoarthritis involving the condyle can be visualized on ultrasound, as demonstrated in Figure 7.

4. Discussion

We introduce an advanced technique for evaluating the temporomandibular joint through ultrasound imaging by positioning the probe parallel to the articular disc throughout dynamic motion. US was presented as a screening tool for TMJ dysfunction due to its ubiquitous nature and relatively inexpensive cost. MRI was chosen as the gold standard for comparison due to its high level of specificity and sensitivity, as well as its role in current standard of practice.

We have limited our description of articular disc pathology to anterior, posterior, medial, and lateral dislocation, based on the most prominent feature only. While this creates labelling bias, this is unlikely to affect the patient outcome as the primary role is screening and subsequent MRI studies were performed for further characterization. Lateral displacement was not visualized in our study; however, this is not unexpected. Based on the 4% prevalence of lateral displacement by Katzberg et al. [17], only a single case is expected within a group of 29, and random chance alone is enough to explain its absence. However, medial and lateral displacements were generally difficult to visualize on US and are likely underestimated based on US alone. Validation of lateral displacement on US will require a much larger sample size given the relative rarity.

Prescreening patients for TMJ symptoms inherently creates a selection bias, with our measured prevalence of 47.5% grossly overestimating prevalence in the general population, but reflecting realistic clinical practice and the likely imaging prevalence. While the power of our study is limited, we believe our results to be sufficient for the initial validation of US as a screening tool to help decide who should proceed with additional MRI. We continue to screen patients with our US technique and have evaluated more than 350 additional patients; however, lack of corresponding MRI evaluation prevented their inclusion in this study.

Ethical management, requiring a definitive diagnosis for treatment to not be delayed, prevented US image acquisition and interpretation prior to MRI evaluation. Potential bias was minimized by limiting the number of MRIs interpreted by the expert radiologist who interpreted the US studies, and keeping him ignorant of MRI results until assessment of the US images was completed. In cases where the MRI was read first by the same radiologist who read the subsequent US, the US interpretation was held for 3-4 weeks to minimize recall bias.

Of the 6 false negative cases obtained using our technique, all cases noted to involve medial disc displacement were included. This is likely due to the limited penetrance of US because of bone and other anatomy, restricting it to the superficial one-third of the disc. Others have also noted that laterally or medially displaced discs are known to be inadequately visualized and evaluated with present ultrasound techniques [13].

Advantages of US over MRI identified during our study include the ability to observe real-time motion, clicking and crepitus, the ability to localize imaging to patient-directed regions of pain, and the ability to evaluate patients who are claustrophobic or have stents and implants that are not MRI compatible. Doppler imaging enabled us to diagnose inflammation by the presence of abnormal blood flow that, while theoretically possible if contrast is used, is unlikely on MRI with standard practices. US is also able to

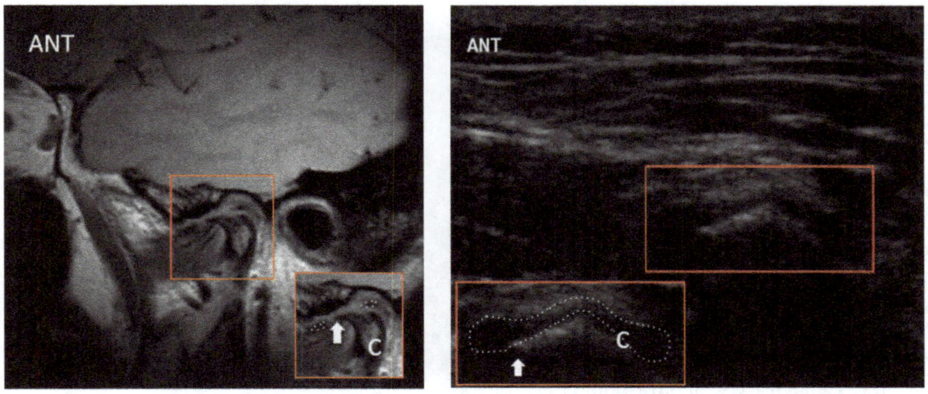

(a) (b)

Figure 7: Osteoarthritis with the deformed articular surface of the condyle with a large anterior marginal osteophyte and deformed disc with central thinning on (a) MR and (b) ultrasound. A focal annotated view was provided to aid visualization with the articular disc outlined with a dotted contour and the osteophyte indicated by an arrow; anterior = "ANT"; condyle = "c."

visualize cortical osseous defects including osteophytes and erosions. Retrodiscal visualization with US may partially be limited by patient body habitus and permitted acoustic windows by the adjacent osseous structures.

Disadvantages of US include the previously mentioned difficulties in visualizing medial and lateral disc displacements. While disc thickness and shape can be assessed with US, perforations and adhesions will not be adequately visualized. Subcortical osseous abnormalities also cannot be visualized. US always carries the inherent operator dependence, and there is necessarily a learning curve before an operator will obtain the expertise required to match the results presented in this paper. Our study is also limited to conventional US and MRI reconstruction algorithms. Others have evaluated enhancement filters for possible improvement of diagnostic efficiency on MRI [18], and similar evaluation on US is a possible topic for future research.

Our referring clinicians have stressed the importance of TMJ imaging to help differentiate between early and late changes. Early changes tend to be limited to disc displacement only, while late changes tend to include osseous remodelling, which may be underestimated or not assessed despite the advanced experience of the clinician. Fixed versus reducible disc displacements were important to them for treatment planning. For fixed disc displacement, our clinicians focus on mobilization of the joint, while reducible displacements are usually treated with bite splints. Surgery was not a common treatment option in their practices.

We believe that US ultimately has a role beyond screening for further MRI evaluation and can be used for definitive diagnosis in the majority of cases; however, definitive validation will likely require further evaluation using a larger sample size and hopefully a randomized prospective study in which patients can be placed in MRI-only and US-only evaluation.

5. Conclusions

US screening is a viable supplement to the more expensive MRI evaluation, especially when MRI access is limited, with the following caveats:

(1) Ultrasound should currently be limited to use as an initial screening tool, and the sonologist needs to only detect if the exam is normal or abnormal.

(2) If found to be normal, and surgery is not contemplated, then no further investigation is deemed necessary.

(3) If found to be abnormal, the patient should be referred for MRI.

(4) Due to poor sensitivity in visualizing medial disc displacement, if suspected, MRI should be performed despite a normal screening US.

Acknowledgments

The authors thank Judy Rubin for the illustration in Figure 2.

References

[1] J. M. H. Dibbets and L. T. van der Weele, "Prevalence of TMJ symptoms and X-ray findings," *European Journal of Orthodontics*, vol. 11, no. 1, pp. 31–36, 1989.

[2] P. L. Westesson and S. L. Bronstein, "Temporomandibular joint: comparison of single- and double-contrast arthrography," *Radiology*, vol. 164, no. 1, pp. 65–70, 1987.

[3] E. L. Christiansen, J. R. Thompson, A. N. Hasso et al., "CT number characteristics of malpositioned TMJ menisci," *Investigative Radiology*, vol. 22, no. 4, pp. 315–321, 1987.

[4] R. W. Katzberg, P. L. Westesson, R. H. Tallents et al., "Temporomandibular joint: MR assessment of rotational and sideways disk displacements," *Radiology*, vol. 169, no. 3, pp. 741–748, 1988.

[5] C. A. Helms and R. C. Fritz, *Magnetics Resonance Imaging of the Body*, C. B. Higgins, H. Hricak, and C. A. Helms, Eds., Raven Press, Ely, MN, USA, 1992.

[6] X. Tomas, J. Pomes, J. Berenguer et al., "MR imaging of temporomandibular joint dysfunction: a pictorial review," *RadioGraphics*, vol. 26, no. 3, pp. 765–781, 2006.

[7] H. Salé, F. Bryndahl, and A. Isberg, "Temporomandibular joints in asymptomatic and symptomatic nonpatient volunteers: a prospective 15-year follow-up clinical and MR imaging study," *Radiology*, vol. 267, no. 1, pp. 183–194, 2013.

[8] V. Stefanoff, J.-E. Hausamen, and P. van den Berghe, "Ultrasound imaging of the TMJ disc in asymptomatic volunteers," *Journal of Cranio-Maxillofacial Surgery*, vol. 20, no. 8, pp. 337–340, 1992.

[9] T. Hayashi, J. Ito, J. Koyama, and K. Yamada, "The accuracy of sonography for evaluation of internal derangement of the temporomandibular joint in asymptomatic elementary school children: comparison with MR and CT," *AJNR: American Journal of Neuroradiology*, vol. 22, no. 4, pp. 728–734, 2001.

[10] R. Emshoff, S. Jank, A. Rudisch, and G. Bodner, "Are high-resolution ultrasonographic signs of disc displacement valid?" *Journal of Oral and Maxillofacial Surgery*, vol. 60, no. 6, pp. 623–628, 2002.

[11] M. Melis, S. Secci, and C. Ceneviz, "Use of ultrasonography for the diagnosis of temporomandibular joint disorders: a review," *American Journal of Dentistry*, vol. 20, no. 2, pp. 73–78, 2007.

[12] R. W. Katzberg, "Is ultrasonography of the temporomandibular joint ready for prime time? Is there a "window" of opportunity?" *Journal of Oral and Maxillofacial Surgery*, vol. 70, no. 6, pp. 1310–1314, 2012.

[13] C. Li, N. Su, X. Yang, X. Yang, Z. Shi, and L. Li, "Ultrasonography for detection of disc displacement of temporomandibular joint: a systematic review and meta-analysis," *Journal of Oral and Maxillofacial Surgery*, vol. 70, no. 6, pp. 1300–1309, 2012.

[14] R. W. Katzberg, W. F. Conway, S. J. Ackerman, T. S. Gonzales, V. Kheyfits, and M. S. Cronan, "Pilot study to show the feasibility of high-resolution sagittal ultrasound imaging of the temporomandibular joint," *Journal of Oral and Maxillofacial Surgery*, vol. 75, no. 6, pp. 1151–1162, 2017.

[15] N. Su, A. J. van Wijk, C. M. Visscher, F. Lobbezoo, and G. J. M. G. van der Heijden, "Diagnostic value of ultrasonography for the detection of disc displacements in the temporomandibular joint: a systematic review and meta-analysis," *Clinical Oral Investigations*, vol. 22, no. 7, pp. 2599–2614, 2018.

[16] S. M. Shaffer, J.-M. Brismée, P. S. Sizer, and C. A. Courtney, "Temporomandibular disorders—part 1: anatomy and examination/diagnosis," *Journal of Manual & Manipulative Therapy*, vol. 22, no. 1, pp. 2–12, 2014.

[17] R. W. Katzberg, P.-L. Westesson, R. H. Tallents, and C. M. Drake, "Anatomic disorders of the temporomandibular joint disc in asymptomatic subjects," *Journal of Oral and Maxillofacial Surgery*, vol. 54, no. 2, pp. 147–153, 1996.

[18] G. A. Montesinos, S. L. P. Castro Lopes, T. Trivino et al., "Subjective analysis of the application of enhancement filters on magnetic resonance imaging of the temporomandibular joint," *Oral Surgery, Oral Medicine, Oral Pathology and Oral Radiology*, vol. 127, no. 6, pp. 552–559, 2019.

20

Perception of Ghanaian Primigravidas Undergoing Their First Antenatal Ultrasonography in Cape Coast

Emmanuel Kobina Mesi Edzie,[1] **Klenam Dzefi-Tettey**,[2] **Philip Narteh Gorleku**,[1] **James William Ampofo**,[3] **Albert Dayor Piersson**,[3] **Abdul Raman Asemah**,[1] **Henry Kusodzi**,[1] **and Richard Ato Edzie**[1]

[1]*Department of Medical Imaging, School of Medical Sciences, College of Health and Allied Sciences, University of Cape Coast, P.M.B. University of Cape Coast, Cape Coast, Ghana*
[2]*Department of Radiology, Korle Bu Teaching Hospital, P.O. Box KB77, Korle Bu, Accra, Ghana*
[3]*Department of Imaging Technology and Sonography, School of Allied Health Sciences, College of Health and Allied Sciences, University of Cape Coast, P.M.B. University of Cape Coast, Cape Coast, Ghana*

Correspondence should be addressed to Emmanuel Kobina Mesi Edzie; emmanuel.edzie@ucc.edu.gh

Academic Editor: Daniele La Forgia

Ultrasound scans have become an essential requirement of pregnancy care in countries with developed health services and increasingly being used in medical practice in Ghana as well. The aim of this study was to find out the perception of primigravidas experiencing antenatal ultrasonography for the first time in Cape Coast. This was a descriptive, prospective study which employed the use of a questionnaire to obtain data from 384 consented respondents, who were primigravidas experiencing antenatal ultrasonography for the first time in three selected public health facilities in Cape Coast Metropolis over a six-month period. Sociodemographic data, reasons for undergoing antenatal ultrasound, their expectations, knowledge in fetal abnormalities, and suggestions to help improve their future experiences were collected. The data were analyzed using SPSS software, version 20.0 (SPSS Inc., Chicago, IL, USA). Out of a total number of 384 respondents, 87.8% of them knew about what ultrasound is used for. 87.5% scanned because a doctor or midwife requested for the scan whilst 53.9% scanned to check for fetal abnormalities. 98.4% indicated that ultrasound scanning has positive effects on pregnancy outcome. An expensive service was stated as a negative reason that would influence the decision to undergo the examination next time; nonetheless, 90.4% would recommend it to other women and suggested showing the fetus on monitor while scanning and providing accurate findings would make their future experiences better. The perception of the primigravidas was largely positive. Checking for fetal abnormalities was a major reason for the scans, although their knowledge in specific fetal abnormalities was low. They expected to know the fetal sex, but that was not a major reason for scanning. Showing them the monitor was the most frequent suggestion to make future experience better.

1. Introduction

Ultrasound technology, initially developed in the advanced world, is now continuously evolving in other parts of the world and has become a crucial part of antenatal care in developing countries [1–4]. Today, the use of ultrasound has become a common practice for routine antenatal care in health centres; consequently, there has been a lot of interventional packages like specialized ultrasound training to improve women's experience with antenatal ultrasonography [5]. Its use has shown benefits for women who perceive antenatal scanning as a means for reassurance about the health and wellbeing of their fetus, while for others, ultrasound might be injurious and can harm or deform the fetus [6, 7]. The importance of ultrasound scanning in prenatal care cannot be overemphasized although there may be variations in the degree of diagnostic accuracy of ultrasound depending on when pregnant women present themselves for an ultrasound examination (in the estimation of gestational age, determination of fetal sex and fetal anomaly, etc.) [8] which can give adequate and timely information for the necessary decisions to be made and also helps in keeping pregnant women informed about the wellbeing of their unborn babies and keeping them reassured [6, 7]. A correct determination of gestational age is needed to distinguish preterm newborns from newborns who are with low birth weight (but not preterm), which is important because the needed interventions may differ [9]. The regular use of ultrasound scan in the management of pregnancy has dramatically improved the detection of high-risk pregnancies and increased prenatal care attendance although there is no consensus about whether the use of obstetric ultrasound has the ability to decrease maternal and child mortality in low- and middle-income countries [10–12].

Across many countries, women have rated ultrasonography as one of the most crucial part of their antenatal care [13]. In view of the overwhelming benefits of ultrasound in women, many women in Africa have not fully taken advantage of this imaging modality partly due to the misconceptions they have or have heard about the procedure elsewhere [14]. In sub-Saharan Africa, the kind of perception women have on antenatal ultrasound varies and greatly depends on the educational status attained [15, 16]. In some African societies, there are some cultural resistances to ultrasound usage in obstetrics, where it runs up against traditional myths and taboos. Some ethnic groups consider it a bad luck to reveal the content of the uterus in pregnancy and to be able to see the fetus [17, 18]. However, in some parts of sub-Saharan Africa, women have positive views about ultrasound services and considered ultrasound as a tool that could make pregnancy and childbirth safer [19]. For instance, in the rural Botswana district hospital, pregnant women showed signs of trusting the ultrasound results more than their own bodily sensations to confirm a live fetus [20].

In Ghana, there are many public and private ultrasound-imaging centres, and antenatal care practitioners are equally increasingly referring their clients for ultrasound evaluation of their pregnancies [21]. Many pregnant women undergo antenatal ultrasound imaging examination daily in Cape Coast and it will be interesting to know how these pregnant women perceive antenatal ultrasonography especially for first-time users. The perception of primigravidas about antenatal ultrasonography has been scarcely described in this locality. Therefore, this study is designed to determine the perception of the primigravidas without prior experience of antenatal ultrasonography scan in Cape Coast.

2. Materials and Methods

This was a cross-sectional prospective study conducted from 1st May to 30th September 2019 in the Cape Coast Metropolis of Ghana using a questionnaire. The questionnaire was designed to address how the primigravidas experiencing their first antenatal ultrasound perceive the use of ultrasonography, with regard to their knowledge and expectations just before their first antenatal ultrasound examination and their suggestions and recommendations just after undergoing the examination. This was done in order to capture the perception of respondents on each variable under consideration.

The respondents were primigravidas experiencing their first antenatal ultrasonography from the Cape Coast Teaching Hospital (CCTH), Adisadel Clinic, and Ankaful General Hospital (AGH) and those who had experienced antenatal ultrasonography before were excluded. CCTH is located in the central part of the Cape Coast Metropolis of the Central Region of Ghana and is the largest public health institution in the region, which offers tertiary services. It also serves as a referral point for both public and private primary and secondary health facilities in the Central Region. Adisadel Clinic and Ankaful General Hospital, both being secondary health facilities, are located in the southern part and the north-western part of Cape Coast Metropolis, respectively. These selected sites are the main public health facilities that offer ultrasound services in Cape Coast Metropolis.

The sample size of 384 was obtained using the population of women in the Central Region of Ghana from the National Census 2010, which was estimated to be about 1,151,751 (2010 Population and Housing Census) [22] and using the statistical software sample size calculator [23] at a confidence level of 95% with an error margin of 5%. The respondents were obtained from outpatients visiting these facilities for antenatal ultrasound imaging. Simple random sampling technique was used to select respondents for the study in each facility after proportionately allocating the number of respondents that were selected from each facility based on how busy the ultrasonography unit was in the past year. CCTH had an annual ultrasound imaging examinations of 8436 for 2018, Adisadel Clinic had 3120, and AGH had 2080 for 2018 from the primary records of the respective facilities giving a total of 13,636 examinations. Using simple proportions, 237, 88, and 59 respondents were obtained from CCTH, Adisadel Clinic, and Ankaful General Hospital, respectively, as shown in Table 1.

Between the hours of 7:00 AM and 8:00 AM each day, pregnant women who reported to the ultrasound unit were approached and those who were primigravidas irrespective of their gestational age and were there for their first scan were identified. The nature of the study was explained to them and all of those willing to participate were recruited and given consent form to sign. Numbers were assigned to these consented participants and a maximum of five were picked through balloting every day. The questionnaires were pretested to check for clarity, reliability, and validity. The pretested questionnaires with both open- and close-ended questions were administered to these five randomly selected participants until the target for each site was attained. The questionnaires were administered in two parts, the first part, which featured questions to elicit their knowledge and views about the procedure, their expectations during the procedure, and the reason why they were there for the ultrasound examinations, before entering the scan room and the second part, which included questions like whether participants would recommend antenatal ultrasound scan to other women and why, and their suggestions to the doctors to

Table 1: Sample size determination for each site.

Facility	Ultrasound throughput 2018	Number of participants at each site
CCTH	8436	237
Adisadel	3120	88
AGH	2080	59
Total	13636	384

make their next experience better, after experiencing the scan.

The questionnaires were retrieved and carefully checked for completeness. The data obtained from both open- and close-ended questions were grouped, organized, coded, and inputted into Excel (2010) and analyzed using SPSS software, version 20.0 (SPSS Inc., Chicago, IL, USA) for Windows to obtain frequencies, charts, and percentages. A Chi-squared test for independence was conducted to establish the association between the levels of education of the participants and various responses regarding their knowledge on congenital abnormalities and reasons for antenatal ultrasonography. The level of significance was specified at $P < 0.05$.

2.1. Ethical Consideration. Ethical clearance for this study was obtained from the Institutional Review Board of the CCTH. Written informed consent was obtained from each participant before the questionnaire was administered. Those who did not consent were excluded. Confidentiality and anonymity were ensured. The questionnaires were safely stored in a locked cabinet at the Department of Radiology of CCTH. This study conformed to the 1975 Declaration of Helsinki.

3. Results

3.1. Sociodemographic Characteristics of Participants. A total of 384 primigravidas attending antenatal ultrasound imaging in Cape Coast met the inclusion criteria and were recruited into the study. The mean age of the primigravidas was 29.1 years (SD 1.14 years). Sociodemographic characteristics (age ranges, educational status, religion, occupation, and marital status) are shown in Table 2.

The majority of the respondents 337 (87.8%) indicated that they knew what ultrasound is used for. Almost all the women 378 (98.4%) indicated that ultrasound has positive effects on pregnancy outcome (generally safe, check fetal wellbeing, position and presentation, etc.) with just few 6 (1.6%) stating ultrasound has negative effects on pregnancy outcome (time wasting, the wrong diagnosis of fetal sex and abnormality, the wrong estimation of date of delivery, etc.). The decision of the women to undergo their next ultrasound scan would be influenced by the cost of the ultrasound scan in 374 (97.4%) of responses and stated the following as reasons: expensive service in 171 (45.7%), free service in 119 (31.8%), and service captured under NHIS in 84 (22.5%) responses. The cost was not a factor for 10 (2.6%) of the respondents (Table 3).

Table 2: Sociodemographic characteristics of participants.

Variable	Frequency (%)
Age of respondents	
11–20 years	41 (10.7)
21–30 years	180 (46.9)
31–40 years	148 (38.5)
41–50 years	15 (3.9)
Level of education	
No formal education	21 (5.5)
Basic education (class 1 to junior high)	181 (47.1)
Secondary education	89 (23.2)
Tertiary education	93 (24.2)
Religion	
Christian	336 (87.5)
Muslim	48 (12.5)
Occupation	
Farmer	5 (1.6)
Trader	132 (41.6)
Civil servant	16 (5.0)
Housewife	6 (1.9)
Self-employed	5 (1.6)
Vocational	69 (21.8)
Professionals	84 (26.5)
Marital status	
Single	85 (22.1)
Married	293 (76.3)
Divorced	1 (0.3)
Widowed	1 (0.3)
Separated	4 (1.0)

3.2. The Women's Views on Frequency of Ultrasound Imaging during the Pregnancy. The majority of the respondents 133 (34.6%) indicated that they wanted antenatal ultrasound imaging done three times in a pregnancy. 93 (24.2%), 70 (18.2%), and 48 (12.5%) of the respondents wanted ultrasound scan performed for them two times, more than three times, and once, respectively. Out of the 384 respondents, 40 (10.4%) did not know the number of times they wanted ultrasound imaging done during a pregnancy.

The commonest reason for women to undergo ultrasound imaging was because a doctor or midwife requested it in 336 (87.5%) of the respondents. 184 (47.9%) had the scan done because they thought it was relevant to the management of their pregnancy, but 200 (52.1%) did not think so. Only 146 (38.0%) of the 384 women would do an ultrasound imaging to check the gender of the fetus. Out of the total of 384 women, 207 (53.9%) of the women were interested in checking for abnormalities in the fetus, 150 (39.1%) wanted to confirm the estimated date of delivery, and 133 (34.6%) were interested in checking for the number of fetuses. None

Table 3: Respondents views about obstetric ultrasound scans.

Variable	Frequency (%)
Do you know what ultrasound is used for?	
Yes	337 (87.8)
No	47 (12.2)
What effects do you think ultrasound can have on your pregnancy outcome?	
Positive effects	378 (98.4)
Negative effects	6 (1.6)
Will the cost of ultrasound scanning influence your decision to undergo the examination next time?	
Yes	374 (97.4)
No	10 (2.6)
Why the cost will influence your decision?	
Expensive services	171 (45.7)
Captured under NHIS	84 (22.5)
Free services	119 (31.8)

NHIS: National Health Insurance Scheme.

of the pregnant women undertook the scan because religious leaders advised them to do so. Regarding expectations of the participants for antenatal ultrasound scan, responses from the participants indicated that 223 (58.1%) expected to know pregnancy-related complications, 224 (58.3%) wanted to know the gender of the fetus, while 221 (57.6%) expected to be informed on any abnormalities in the fetus during their scan. However, 184 (47.9%) expected to be informed on whether the placenta is located normally, 141 (36.7%) wanted to be informed on the number of fetuses they were carrying, and 126 (32.8%) indicated that they wanted to see their fetus before birth (Table 4).

The majority of the respondents 135 (35.2%) suggested that they should be allowed to view the scan monitor during the scanning process; the other suggestions are shown in Figure 1.

The degree to which respondents agreed or disagreed with the benefits of antenatal ultrasound imaging showed that the majority 354 (92.2%) of the participants, comprising 190 (49.5%) strongly agreeing and 164 (42.7%) agreeing that ultrasound can help in diagnosing some congenital abnormalities, while only 13 (3.4%) strongly or just disagreed that ultrasound can help in diagnosing some congenital abnormalities. 17 (4.4%) were neutral. Almost all the respondents 382 (99.5%) further affirmed that ultrasound imaging is necessary in pregnancy comprising 284 (74.0%) and 98 (25.5%) strongly agreeing and just agreeing, respectively. None strongly disagreed that ultrasound was necessary in pregnancy with only 1 (0.3%) just disagreeing, and 1 (0.3%) was neutral. Also 209 (54.4%) and 113 (29.4%) strongly agreed and agreed, respectively, that ultrasound can help determine the gender of the fetus with a composite 322 (83.8%) agreeing, whereas 30 (7.8%) were neutral and 27 (7.0%) and 5 (1.3%) disagreed and strongly disagreed, respectively. 374 (97.4%) of the respondents indicated that they strongly agreed and agreed that ultrasound can determine the position of the fetus; 3 (0.8%) disagreed and 7 (1.8%) were neutral. With respect to the ability of antenatal ultrasound imaging to determine the presentation of the fetus, a majority of the women 336 (90.1%), comprising 224 (58.3%) who strongly agreed and 112 (31.8%) agreed, 25

Table 4: The women's reasons for undergoing ultrasound and expectations for the scan.

Variable	Frequency (%)
Reasons	
Requested by doctor	
Yes	336 (87.5)
No	48 (12.5)
Relevant to management of pregnancy	
Yes	184 (47.9)
No	200 (52.1)
To estimate date of delivery	
Yes	150 (39.1)
No	234 (60.9)
To check the number of fetuses	
Yes	133 (34.6)
No	251 (65.4)
To check the gender of fetus	
Yes	146 (38.0)
No	238 (62.0)
To check for abnormalities in the fetus	
Yes	207 (53.9)
No	177 (46.1)
A religious leader advised me to do it	
Yes	0 (0.0)
No	384 (100.0)
Expectations	
Know gender of fetus	
Yes	224 (58.3)
No	160 (41.7)
See fetus before birth	
Yes	126 (32.8)
No	258 (67.2)
Pregnancy-related complications	
Yes	223 (58.1)
No	161 (41.9)
Know placenta is located normally	
Yes	184 (47.9)
No	200 (52.1)
Know any abnormalities in fetus	
Yes	221 (57.6)
No	163 (42.4)
Know the number of fetuses	
Yes	141 (36.7)
No	243 (63.3)

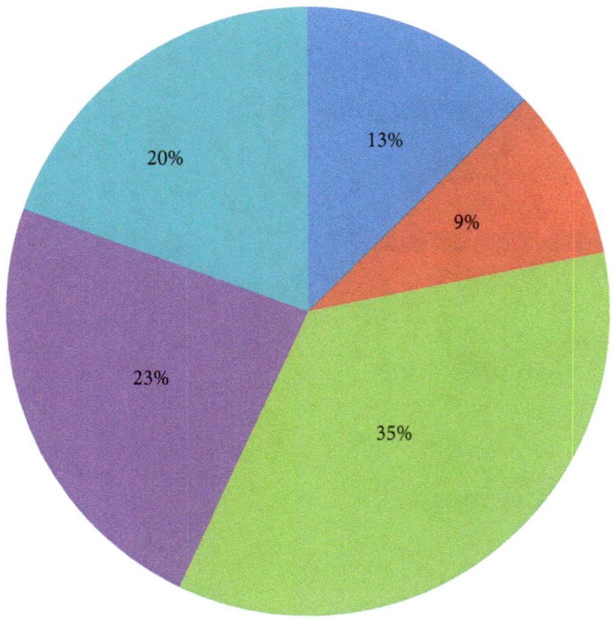

FIGURE 1: Participants' suggestions to doctors to make their experience better during their next ultrasound imaging.

(6.5%) were neutral, 11 (2.9%) disagreed, and 2 (0.5%) strongly disagreed as shown in Figure 2.

Out of the total number of 384 respondents, 246 (64.1%) agreed that ultrasound can diagnose abnormal head development and the rest did not. 201 (52.3%) also indicated that it could help diagnose cardiac developmental abnormalities whereas 151 (39.3%) stated that it can diagnose cleft palate. The responses further showed that 165 (43.0%), 121 (31.5%), and 67 (17.4%) of the respondents specified that ultrasound could help diagnose limb abnormalities, fetal organ abnormalities, and Down's syndrome, respectively (Figure 3).

A high number, 347 (90.4%), of the participants would recommend antenatal ultrasound imaging to other women; the rest 37 (9.6%) would not. The majority of the 347 respondents, 107 (30.8%), cited that their main reasons for recommending the antenatal ultrasonography were to ensure the detection of the fetal position, development, and pregnancy-related complications. Detection of congenital abnormalities was also indicated by 97 (28.0%) respondents as another reason for their recommendation of ultrasound scan followed by 86 (24.8%) that stated the management of pregnancy and planning for recommending ultrasonography scan. It was also stated by 57 (16.4%) of the respondents that knowing the estimated date of delivery and confirming pregnancy was also a reason for recommending the scan (Table 5).

4. Discussion

Since its perfected clinical use in the 1950s, ultrasound plays an essential role in antenatal care around the world [24]. The modal age range for this study was 21–30 years. This agrees with the same age range reported by Saleh et al. [15]. The mean age for the participants was 29.1 (SD 1.14) years, which is similar to the 29.4 years reported in Sweden by Georgsson Öhman and Waldenström [25] and deviated from the 27.7 years reported in Nottingham by Whynes [26] and 28.1 years in Ghana by Mensah et al. [21]. The majority of the primigravidas (76.3%) in the study were married, which is expected in our setting where most gravid women are usually married corroborated by Mensah et al. [21] and Adekanmi et al. [6].

The majority of the participants (98.4%) stated that ultrasound has mainly positive effects on pregnancy outcome (generally safe, check fetal wellbeing, position and presentation, etc.). Saleh et al. [15] reported that the ultrasound procedure is safe, which is one of the positive effects found in this study. This finding is encouraging, as it will not deter them from undergoing the examination. The decision of the respondents to undergo the scan the next time would be influenced by the cost of the examination in 97.4% of cases and most of them stated expensive cost as their main reason in this study. Most of the participants (34.6%) indicated that the scans should be done three times during the course of a pregnancy contrary to what was found in Nigeria by Saleh et al. [15] that showed that most (41.0%) wanted it twice. This study found that the modal number of scans the women wanted to undergo was 3.0 which is higher than the 2.0 reported in Ghana by Mensah et al. [21] and in UK by Whynes [26]. These differences may be due to the fact that we looked at the expected number of scans per pregnancy while the studies done in Ghana and UK above looked at the actual number of scans that were done.

The main reasons why the respondents had their antenatal scans were that a doctor or midwife requested for it in 87.5% of responses. This agrees with a study conducted by Mensah et al. [21] which reported that 100% of the requests were from the doctor or midwife. This may be explained by the fact that in Ghana, requests are made by practitioners for antenatal ultrasonography during routine antenatal care in order to monitor the progress of pregnancy. Irrespective of their educational background (Table 6), the majority of the participants from this study (53.9%) wanted to know if there were any fetal abnormalities (Table 4). This is similar to a study conducted in Sweden, which also reported the majority of respondents who wanted confirmation of normality [25]. The knowledge about the normality status of the fetus turns to reassure pregnant women about the health and safety of the fetus.

39.1%, 38.0%, and 34.6% indicated they wanted to know their estimated date of delivery, gender of the fetus, and the number of the fetuses, respectively. These may be low due to the fact that those variables are out of control of the women and therefore were not the main reasons they considered for undergoing the scans. Nonetheless, a higher percentage (83.8%) of the women knew the capability of ultrasound in detecting the gender of the fetus even though it was not a major reason for the scan. A reason that may account for this disparity may be sociocultural, since inheritance and lineage may be maternal or paternal in various parts of the country

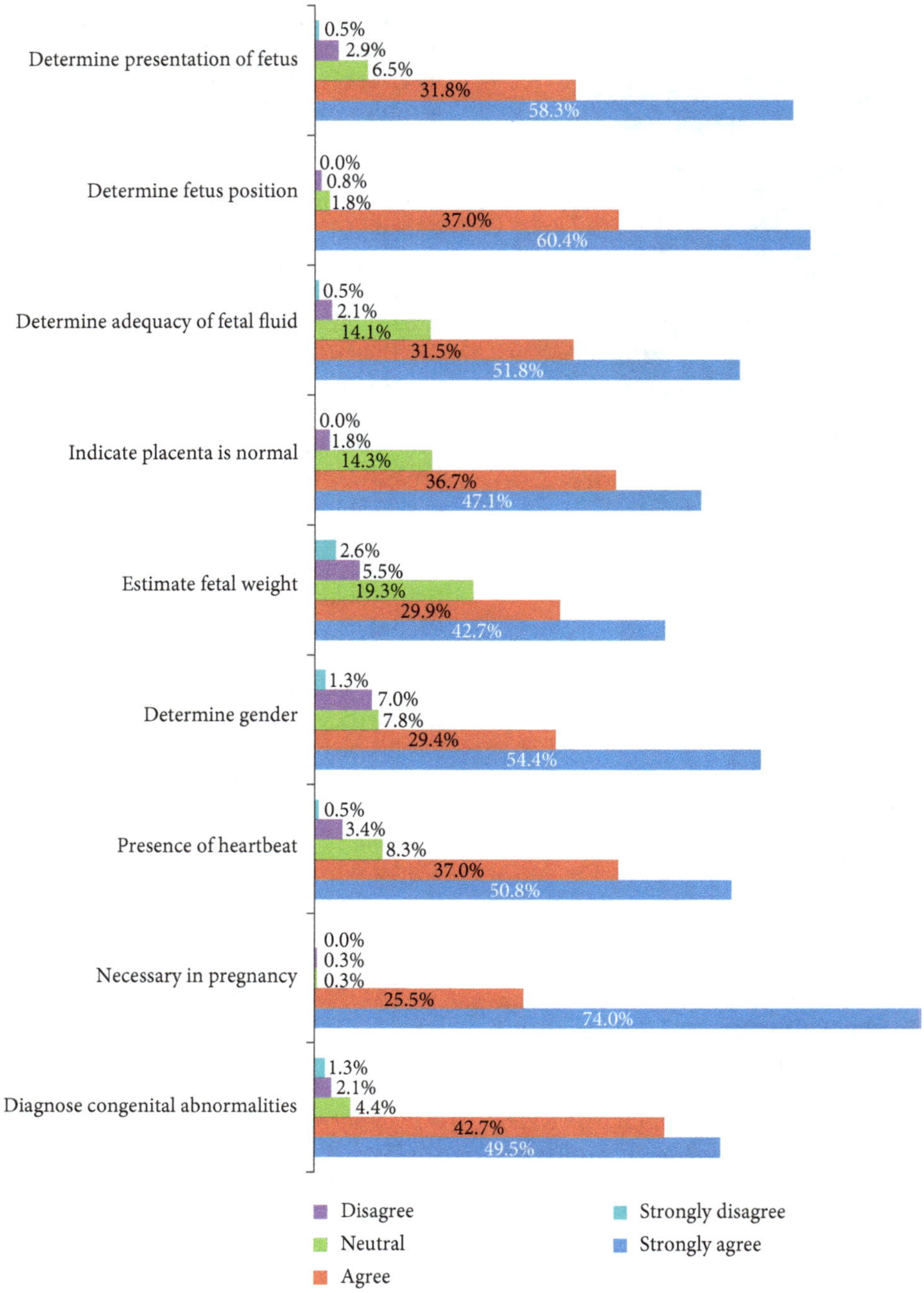

Figure 2: Knowledge of respondents about the ultrasound imaging.

and also, Ghanaian custom views children as members of either their mother's or father's lineage (extended family), but not both. The patrilineal custom charges a man's lineage with caring for his widow and children, while matrilineal custom places this burden on the widows' lineage—her father, brother, and uncles—and hence there is no emphasis placed on gender [27].

Religious considerations did not influence the participants in their decision to undergo the scanning, though all the respondents were either Christians or Muslims. This is interesting to note because Ghanaian societies are highly influenced by religion in almost all spheres of life, which corroborates with a study in Ghana, which reported prayers and revelation, reversing negative dreams, laying of hands, and anointing pregnant women as pastor's spiritual interventions in pregnancies by Aziato et al. [28].

It was noted that even before undergoing ultrasound scan for the first time, these primigravidas had a wide range of expectations for the ultrasound examination including knowing gender of the fetus (58.3%), fetal abnormalities (57.6%), seeing of the fetus before birth (32.8%), knowing the number of fetuses (36.7%), etc. as shown in Table 4 which were much lower than that of Irish counterparts (90%, 85%, 62%, and 99%, respectively), as reported by [29]. The higher degree of expectation of the Irish respondents may be because all the

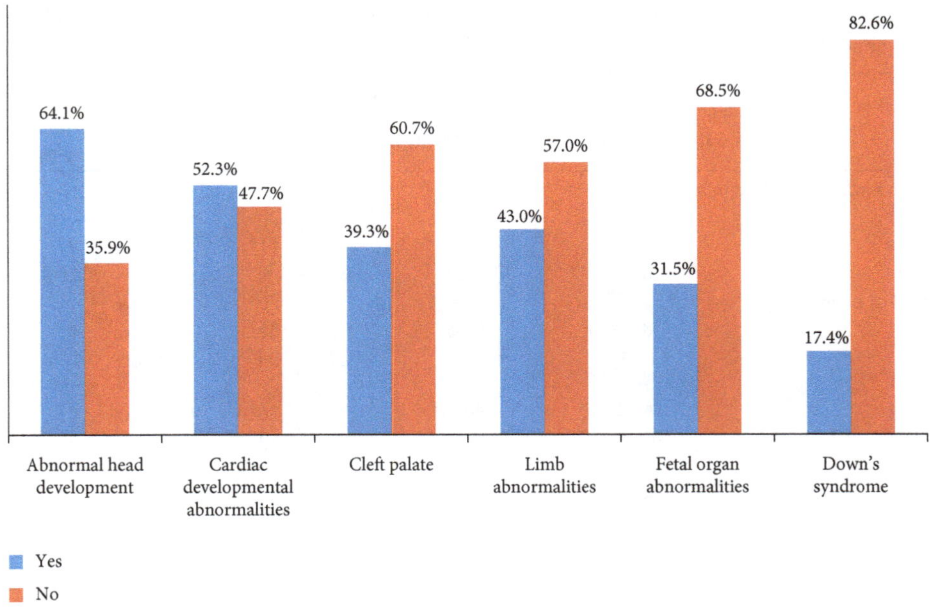

FIGURE 3: Knowledge of congenital abnormalities that ultrasound can diagnose.

TABLE 5: The women's reasons for recommending ultrasound scanning to other women.

Variable	Frequency (%)
Will you recommend ultrasound to other women?	
Yes	347 (90.4)
No	37 (9.6)
Reasons for the recommendations	
Detect congenital abnormalities	97 (28.0)
Detect fetal position, development, and pregnancy-related complication	107 (30.8)
Management of pregnancy and planning	86 (24.8)
To know the estimated date of delivery and confirm pregnancy	57 (16.4)

participants were literates whilst in our study the literacy level of most of the respondents was low.

With regards to the knowledge of the respondents, 87.8% of the respondents had knowledge about what ultrasound is used for, similar to what was found in Nigeria by Agbata et al. [30] who reported that a high percentage of respondents had knowledge on the use of ultrasound in pregnancy. This is consistent with the report showing that knowledge on ultrasound is high, since there is an extensive use of ultrasound in health care today as part of routine antenatal care as well as unlimited access to information, according to Saleh et al. [15]. The majority (above 80%) agreed that ultrasound can determine the presentation of the fetus, the presence of a heartbeat, indicate whether the placenta is normal, congenital abnormalities, the fetal gender, the position of the fetus, estimate fetal weight, adequacy of fluid around the fetus, and is necessary in pregnancy (Figure 2). This is comparable to the findings with some similar parameters as reported by [29]. This confirms that the women exhibited a high degree of knowledge about obstetric ultrasonography, which is laudable. Our study found that the expressed knowledge of the participants on specific congenital and chromosomal abnormalities was varied, but generally low (Figure 2), even though we found a significant association between their level of education and knowledge on some specific congenital abnormalities like cleft palates, fetal organ abnormalities, and Down's syndrome. This result is comparable to the varied results reported in Ireland with regards to fetal malformations and chromosomal abnormalities [29]. This may be due to the varying depth of technical knowledge.

The percentages of suggestions made by our respondents to make their next experience better in this study were generally higher than what was reported by a study in Nottingham which reported only 6.6% of respondents suggesting information flow as the area for improvement and 4.1% suggesting more detailed interpretation of the screen images (Whynes [26]) as compared to 12.8% and 23.4%, respectively, in our study (Figure 1). This may be due to the fact that Nottingham respondents were more satisfied with the ultrasound services provided and hence did not offer too many suggestions. Generally, the women considered antenatal ultrasound an essential part of antenatal care with most (90.4%) indicating that they would recommend it to other women and cited detection of the fetal position, fetal development, and pregnancy-related complications as their reasons for the recommendation.

Table 6: A cross-tabulation of the levels of education of participants against women's reasons for undergoing ultrasound scanning and knowledge of congenital abnormalities that ultrasound can diagnose.

Variable	Levels of education				χ^2	*P* value
	No formal education	Basic education	Secondary education	Tertiary education		
The women's reasons for undergoing ultrasound						
Requested by doctor						
Yes	15	157	81	83	6.317	0.097
No	6	24	8	10		
Relevant to management of pregnancy						
Yes	8	78	35	63	19.777	**0.000***
No	13	103	54	30		
Estimate date of delivery						
Yes	5	54	36	55	24.349	**0.000***
No	16	127	53	38		
Check number of fetuses						
Yes	5	50	30	48	16.891	**0.001***
No	16	131	59	45		
Check gender of fetus						
Yes	4	61	36	45	9.105	**0.028***
No	17	120	53	48		
Abnormalities in fetus						
Yes	9	88	51	59	6.884	0.076
No	12	93	38	34		
Knowledge of congenital abnormalities that ultrasound can diagnose						
Abnormal head development						
Yes	13	112	63	58	2.282	0.516
No	8	69	26	35		
Cardiac developmental abnormalities						
Yes	9	93	47	52	1.308	0.727
No	12	88	42	41		
Cleft palate						
Yes	7	85	30	29	8.501	**0.037***
No	14	96	59	64		
Limb abnormalities						
Yes	8	77	35	45	1.813	0.612
No	13	104	54	48		
Fetal organ abnormalities						
Yes	5	45	25	46	18.654	**0.000***
No	16	136	64	47		
Down's syndrome						
Yes	0	27	13	27	14.407	**0.002***
No	21	154	76	66		

*Statistically significant. Pearson's Chi-square (χ^2) was used to examine the relationship between levels of education of participants against women's reasons for undergoing ultrasound scanning and their knowledge of congenital abnormalities that ultrasound can help diagnose. *P* value ≤0.05 is statistically significant.

4.1. Limitation of the Study. Interpretation of questionnaires to nonliterate clients may introduce interviewer bias. Although responses from the open-ended questions were checked and grouped under common themes, certain opinions may have been suppressed.

5. Conclusion

The main reasons for the Ghanaian primigravidas to undergo ultrasound imaging were because the doctor or midwife requested for the scan and also to check for fetal abnormalities. The general knowledge on ultrasound use in pregnancy was high but the knowledge of specific congenital fetal abnormalities that can be detected by ultrasound imaging was generally low. Religious considerations did not influence the participants in their decision to undergo the ultrasound scanning, which is encouraging in the Ghanaian/African setting where religion plays a key role in the way things are done. The main expectations of the respondents in this study were to know gender, pregnancy-related complications, and abnormalities in the fetus. The most common suggestions stated by the participants to make their future experiences with ultrasound better were that the practitioners should allow them to view the scan monitor during the procedure, be provided with more accurate ultrasound findings, and the ultrasound examination be made affordable in terms of pricing. The perception of the respondents on ultrasound imaging during pregnancy was largely positive.

5.1. Implications for Practice. Expectations from the women to diagnose congenital abnormalities were moderate and hence practitioners must be skilled enough to meet such expectations. Low knowledge about specific fetal abnormalities that ultrasound can help diagnose means practitioners must give more education. Provision of modern equipment to improve detection of more complications and to improve accuracy of findings is encouraged.

Authors' Contributions

E. K. M. Edzie, K. Dzefi-Tettey, P. N. Gorleku, J. W. Ampofo, A. D. Piersson, A. R. Asemah, H. Kusodzi, and R. A. Edzie made substantial contributions to conception, literature search, design, acquisition of data, analysis, interpretation of the data, drafting, revision, and approval of the manuscript for publication.

Acknowledgments

The authors are grateful to the pregnant women attending Antenatal Care at the Cape Coast Teaching Hospital, Adisadel Clinic, and Ankaful General Hospital. The authors are grateful to the doctors, sonographers, and nurses at the obstetric ultrasound units of these hospitals for their co-operation and making this study a success.

References

[1] T. Gammeltoft, H. T. T. Nguyên, and T. Nguyen, "The commodification of obstetric ultrasound scanning in hanoi, Viet Nam," *Reproductive Health Matters*, vol. 15, no. 29, pp. 163–171, 2007.

[2] J. Garcia, L. Bricker, J. Henderson et al., "Women's views of pregnancy ultrasound: a systematic review," *Birth*, vol. 29, no. 4, pp. 225–250, 2002.

[3] H. Bashour, R. Hafez, and A. Abdulsalam, "Syrian women's perceptions and experiences of ultrasound screening in pregnancy: implications for antenatal policy," *Reproductive Health Matters*, vol. 13, no. 25, pp. 147–154, 2005.

[4] J. A. Akinmoladun, G. I. Ogbole, T. A. Lawal, and O. A. Adesina, "Routine prenatal ultrasound anomaly screening program in a Nigerian University Hospital: redefining obstetrics practice in a developing African country," *Nigerian Medical Journal*, vol. 56, no. 4, pp. 263–267, 2015.

[5] E. T. Kim, K. Singh, A. Moran, D. Armbruster, and N. Kozuki, "Obstetric ultrasound use in low and middle income countries: a narrative review," *Reproductive Health*, vol. 15, no. 1, p. 129, 2018.

[6] A. J. Adekanmi, I. O. Morhason-Bello, O. M. Atalabi, B. O. Adedokun, A. A. Adeniji-Sofoluwe, and A. O. Marinho, "Misconception about ultrasound among Nigerian women attending specialist and tertiary health institutions in Ibadan," *Tropical Journal of Obstetrics and Gynaecology*, vol. 29, no. 2, 2012.

[7] P. L. Rice and C. Naksook, "Pregnancy and technology: Thai women's perceptions and experience of prenatal testing," *Health Care for Women International*, vol. 20, no. 3, pp. 259–278, 1999.

[8] K. Stanton and L. Mwanri, "Global maternal and child health outcomes: the role of obstetric ultrasound in low resource settings," *World Journal of Preventive Medicine*, vol. 1, no. 3, pp. 22–29, 2013.

[9] B. J. Wylie, L. Kalilani-Phiri, M. Madanitsa et al., "Gestational age assessment in malaria pregnancy cohorts: a prospective ultrasound demonstration project in Malawi," *Malaria Journal*, vol. 12, no. 1, p. 183, 2013.

[10] M. G. Kawooya, R. O. Nathan, J. Swanson et al., "Impact of introducing routine antenatal ultrasound services on reproductive health indicators in mpigi district, Central Uganda," *Ultrasound Quarterly*, vol. 31, no. 4, pp. 285–289, 2015.

[11] E. M. McClure, R. O. Nathan, S. Saleem et al., "First look: a cluster-randomized trial of ultrasound to improve pregnancy outcomes in low income country settings," *BMC Pregnancy and Childbirth*, vol. 14, no. 1, p. 73, 2014.

[12] R. O. Nathan, J. O. Swanson, D. L. Swanson et al., "Evaluation of focused obstetric ultrasound examinations by health care personnel in the democratic republic of Congo, Guatemala, Kenya, Pakistan, and Zambia," *Current Problems in Diagnostic Radiology*, vol. 46, no. 3, pp. 210–215, 2017.

[13] K. Huang, F. Tao, J. Raven, L. Liu, X. Wu, and S. Tang, "Utilization of antenatal ultrasound scan and implications for caesarean section: a cross-sectional study in rural Eastern China," *BMC Health Services Research*, vol. 12, no. 1, 2012.

[14] H. H. Bijma, A. van der Heide, and H. I. J. Wildschut, "Decision-making after ultrasound diagnosis of fetal abnormality," *European Clinics in Obstetrics and Gynaecology*, vol. 3, no. 2, pp. 89–95, 2007.

[15] A. Saleh, G. Idris, A. Dare, M. Yahuza, M. Suwaid, and S. Idris, "Awareness and perception of pregnant women about obstetrics ultrasound at Aminu Kano Teaching Hospital," *Sahel Medical Journal*, vol. 20, no. 1, p. 38, 2017.

[16] C. A. Enakpene, I. O. Morhason-Bello, A. O. Marinho et al., "Clients' reasons for prenatal ultrasonography in Ibadan, south west of Nigeria," *BMC Women's Health*, vol. 9, no. 1, p. 12, 2009.

[17] R. D. Harris and W. M. Marks, "Compact ultrasound for improving maternal and perinatal care in low-resource settings," *Journal of Ultrasound in Medicine*, vol. 28, no. 8, pp. 1067–1076, 2009.

[18] J. M. Carrera, "Obstetric ultrasounds in Africa: is it necessary to promote their appropriate use?" *Donald School Journal of Ultrasound in Obstetrics and Gynecology*, vol. 5, no. 3, pp. 289–296, 2011.

[19] A. B. Ross, K. K. DeStigter, M. Rielly et al., "A low-cost ultrasound program leads to increased antenatal clinic visits and attended deliveries at a health care clinic in rural Uganda," *PLoS One*, vol. 8, no. 10, Article ID e78450, 2013.

[20] S. Tautz, A. Jahn, I. Molokomme, and R. Görgen, "Between fear and relief: how rural pregnant women experience foetal ultrasound in a Botswana district hospital," *Social Science & Medicine*, vol. 50, no. 5, pp. 689–701, 2000.

[21] Y. Mensah, K. Nkyekyer, and K. Mensah, "The Ghanaian woman's experience and perception of ultrasound use in

antenatal care," *Ghana Medical Journal*, vol. 48, no. 1, p. 31, 2014.

[22] Ghana Statistical Service, *2010 Population & Housing Census*, Ghana Statistical Service, Accra, Ghana, 2012.

[23] Raosoft, "Sample Size Calculator by Raosoft, Inc. Sample Size," 2004, https://www.raosft.com/samplesize.html.

[24] The History of Fetal Ultrasound|Pregnancy Imaging|Live Science, https://www.livescience.com/32071-history-of-fetal-ultrasound.html.

[25] S. Georgsson Öhman and U. Waldenström, "Second-trimester routine ultrasound screening: expectations and experiences in a nationwide Swedish sample," *Ultrasound in Obstetrics and Gynecology*, vol. 32, no. 1, pp. 15–22, 2008.

[26] D. K. Whynes, "Receipt of information and women's attitudes towards ultrasound scanning during pregnancy," *Ultrasound in Obstetrics and Gynecology*, vol. 19, no. 1, pp. 7–12, 2002.

[27] E. Kutsoati and R. K. Morck, "Family ties, inheritance rights, and successful poverty alleviation: evidence from Ghana," *SSRN Electronic Journal*, vol. 2, pp. 215–252, 2012.

[28] L. Aziato, P. N. A. Odai, and C. N. Omenyo, "Religious beliefs and practices in pregnancy and labour: an inductive qualitative study among post-partum women in Ghana," *BMC Pregnancy and Childbirth*, vol. 16, no. 1, 2016.

[29] J. G. Lalor and D. Devane, "Information, knowledge and expectations of the routine ultrasound scan," *Midwifery*, vol. 23, no. 1, pp. 13–22, 2007.

[30] A. T. Agbata, C. I. Ukaegbe, L. O. Lawani, K. C. Ekwedigwe, and L. O. Ajah, "Women's views on routine antenatal ultrasound scan in a low resource Nigerian setting," *Journal of Clinical and Diagnostic Research*, vol. 12, no. 6, 2018.

21

Quantitative Evaluation of Display Contrast of Gd-EOB-DTPA-Enhanced Magnetic Resonance Images: Effects of the Flip Angle and Grayscale Gamma Value

Yusuke Inoue,[1] Hirofumi Hata,[2] Ai Nakajima,[2] Keiji Matsunaga,[1] Yusuke Ohzeki,[2] Tetsuya Hashimoto,[2] and Hiroki Haradome[3]

[1] *Department of Diagnostic Radiology, Kitasato University School of Medicine, Sagamihara, Kanagawa, Japan*
[2] *Department of Radiology, Kitasato University Hospital, Sagamihara, Kanagawa, Japan*
[3] *Department of Diagnostic Radiology, Kitasato University Hospital, Sagamihara, Kanagawa, Japan*

Correspondence should be addressed to Yusuke Inoue; inoueys34@gmail.com

Academic Editor: Paul Sijens

Introduction. Display contrast can be changed nonlinearly by manipulating the gamma value of the grayscale. We investigated the contrast of the hepatobiliary-phase images acquired with different flip angles (FAs) and displayed with different gamma values in Gd-EOB-DTPA-enhanced magnetic resonance imaging. *Material and Methods*. Twenty patients with liver tumors were studied. Hepatobiliary-phase images were acquired at low (12°) and high (30°) FAs. Low-FA images were converted to simulate images displayed with different gamma values, using ImageJ software. To assess image contrast, the liver-to-muscle signal ratio (LMR), liver-to-spleen signal ratio (LSR), contrast ratio (CR), liver signal-to-noise ratio (SNR), and contrast-to-noise ratio (CNR) were calculated. *Results*. The LMR, LSR, and CR were higher in the high-FA images than in the low-FA original images. Although the SNR was lower in the high-FA images, indicating an increase in noise, the CNR was higher. Raising the gamma value increased the LMR, LSR, and CR, notably decreased the SNR, and slightly decreased the CNR. *Conclusion*. Increasing the FA enhanced image contrast, supporting its usefulness for improving the delineation of focal liver lesions. Although the associated increase in noise may be problematic, raising the grayscale gamma value enhances the display contrast of low-FA images.

1. Introduction

Gadolinium ethoxybenzyl-diethylenetriamine pentaacetic acid (Gd-EOB-DTPA) is a hepatobiliary contrast agent for magnetic resonance (MR) imaging. The agent is selectively taken up by hepatocytes and excreted via the biliary system. Typically, in addition to acquisition of dynamic images at the time of intravenous administration, hepatobiliary-phase imaging is performed 20 min later. Gd-EOB-DTPA enhances the signal of liver parenchyma on the hepatobiliary-phase images and increase the contrast between liver parenchyma and focal liver lesions, facilitating lesion detection [1, 2].

Gd-EOB-DTPA-enhanced MR imaging usually utilizes a T1-weighted gradient echo sequence, in which the flip angle (FA), together with the repetition time, is a key parameter to determine image contrast. Increasing the FA has been demonstrated to increase the contrast of the hepatobiliary-phase images and to improve the detectability and conspicuity of focal liver lesions [3, 4]. Acquisition of high-FA hepatobiliary-phase images is accepted to be a useful adjunct to the acquisition of dynamic and hepatobiliary-phase images using a low FA.

Medical images, including MR images, are displayed on the monitors of picture archiving and communication system (PACS) viewers for visual image interpretation. The interpreter can adjust the display conditions, which are crucial for visual interpretation and thus for clinical diagnosis. Display conditions are usually manipulated using the window width and window level. The window width is the difference between the upper and lower limits of the display window; display contrast can be enhanced by narrowing it, with no need for additional data acquisition. In computed tomography, the pixel values expressed in Hounsfield units are calibrated and the optimal window setting can be standardized. In contrast, the signal intensities of MR images vary greatly depending on scanners, imaging parameters, and patients [5]. Although standardization of window settings has been attempted [6–8], interpreters commonly adjust the display conditions during interpretation manually and subjectively, which increases interpreter's burden and dependency on interpreter's skill.

Manipulating the gamma value of the grayscale also changes image appearance on the monitors. The gamma value determines the grayscale pattern, and the relationship between the pixel value and brightness on the monitor can be changed nonlinearly by manipulating the gamma value. A gamma value of 1 corresponds to an ordinary linear scale. Raising the gamma value increases the contrast between regions with high and medium pixel values, while decreasing the contrast between regions with medium and low pixels values, and would be expected to enhance the contrast between liver parenchyma and focal liver lesions. Although the grayscale pattern of the display device itself is usually fixed to the Grayscale Standard Display Function (GSDF), defined in Digital Imaging and Communications in. Medicine (DICOM) part 14, in the PACS viewer, software-based manipulation of each image set is possible using software of the viewer.

We routinely acquire low-FA images during the dynamic phase and both low-FA and high-FA images during the hepatobiliary phase in Gd-EOB-DTPA-enhanced MR imaging. In the present preliminary study, we quantitatively evaluated the contrast of the hepatobiliary-phase images acquired at low and high FAs. The contrast of low-FA images was assessed in relation to the grayscale gamma value. The aim of this study was to examine the potential of high-gamma display as a method of improving image contrast in Gd-EOB-DTPA-enhanced MR imaging.

2. Material and Methods

2.1. Patients. Data from 20 patients (17 men and 3 women; 68.0 ± 11.1 years, mean ± SD) who underwent Gd-EOB-DTPA-enhanced MR imaging using a 1.5T scanner for clinical indications from January 2015 to July 2015 were analyzed retrospectively. Patients in whom untreated liver tumors (hepatocellular carcinoma 13, metastatic liver tumor 7) of 2 cm or larger were identified on hepatobiliary-phase images were included. The exclusion criteria were (1) poor breath holding, (2) prior liver resection, (3) extensive liver tumors, (4) prior splenectomy, and (5) severe atrophy of the erector muscles of spine, and otherwise, patients were enrolled consecutively. The criteria (2)-(5) were defined to allow appropriate setting of regions of interest (ROIs). Of the 20 patients, ten had liver cirrhosis, one had chronic hepatitis, one had primary biliary cirrhosis, and eight normal background livers. The study protocol was approved by the Institutional Review Board, and the need for informed consent was waived.

2.2. Imaging Procedures. MR imaging was performed using a 1.5T clinical scanner (Signa HDxt; GE Healthcare, Waukesha, WI) with a 12-channel phased-array coil. With intravenous administration of Gd-EOB-DTPA (0.025 mmol/kg; Bayer Yakuhin, Osaka, Japan), dynamic and hepatobiliary-phase images were acquired in the axial plane using liver acquisition with volume acceleration (LAVA) sequence, during a single breath hold at expiration.

Hepatobiliary-phase images were obtained at an FA of 12° (low FA) and then at an FA of 30° (high FA). Other imaging parameters were typically as follows: repetition time = 4.3 ms (low FA) or 5.6 ms (high FA), echo time = 2.0 ms (low FA) or 2.2 ms (high FA), field of view = 360 mm, matrix = 320 × 192, slice thickness = 5 mm, slice number = 44, and acquisition time = 16 s (low FA) or 21 s (high FA). Repetition time and echo time differed between low-FA and high-FA imagings because they were determined automatically depending on the FA. True spatial resolution was 1.1 × 1.9 × 5.0 mm^3, and reconstructed spatial resolution was 0.7 × 0.7 × 2.5 mm^3. Field of view and slice number were increased as required in large patients. A parallel imaging technique (array spatial sensitivity encoding technique [ASSET]) was used with a reduction factor of 2. Image uniformity correction was performed using phased-array uniformity enhancement (PURE).

2.3. Image Analysis. Images were analyzed using ImageJ software ver. 1.48v (National Institutes of Health, Bethesda, MD). The pixel values of low-FA images were converted using the gamma correction function of the software, and stored. The gamma values were set at 1.2, 1.5, and 1.8 to produce gamma-1.2, gamma-1.5, and gamma-1.8 images, respectively. The original images corresponds to images with a gamma value of 1.0. Although image display can be changed on a PACS monitor by manipulating the gamma value of the grayscale, the pixel values are not affected by such manipulation. We created and stored images after gamma correction, simulating images displayed with different gamma values, to quantitatively assess image contrast.

Signal intensities were measured in the low-FA images with different gamma values and in the high-FA original images. ROIs were placed in the liver parenchyma, spleen, muscle, and liver tumors. For the liver parenchyma, a circular ROI of 100 mm^2 was placed in each of the anterior segment of the right hepatic lobe, the posterior segment of the right lobe, and the medial segment of the left lobe, avoiding vessels, focal liver lesions, and imaging artifacts, on the slice exhibiting the right main branch of the portal vein. The means and SDs of the signal intensities in the ROIs were averaged among the three ROIs to obtain liver signal and liver noise, respectively. For the muscle, an elliptical ROI of 100 mm^2 was placed in each of the right and left paravertebral muscles, minimizing inclusion of fat, on the slice used to assess liver signals. Muscle signal was defined as the average of the mean signal intensities in the right and left ROIs. A circular ROI of 200 mm^2 was placed in the spleen, and spleen signal was defined as the mean signal intensity in the ROI. As for the liver tumor, the largest tumor was selected for analysis when two

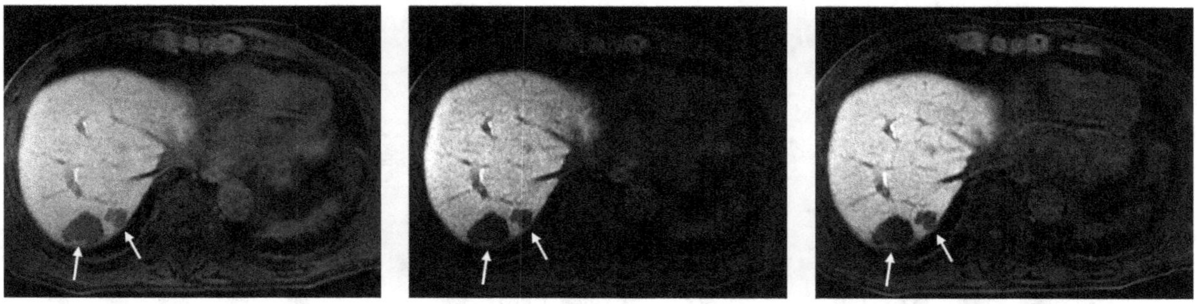

(a) (b) (c)

FIGURE 1: A low-FA original image (a), a low-FA gamma-1.8 image (b), and a high-FA image (c) in a 66-year-old man with metastatic liver tumor (arrows).

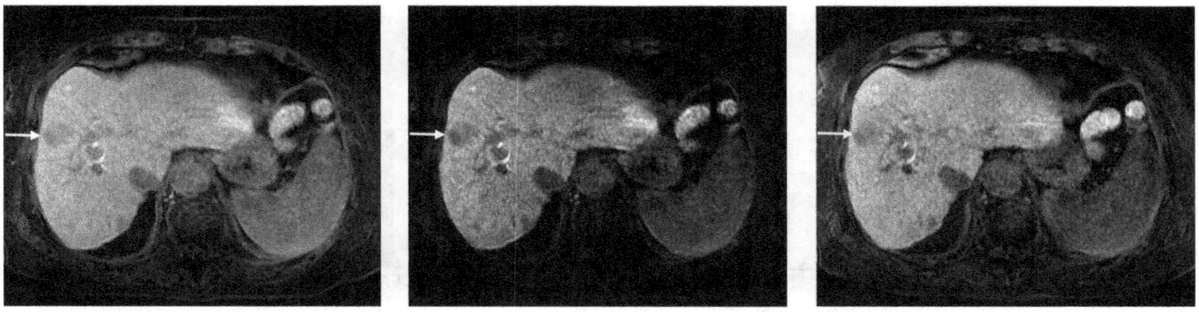

(a) (b) (c)

FIGURE 2: A low-FA original image (a), a low-FA gamma-1.8 image (b), and a high-FA image (c) in a 73-year-old woman with hepatocellular carcinoma (arrows) and liver cirrhosis.

or more tumors were present in a given patient, and an ROI of 100 mm^2 was placed on a slice exhibiting the largest cross-section of the tumor. The dominant component showing homogenous intensity was assessed when the signal intensity of the tumor was heterogeneous. Tumor signal was defined as the mean signal intensity in the ROI.

To assess image contrast, the liver-to-muscle signal ratio (LMR), liver-to-spleen signal ratio (LSR), contrast ratio (CR), liver signal-to-noise ratio (SNR), and contrast-to-noise ratio (CNR) were calculated for each image set as follows:

$$\text{LMR} = \text{liver signal/muscle signal}$$

$$\text{LSR} = \text{liver signal/spleen signal}$$

$$\text{CR} = (\text{liver signal} - \text{tumor signal})/\text{liver signal}$$

$$\text{SNR} = \text{liver signal/liver noise}$$

$$\text{CNR} = (\text{liver signal} - \text{tumor signal})/\text{liver noise}.$$

2.4. Statistical Analysis. Values are expressed as means ± SDs. Indices of image contrast were compared statistically among low-FA original images, low-FA gamma-1.8 images, and high-FA original images. For parametric distribution, comparison was made by one-way repeated analysis of variance, and post hoc analysis was performed by the paired t test with Holm's correction. For nonparametric distribution, the Friedman's test was used, followed by the Wilcoxon signed rank test with Holm's correction for post hoc analysis. A p value of less than 0.05 was deemed to be statistically significant.

3. Results

The high-FA images provided higher image contrast visually between the liver and muscle, the liver and spleen, and liver parenchyma and liver tumor, when compared with the low-FA original images (Figures 1 and 2). On quantitative analysis, the LMR, LSR, and CR were higher in the high-FA images than in the low-FA original images (Figure 3). Although the SNR was lower in the high-FA images, indicating an increase in noise, the CNR was higher.

Raising the gamma value of the grayscale enhanced image contrast visually. The LMR, LSR, and CR increased with the gamma value. As the gamma value increased, the SNR decreased notably, indicating an increase in noise, and the CNR decreased slightly.

The CR in the low-FA gamma-1.8 images was comparable to that in the high-FA images, and this value was selected for further analysis. The low-FA original images, and low-FA gamma-1.8 images, and high-FA images were subjected to statistical evaluation. The differences in all five indices between the high-FA images and low-FA original images were statistically significant. The CR did not differ significantly between the high-FA images and low-FA gamma-1.8 images, and was lower in the low-FA original images (Figure 4).

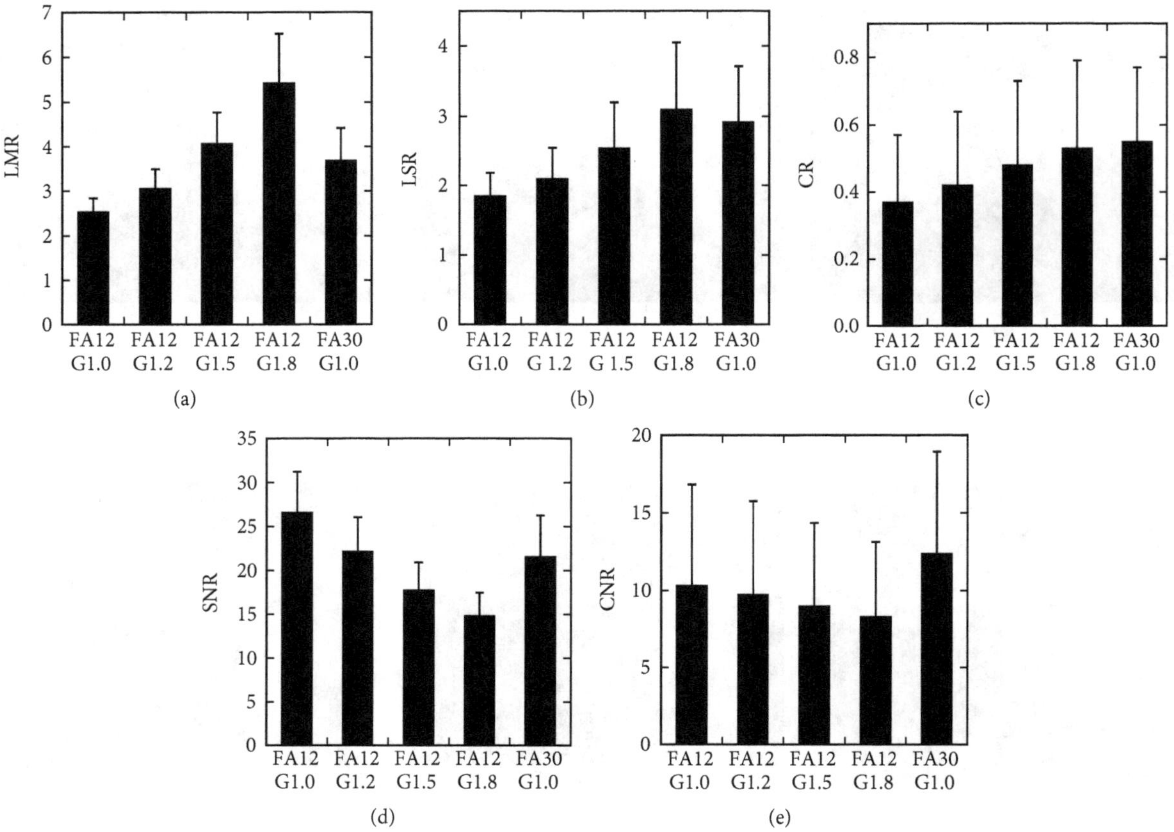

FIGURE 3: Results of quantitative indices: LMR (a), LSR (b), CR (c), SNR (d), and CNR (e). Error bars indicate SDs. FA12 and FA30 represent FAs of 12° and 30°, respectively. G1.0, G1.2, G1.5, and G1.8 represent the gamma values of 1.0, 1.2, 1.5, and 1.8, respectively.

The LMR and LSR was greatly and slightly higher in the low-FA gamma-1.8 images than in the high-FA images, respectively, with statistical significance. The SNR and CNR were significantly lower in the low-FA gamma-1.8 images.

4. Discussion

We quantitatively evaluated the image contrast of hepatobiliary-phase images in Gd-EOB-DTPA-enhanced MR imaging, with special reference to the potential usefulness of manipulating the gamma value of the grayscale for monitor display. Increasing the FA in image acquisition has been demonstrated to increase image contrast and to improve the delineation of focal liver lesions [3, 4]. In the present study, increasing the FA from 12° to 30° increased image contrast, as indicated by higher LMR, LSR and CR values, in line with the previous studies. Increasing the FA reduced the CR because of an increase in noise; however, the increase in contrast overrode the noise increase, resulting in a higher CNR. These results, increase in both the CR and CNR, supports usefulness of high-FA imaging to improve the delineation of focal liver lesions in hepatobiliary-phase images.

Imaging at a different FA provides a different image set. Even a given image set has a different appearance on the monitor when a different grayscale is used. The gamma value of the grayscale defines the relationship between the pixel value and brightness on the monitor, which can be changed nonlinearly by manipulating the gamma value. In the present study, raising the gamma value increased the LMR, LSR, and CR, indicating an increase in contrast. Application of a gamma value of 1.8, instead of 1.0, to low-FA images yielded LSR and CR values comparable to, and an LMR value higher than, those in the high-FA images. On the other hand, because raising the gamma value increases differences in brightness between high-value and medium-value pixels nonspecifically, this manipulation caused evident noise increase, as indicated by the reduction in the SNR. Unlike increasing the FA, raising the gamma value decreased the CNR. The CNR was lower in low-FA gamma-1.8 images than in high-FA images. Display of low-FA images with the gamma value of 1.8 is indicated to provide image contrast comparable to that of high-FA images, with no need for additional data acquisition; however, poorer noise property may hamper image interpretation. The usefulness of this display method may depend on various factors such as the MR scanner, imaging sequence, status of background liver, and nature of focal liver lesions. The quantitative analysis of image characteristics in this preliminary study employing a small number of patients indicates that the method may be useful but the usefulness is not conclusive, and further studies using visual interpretation of many clinical images are warranted.

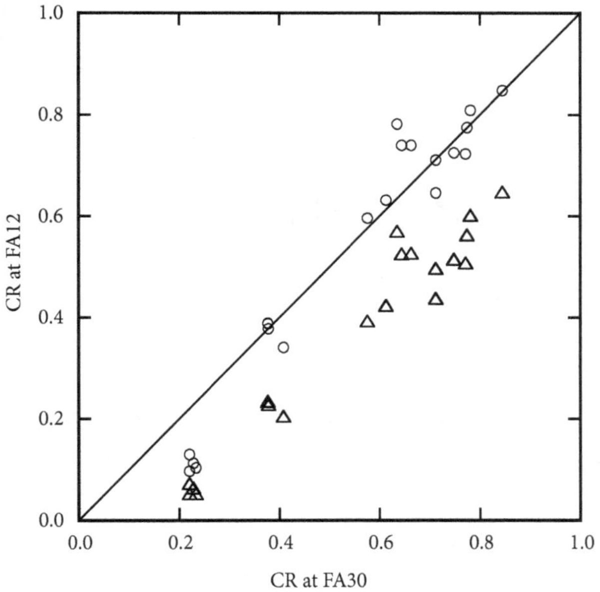

FIGURE 4: Relationship between CRs determined at FAs of 30° (FA30) and 12° (FA12). CRs obtained at an FA of 12° are presented for gamma values of 1.0 (open triangles) and 1.8 (open circles), respectively. The solid line represents the line of identity.

In this study, we created and stored additional images using the gamma correction function of ImageJ software to assess image characteristics quantitatively. Such processing is not required when high-gamma display is used for visual interpretation. Enhancement of the display contrast of low-FA images is easily achieved on a PACS viewer by manipulating the gamma value; it is unnecessary to process the original data. This is similar to adjustment of display conditions using the window width and window level. Adjustment using the width and level requires trial and error by the image interpreter to find an optimal combination of these two parameters and may be troublesome especially for inexperienced interpreters [9]. Since the signal intensities are affected by various factors, an optimal combination of the width and level cannot be fixed. Application of a fixed gamma value for enhancement of display contrast may contribute to improving efficiency and reproducibility in optimizing image display, which would have a substantial impact on clinical radiology practice. High-FA imaging offers better contrast than low-FA imaging and the hepatobiliary-phase imaging is often performed at both high and low FAs. However, repetitive imaging at different FAs is not applicable to dynamic imaging because of rapid changes in Gd-EOB-DTPA distribution early after injection. Only conventional low-FA images are usually acquired during the dynamic phase. Manipulation of the gamma value does not require an additional data acquisition and is expected to have a potential of improving assessment of vascularity on dynamic images.

5. Conclusions

We investigated methods for improving the contrast of hepatobiliary-phase images in Gd-EOB-DTPA-enhanced MR imaging. Increasing the FA increased image contrast, supporting its usefulness in improving the delineation of focal liver lesions. Although the increase in noise may be problematic, raising the gamma value of the grayscale is indicated to improve the display contrast of low-FA images conveniently. Manipulation of display contrast using the grayscale gamma value may aid in visual evaluation of focal liver lesion and is worth further evaluation.

Acknowledgments

The authors thank Mr. Hiroki Miyatake for his support in data analysis.

References

[1] C. J. Zech, C. Bartolozzi, P. Bioulac-Sage et al., "Consensus report of the fifth international forum for liver MRI," *American Journal of Roentgenology*, vol. 201, no. 1, pp. 97–107, 2013.

[2] M. Kudo, O. Matsui, M. Sakamoto et al., "Role of gadolinium-ethoxybenzyl-diethylenetriamine pentaacetic acid-enhanced magnetic resonance imaging in the management of hepatocellular carcinoma: Consensus at the symposium of the 48th annual meeting of the liver cancer study group of Japan," *Oncology (Switzerland)*, vol. 84, pp. 21–27, 2013.

[3] H. Haradome, L. Grazioli, K. Al Manea et al., "Gadoxetic acid disodium-enhanced hepatocyte phase MRI: Can increasing the flip angle improve focal liver lesion detection?" *Journal of Magnetic Resonance Imaging*, vol. 35, no. 1, pp. 132–139, 2012.

[4] M. R. Bashir, D. B. Husarik, T. J. Ziemlewicz, R. T. Gupta, D. T. Boll, and E. M. Merkle, "Liver MRI in the hepatocyte phase with gadolinium-EOB-DTPA: Does increasing the flip angle improve conspicuity and detection rate of hypointense lesions?" *Journal of Magnetic Resonance Imaging*, vol. 35, no. 3, pp. 611–616, 2012.

[5] L. G. Nyúl and J. K. Udupa, "On standardizing the MR image intensity scale," *Magnetic Resonance in Medicine*, vol. 42, no. 6, pp. 1072–1081, 1999.

[6] M. Sasaki, M. Ida, K. Yamada, Y. Watanabe, and M. Matsui, "Standardizing display conditions of diffusion-weighted images using concurrent b0 images: A multi-vendor multi-institutional study," *Magnetic Resonance in Medical Sciences*, vol. 6, no. 3, pp. 133–137, 2007.

[7] T. Hirai, M. Sasaki, M. Maeda et al., "Diffusion-weighted Imaging in Ischemic Stroke. Effect of Display Method on Observers' Diagnostic Performance," *Academic Radiology*, vol. 16, no. 3, pp. 305–312, 2009.

[8] H. Nagashima, K. Doi, T. Ogura, and H. Fujita, "Automated adjustment of display conditions in brain MR images: Diffusion-weighted MRIs and apparent diffusion coefficient maps for hyperacute ischemic stroke," *Radiological Physics and Technology*, vol. 6, no. 1, pp. 202–209, 2013.

[9] T. Hara, Y. Inoue, R. Ukisu, and H. Hata, "Methods for optimizing the display conditions of brain magnetic resonance images," *Japanese Journal of Radiology*, vol. 35, no. 10, pp. 622–627, 2017.

22

Safety of 3 Tesla Magnetic Resonance Imaging in Patients with Sickle Cell Disease

Olivia Justice,[1] **Lori C. Jordan**,[1,2,3] **Chelsea A. Lee**,[1,2] **Niral J. Patel**,[1,2] **Spencer Waddle**,[1] **Sumit Pruthi**,[1] **L. Taylor Davis**,[1] **Adetola A. Kassim**,[4,5] **and Manus J. Donahue**[1,3,6]

[1]*Department of Radiology, Vanderbilt University Medical Center, Nashville, TN, USA*
[2]*Department of Pediatrics, Division of Pediatric Neurology, Vanderbilt University Medical Center, Nashville, TN, USA*
[3]*Department of Neurology, Vanderbilt University Medical Center, Nashville, TN, USA*
[4]*Department of Pediatrics, Vanderbilt-Meharry Center for Excellence, Sickle Cell Disease, Vanderbilt University Medical Center, Nashville, TN, USA*
[5]*Department of Internal Medicine, Division of Hematology/Oncology, Vanderbilt University Medical Center, Nashville, TN, USA*
[6]*Department of Psychiatry, Vanderbilt University Medical Center, Nashville, TN, USA*

Correspondence should be addressed to Manus J. Donahue; mj.donahue@vumc.org

Academic Editor: André Luiz Ferreira COSTA

Sickle cell disease (SCD) is a well-characterized hemoglobinopathy affecting more than 20 million individuals worldwide and carries an increased risk of cerebral vasculopathy, cerebral infarct, and stroke. As mechanisms of cerebral infarction in SCD are partly attributable to microvascular vaso-occlusive crises, manifesting as altered cerebral blood flow and associated impaired oxygen delivery, magnetic resonance imaging (MRI) methods that can quickly provide a comprehensive perspective on structural and functional disease status, without exogenous contrast administration or ionizing radiation, have emerged as crucial clinical tools for surveillance. However, early *ex vivo* MRI work in suspended erythrocytes containing hemoglobin S at 0.35 Tesla (T) suggested that sickled erythrocytes can orient preferentially in the presence of an external magnetic field, and as such, it was suggested that MRI exams in sickle cell hemoglobinopathy could induce vaso-occlusion. While this observation has generally not impacted clinical imaging in individuals with SCD, it has led to resistance for some sickle cell studies within the engineering community among some imaging scientists as this early observation has never been rigorously shown to be unconcerning. Here, we performed MRI at the clinical field strength of 3 T in 172 patients with SCD, which included standard anatomical and angiographic assessments together with gold standard diffusion-weighted imaging (DWI; spatial resolution = $1.8 \times 1.8 \times 4$ mm; *b*-value = 1000 s/mm^2) for acute infarct assessment (performed approximately 20 min after patient introduction to the field iso-center). The presence of vasculopathy, as well as chronic and acute infarcts, was evaluated by two independent board-certified radiologists using standard clinical criteria. In these patients (52.3% female; mean age = 19.6 years; age range = 6–44 years), hematocrit (mean = 25.8%; range = 15–36%), hemoglobin phenotype (87.8% HbSS variant), presence of silent infarct (44.2%), and overt chronic infarct (13.4%) were consistent with a typical SCD population; however, no participants exhibited evidence of acute infarction. These findings are consistent with 3 T MRI not inducing acute infarction or vaso-occlusion in individuals with SCD and suggest that earlier low-field *ex vivo* work of erythrocytes in suspension is not a sufficient cause to discourage MRI scans in patients with SCD.

1. Introduction

Sickle cell disease (SCD) is a genetically inherited blood disorder affecting approximately 300,000 new cases annually worldwide [1, 2]. SCD comprises a range of sickle phenotypes (HbSC, HbSS, HbSβ^0, HbSβ^+, HbSE, and HbSD) [3, 4], whereby the most common and severe is sickle cell anemia (SCA) characterized by the presence of hemoglobin (Hb)-S (HbSS). The presence of the HbSS mutation contributes to both vaso-occlusion as clustered, sickled erythrocytes restrict blood delivery through primarily microvasculature and also hemolysis, resulting in anemia and reduced oxygen delivery to tissues. These factors can manifest as pain crises, organ failure, and chronic anemia and neurologically as cerebral infarction and/or cognitive impairment [1, 5].

Magnetic resonance imaging (MRI), most commonly performed at a field strength of 1.5–3.0 Tesla (T), is often used in patients with SCD to evaluate prior infarct and more recently to evaluate mechanisms that subserve tissue oxygen [5]. MRI does not require exogenous contrast or ionizing radiation and therefore is well suited for surveillance imaging or therapy response evaluation. MRI is used frequently in both children and adults for infarct [5–7] and vasculopathy [8, 9] assessment, to evaluate iron loading and accumulation [10, 11], and studies have also reported evidence of acute infarcts visible on MRI in a small subset of children with SCD, which occurred with or without recent clinical symptoms [12, 13].

Some resistance, largely with imaging scientists, remains regarding the safety of MRI in patients with SCD despite widespread acceptance of MRI amongst clinicians and clinical researchers. This resistance is attributable to a study published in 1985 in *Investigative Radiology*, in which it was reported that erythrocytes drawn from individuals with SCA and scanned *ex vivo* in suspension at a field strength of 0.35 T align orthogonal to the external magnetic field, and as such, it is possible that this preferential orientation could contribute to an elevated risk of steno-occlusion if similar effects are present *in vivo* [14]. Despite more than three decades passing since this original work, no study has provided *in vivo* data on the potential safety of MRI in patients with SCD for not inducing acute infarcts. Importantly, large clinical trials that include neuroimaging in asymptomatic participants, such as the pediatric silent cerebral infarct transfusion (SIT) trial [13, 15], found that 10 out of 771 children with MRI had evidence of acute silent cerebral ischemia (confirmed by diffusion-weighted imaging, DWI) during scheduled, study-related MRIs not obtained for clinical indications and without stroke symptoms. These were termed acute silent cerebral ischemic events [13]. While 90% of these patients did not have a document report of medical illness two weeks prior to the MRI, some patients may have been in acute vaso-occlusive crises, and as such, it was not possible to discern whether these infarcts were due to the imaging procedure or had initiated before the procedure. A separate study also reported evidence of acute silent cerebral infarcts in seven children scanned with MRI [12]. The overarching assumption is that these observed acute infarcts are coincidental with the MRI as silent cerebral infarcts are common in individuals with sickle cell disease [15], and the imaging exam simply corresponded with the time of an ischemic event.

However, no prospective study has rigorously evaluated the presence of acute ischemic events in adults and children with SCD. To gain additional objective information on MRI safety in participants with SCD, here we apply DWI-MRI in stable pediatric and adult SCD participants to evaluate the primary study hypothesis that MRI performed at the highest clinical field strength of 3 T does not induce acute infarction *in vivo* in patients with SCD.

2. Methods

2.1. Demographics and Recruitment. All participants ($n = 172$) provided informed, written consent in accordance with the ethical standards and approval of the Vanderbilt University Medical Center Institutional Review Board. Participants comprised both adults (≥18 years of age) and children (6–17 years of age) with SCD (including phenotype HbSS, HbSC, or HbSβ^0) and were recruited from a comprehensive SCD clinic as part of a larger prospective study of hemometabolic imaging indicators of stroke risk. Participants were required not to have received medical attention for vaso-occlusive crises within the past seven days, and, if on chronic transfusion, to have been scanned at least three weeks since their last transfusion when their hematocrit was near nadir. Hematocrit and hemoglobin phenotype were evaluated via venipuncture within seven days of the MRI protocol.

2.2. Acquisition. DWI was applied to evaluate the primary study hypothesis, whereas standard anatomical T_2-weighted fluid-attenuated inversion recovery (FLAIR) and T_1-weighted MRI and time-of-flight magnetic resonance angiography (MRA) were applied in sequence to evaluate chronic infarct and vasculopathy extent, respectively. All imaging was performed using body coil radiofrequency transmission and phased-array SENSE reception at a field strength of 3 Tesla (Philips Healthcare, Best, Netherlands).

DWI was performed approximately 20 min after introducing the participant to the isocenter of the scanner and with a standard protocol with field view (FOV) = 230 × 230 × 129 mm, spatial resolution = 1.8 × 1.8 × 4 mm, and *b*-values of 0 and 1000 s/mm^2. Acute lesions will appear on DWI minutes after a stroke occurs [16, 17]. In addition, FLAIR MRI was performed in the axial (FOV = 184 × 230 × 134 mm) and coronal (FOV = 161 × 199 × 200 mm) planes with a common spatial resolution of 0.9 × 1.1 × 3 mm for chronic infarct determination. Intracranial time-of-flight magnetic resonance angiography (spatial resolution = 0.6 × 0.6 × 1.4 mm^3; 3D gradient echo; repetition time/echo time = 23/3.5 ms) and cervical time-of-flight magnetic resonance angiography (spatial resolution = 0.9 × 0.9 × 3.0 mm^3; 2D gradient echo; repetition time/echo time = 18.6/3.2 ms) were performed for vasculopathy determination.

2.3. Analysis. Cervical and major intracranial vessels for each participant were assessed for vasculopathy by two board-certified radiologists as previously described [18]. Each vessel was graded as mild stenosis (0–50%), moderate stenosis (51–69%), severe stenosis (70–99%), or occlusion. Severity of intracranial vasculopathy was graded by the worst vessel seen as mild, moderate, severe, or occluded. Disagreements were resolved by consensus.

Infarcts were classified by the same radiologists. First, the scan was judged as normal or abnormal. If abnormal, the lesions were assigned as either (i) nonspecific white matter hyperintensity if <3 mm in diameter [19] or (ii) focal, discrete ischemic infarcts if ≥3 mm and visible in at least two planes of T_2-weighted FLAIR MRI (axial and coronal). Infarcts were classified as silent using clinical radiological criteria defined above and if no neurological symptoms or signs corresponding to the location of infarcts were detectable following a neurological history or exam by a board-certified neurologist (LCJ; experience >15 years) [13, 15].

2.4. Statistical Considerations. The goal of this study was to report the prevalence of acute silent infarction in a cohort of SCD participants without acute vaso-occlusive crises. Descriptive statistics including mean and ranges for continuous variables (i.e., age and hematocrit) were calculated, along with percent for categorical variables (i.e., sex, acute infarct on DWI MRI, chronic infarct on FLAIR MRI, vasculopathy extent, children or adults, and hemoglobin phenotype). Results are presented both in a stratified manner for biological sex and in a cumulative (i.e., all volunteers) manner. An unpaired Student's *t*-test and chi-squared test were used for evaluating differences in continuous and categorical variables, respectively, between groups. In all cases, two-sided $p < 0.05$ was required for reporting significance.

Finally, because prior infarcts and cerebral vasculopathy are risk factors for new infarcts [6, 18], to provide a description of how the prevalence of these risk factors changed with age, we plotted the cumulative presence of participants with silent cerebral infarct, acute infarct, chronic overt stroke, and vasculopathy with age. This subanalysis provided information on the approximate prevalence of these risk factors across the SCD lifespan.

3. Results

The enrolled cohort consisted of 172 SCD participants, comprised primarily sickle cell anemia (88% HbSS), with a smaller subset that comprised HbS β^0thalassemia (10% HbSβ^0) and milder sickling (2% HbSC). Of these, 52.9% of participants were adults, and 47.1% were children. The mean age of participants in the study was 19.6 years (age range = 6–44 years). 97% of participants were Black, and 3% were Middle Eastern or Asian Indian. Summary statistics for all measures are provided in Table 1.

As required by the inclusion criteria, no participants reported a vaso-occlusive crisis within the past seven days, and none were hospitalized for related indications, including blood transfusion, within seven days before the scan. As such, all participants met criteria for being stable without known, recent acute events.

Of these participants, the mean hematocrit was 25.8% (range = 15%–36%). Hematocrit was mild but significantly reduced in female vs. male patients ($p = 0.002$). This breakdown is consistent with typical ranges and hemoglobin phenotypes present in most North American sickle cell disease clinics. Of these participants, 9.3% met criteria for vasculopathy on MRA. On T_1-weighted and T_2-weighted FLAIR MRI, 76 participants had evidence of SCIs, and 23 participants had evidence of chronic infarcts from overt stroke. The number of chronic silent infarcts was statistically higher in the male vs. female participants (chi-square test; $p = 0.018$).

No participants met criteria for radiological indicators of acute stroke on DWI. Figure 1 displays the quality of imaging data used in the study, summarized from a representative participant with chronic silent infarcts but without evidence of acute infarct. These data are consistent with MRI, performed at the highest clinical field strength of 3 Tesla, not inducing acute infarction in individuals with SCD.

Figure 2 summarizes the cumulative incidence of an event (SCI, overt stroke, observed acute infarct, or vasculopathy) with age. While SCI, overt stroke, and vasculopathy were all observed to increase with increasing age, with the slope being highest for SCIs, there was no evidence of an increase in acute infarct prevalence with increasing age.

4. Discussion

Despite the relative routine use of MRI in patients with SCD, prior large studies have observed limited evidence of DWI lesions [13], and one earlier *ex vivo* evidence suggests that sickle red blood cells' orientation in the presence of an external magnetic field may lead to vaso-occlusive crises [14] However, these prior studies have not controlled for whether patients were in or had recent vaso-occlusive crises that may have led to the DWI being positive for acute infarct, and as such, it was not possible to definitively determine if it was the MRI or the recent clinical history and underlying disease process that accounted for the acute infarct. Given the low prevalence of these acute infarcts, it has been commonly assumed that the MRI itself was not the cause of these events; however, this has not been definitively shown, and prior work suggesting this possibility has not been directly addressed [14]. Here, we performed 3 Tesla MRI in 172 SCD patients in stable conditions without known vaso-occlusive crises. The findings are that in no patients were acute lesions detectable on MRI. These findings provide support for the safety of MRI, performed at the highest available clinical strength of 3 Tesla, in patients with sickle cell disease.

These findings should be considered in light of the original study from 1985 which suggested that MRI may be unsafe in patients with SCD [14]. In this original study, *in vivo* measurements were not performed, and rather, it was only determined *ex vivo* that sickled erythrocytes in suspension have a preferential orientation at a low magnetic field strength of 0.35 T. While it is logical that this orientation should also exist at higher magnetic field strengths, the current data suggest that this biophysical phenomenon does not translate *in vivo* to vaso-occlusion and infarction. The likely reason for this is that the flow characteristics *in vivo* and the associated vascular orientation determine the erythrocyte orientation much more than the static magnetic field, and as such, infarction secondary to the magnetic field is not observed.

The study should also be considered in light of several limitations. First, the study included only 172 total participants. However, thousands of clinical MRIs are performed annually in individuals with SCD without incident as the American Society of Hematology guidelines recommend screening MRI to assess for silent cerebral infarcts in SCD at least once in childhood and adulthood [20]. Second, we did

TABLE 1: Sickle cell disease (SCD) participant demographics and percentage with acute, overt, and silent stroke.

	Female	Male	Combined
Mean age (range) (years)	19 (6–44)	20 (6–37)	19.6 (6–44)
Total number of participants	90 (52.3)	82 (47.7)	172
Number of adults ≥18 years (percent)	43 (47.8)	48 (58.5)	91 (52.9)
Number of children <18 years (percent)	47 (52.2)	34 (41.5)	81 (47.1)
Total hematocrit (range) (percent)	26.1 (15–36)	26.7 (17–35)	25.8 (15–36)
Number with acute infarct present (percent)	0	0	0
Number with chronic silent infarct present (percent)	32 (35.6)	44 (53.7)	76 (44.2)
Number with chronic overt stroke present (percent)	14 (15.6)	9 (11.0)	23 (13.4)
Number with vasculopathy present (percent)	9 (10.0)	7 (8.5)	16 (8.5)
Number with HbSS phenotype (percent)	77 (85.6)	74 (90.2)	151 (87.8)
Number with HbSβ^0 phenotype (percent)	10 (11.1)	7 (8.5)	17 (9.9)
Number with HbSC phenotype (percent)	3 (3.3)	1 (1.2)	4 (2.3)

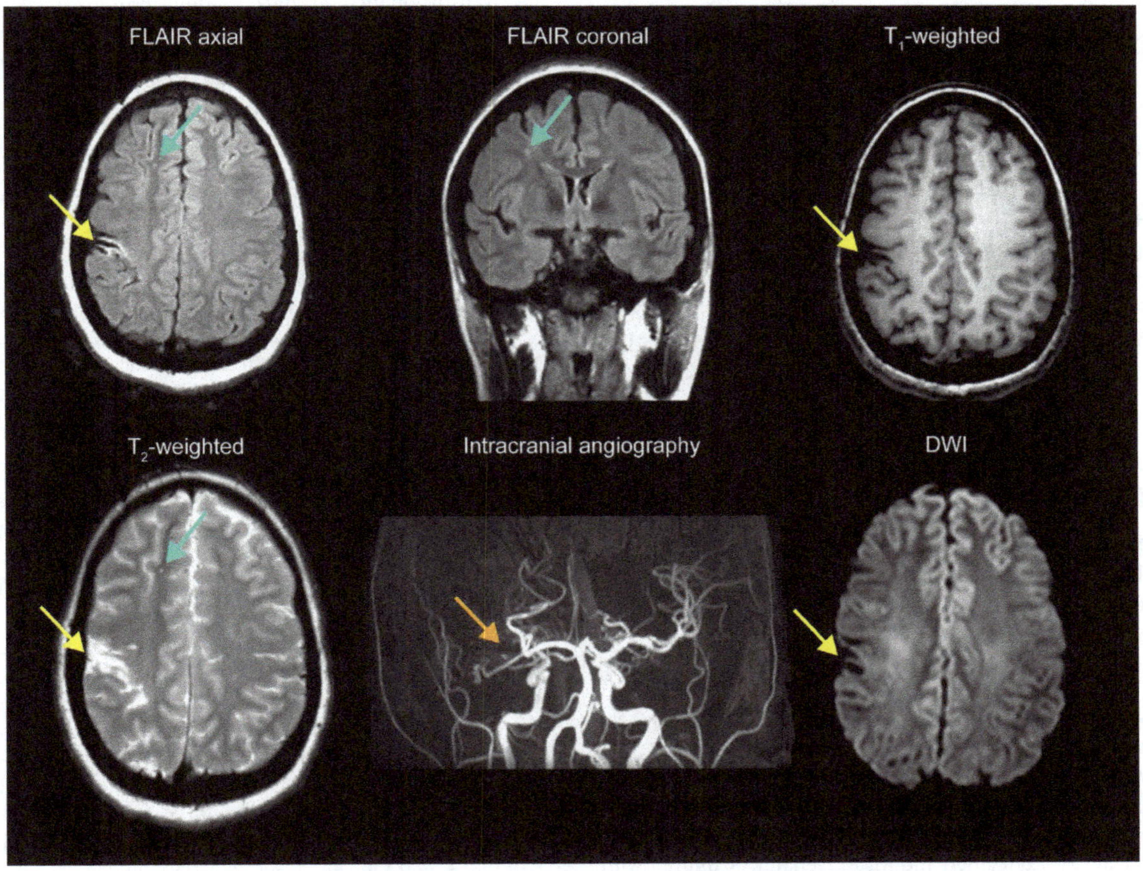

FIGURE 1: Representative scans from the multimodal magnetic resonance imaging protocol from a Black 9-year-old female with hemoglobin SS phenotype. Chronic stroke is apparent (yellow arrows), with additional right parietal and frontal lobe chronic silent cerebral infarcts (blue arrows), which largely colocalize with patchy T_2-hyperintense foci. On intracranial angiography, there is near-complete occlusion of the terminus of the right internal carotid artery with a very short proximal portion of the right M1 segment visible (orange arrow). Extensive collateral vessels are identified extending into the basal ganglia region on the right side. No evidence of acute infarct is visible on diffusion-weighted imaging (DWI).

not find any difference between participants with different sickle cell phenotypes. However, as sickle phenotypes beyond HbSS are relatively rare, the sample size for these other phenotypes is largely insufficient to make claims regarding specific phenotypes. Finally, DWI was performed approximately 20 min after introducing the patient to the isocenter of the scanner. While infarction on DWI should be apparent within several minutes, we cannot rule out that longer waiting times may have yielded different results if ischemia was more mild or collateral flow more robust. However, it should be noted that typical noncontrast head MRI protocols, as are performed in SCD patients, have a duration of approximately 20–25 minutes, and therefore, this time is roughly indicative of a clinical exam.

In conclusion, we performed 3 Tesla MRI in 172 stable SCD participants with no recent history of vaso-occlusive

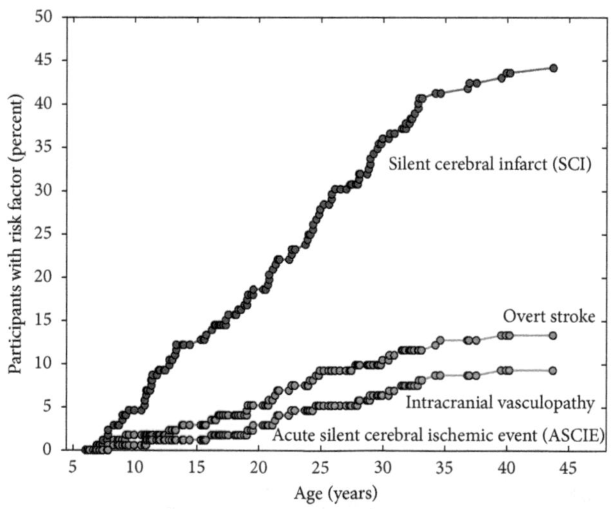

FIGURE 2: Cumulative incidence of radiological risk factors with age over the 172 participants. Note that no participants exhibited evidence of acute silent cerebral ischemic events on diffusion-weighted imaging (DWI).

crisis and representative of a typical cohort of pediatric and adult patients; findings are consistent with 3 T MRI not inducing acute infarction or vaso-occlusion in individuals with SCD and suggest that earlier low-field *ex vivo* work should not discourage MRI scans from being performed in either children or adults with SCD.

Acknowledgments

This study was supported by NIH/NINDS (5R01NS096127 and 5R01NS097763) and the American Heart Association (14CSA20380466).

References

[1] J. Strouse, "Sickle cell disease," *Neuroepidemiology*, vol. 138, pp. 311–324, 2016.

[2] M. R. DeBaun and F. J. Kirkham, "Central nervous system complications and management in sickle cell disease," *Blood*, vol. 127, no. 7, pp. 829–838, 2016.

[3] M. E. Day, M. Rodeghier, and M. R. DeBaun, "Children with HbSβ0 thalassemia have higher hemoglobin levels and lower incidence rate of acute chest syndrome compared to children with HbSS," *Pediatric Blood & Cancer*, vol. 65, no. 11, Article ID e27352, 2018.

[4] I. Ikwuanusi, L. C. Jordan, C. A. Lee et al., "Cerebral hemodynamics and metabolism are similar in sickle cell disease patients with hemoglobin SS and Sβ 0 thalassemia phenotypes," *American Journal of Hematology*, vol. 95, no. 3, pp. E66–E68, 2020.

[5] A. T. Farrell, J. Panepinto, C. P. Carroll et al., "End points for sickle cell disease clinical trials: patient-reported outcomes, pain, and the brain," *Blood Advances*, vol. 3, no. 23, pp. 3982–4001, 2019.

[6] L. C. Jordan, A. A. Kassim, M. J. Donahue et al., "Silent infarct is a risk factor for infarct recurrence in adults with sickle cell anemia," *Neurology*, vol. 91, no. 8, pp. e781–e784, 2018.

[7] M. E. Fields, K. P. Guilliams, D. K. Ragan et al., "Regional oxygen extraction predicts border zone vulnerability to stroke in sickle cell disease," *Neurology*, vol. 90, no. 13, pp. e1134–e1142, 2018.

[8] N. A. Choudhury, M. R. DeBaun, M. R. Ponisio et al., "Intracranial vasculopathy and infarct recurrence in children with sickle cell anaemia, silent cerebral infarcts and normal transcranial doppler velocities," *British Journal of Haematology*, vol. 183, no. 2, pp. 324–326, 2018.

[9] A. A. Schlotman, M. J. Donahue, A. A. Kassim et al., "Intracranial and extracranial vascular stenosis as risk factors for stroke in sickle cell disease," *Pediatric Neurology*, vol. 114, pp. 29–34, 2021.

[10] H. M. Stanley, D. F. Friedman, J. Webb, and J. L. Kwiatkowski, "Transfusional iron overload in a cohort of children with sickle cell disease: impact of magnetic resonance imaging, transfusion method, and chelation," *Pediatric Blood & Cancer*, vol. 63, no. 8, pp. 1414–1418, 2016.

[11] X. Miao, S. Choi, B. Tamrazi et al., "Increased brain iron deposition in patients with sickle cell disease: an MRI quantitative susceptibility mapping study," *Blood*, vol. 132, no. 15, pp. 1618–1621, 2018.

[12] M. M. Dowling, C. T. Quinn, Z. R. Rogers, and G. R. Buchanan, "Acute silent cerebral infarction in children with sickle cell anemia," *Pediatric Blood & Cancer*, vol. 54, no. 3, pp. 461–464, 2010.

[13] C. T. Quinn, R. C. McKinstry, M. M. Dowling et al., "Acute silent cerebral ischemic events in children with sickle cell anemia," *JAMA Neurology*, vol. 70, no. 1, pp. 58–65, 2013.

[14] A. S. Brody, M. P. Sorette, C. A. Gooding et al., "Induced alignment of flowing sickle erythrocytes in a magnetic field A preliminary report," *Investigative Radiology*, vol. 20, no. 6, pp. 560–565, 1985.

[15] M. R. DeBaun, M. Gordon, R. C. McKinstry et al., "Controlled trial of transfusions for silent cerebral infarcts in sickle cell anemia," *New England Journal of Medicine*, vol. 371, no. 8, pp. 699–710, 2014.

[16] L. M. Allen, A. N. Hasso, J. Handwerker, and H. Farid, "Sequence-specific MR imaging findings that are useful in dating ischemic stroke," *RadioGraphics*, vol. 32, no. 5, pp. 1285–1297, 2012.

[17] P. E. Grant, J. He, E. F. Halpern et al., "Frequency and clinical context of decreased apparent diffusion coefficient reversal in the human brain," *Radiology*, vol. 221, no. 1, pp. 43–50, 2001.

[18] M. L. Hulbert, R. C. McKinstry, J. L. Lacey et al., "Silent cerebral infarcts occur despite regular blood transfusion therapy after first strokes in children with sickle cell disease," *Blood*, vol. 117, no. 3, pp. 772–779, 2011.

[19] J. F. Casella, A. A. King, B. Barton et al., "Design of the silent cerebral infarct transfusion (SIT) trial," *Pediatric Hematology and Oncology*, vol. 27, no. 2, pp. 69–89, 2010.

[20] M. R. DeBaun, L. C. Jordan, A. A. King et al., "American Society of Hematology 2020 guidelines for sickle cell disease: prevention, diagnosis, and treatment of cerebrovascular disease in children and adults," *Blood Advances*, vol. 4, no. 8, pp. 1554–1588, 2020.

23

Clinical Application of Magnetic Resonance Spectroscopy in Diagnosis of Intracranial Mass Lesions

Callen Kwamboka Onyambu,[1] **Mufaddal Nuruddin Wajihi**,[2] **and Alfred Otieno Odhiambo**[1]

[1]*Department of Diagnostic Imaging and Radiation Medicine, University of Nairobi, Box 19676-00202, Nairobi, Kenya*
[2]*Nairobi West Hospital, Box 15695-00509, Nairobi, Kenya*

Correspondence should be addressed to Callen Kwamboka Onyambu; callen.onyambu@uonbi.ac.ke

Academic Editor: André Luiz Ferreira Costa

Introduction. Conventional MR imaging provides highly detailed anatomic information with unrivalled soft tissue contrast making it the mainstay in the diagnosis of suspected brain lesions. Despite this, MRI alone at times cannot answer the diagnostic questions in quite a few patients. Proton MR Spectroscopy (H-MRS) provides information on the metabolic composition within an area under interrogation. By comparing the relative concentrations of specific metabolites, the neuroradiologist can deduce critical information regarding neuronal cell density and integrity, cell membrane turnover, metabolic fuel, and possible necrosis in the region of interest. This provides a biochemical picture of the underlying pathology and thus aids in the diagnosis. *Methods.* This was a cross-sectional comparative study. *Results.* Of the 63 patients examined by MRI and MRS for intracranial mass lesions, the radiologists were able to offer a single imaging diagnosis based on MRI alone in only 15 patients (23.8%) while when MRI imaging was combined with MR spectroscopy, a single imaging diagnosis was offered in 47 patients (74.6%). This was an overall statistically significant improvement. *Conclusion.* MRS aided the radiologist in offering a single diagnosis in high versus low-grade gliomas, high-grade gliomas versus tuberculomas, and recurrent tumours versus radiation necrosis.

1. Introduction

Conventional MR imaging provides a highly detailed anatomic depiction of the human body with unrivalled soft tissue contrast and has become the mainstay in the diagnosis of suspected brain lesions [1–3] Advances in MRI technology–including, but not limited to, Gadolinium enhanced imaging, diffusion weighted imaging, perfusion studies, and susceptibility weighted imaging–have improved the accuracy of MRI diagnoses considerably. In spite of these advancements and improved sensitivity, many brain lesions remain a diagnostic problem because of poor specificity [4]. Proton MR Spectroscopy (^{1}H-MRS) provides complementary information, specifically the metabolic composition of the tissue under interrogation. While no less than 200 metabolites are generated in the brain, we are blinded to most. Proton MRS however employs mainly seven metabolites which are metabolically important and easily detectable. These principal metabolites and what they represent include lipids (Lip), lactate (Lac), N-acetyl aspartate (NAA), glutamine/GABA (Glx), creatine (Cr), choline (Cho), and myo-Inositol (mI).

By comparing the relative concentrations of these metabolites, the neuroradiologist can deduce critical information regarding neuronal cell density and integrity, cell membrane turnover, metabolic fuel, and possible necrosis in the region of interest, thereby, the likely underlying pathology [5]. The acquisition of MR spectroscopy only requires the relevant additional software and pulse sequences and an extended imaging time of only 10–12 minutes per patient. ^{1}H-MR spectroscopy is a useful noninvasive add-on to MR imaging.

Using conventional MRI, an experienced neuroradiologist can accurately propose the likely histological diagnosis in 70–90% of brain lesions based on a variety of rather indirect imaging criteria and clinical data [1, 2]. These include age and clinical presentation, location, calcification, cyst formation, and contrast enhancement among others [6]. In the remaining 10–30%, the differentiation of ischaemic mass lesions, intra- and extra-axial brain tumours, discrimination between high- and low-grade tumours, and discrimination between neoplastic and nonneoplastic lesions, however, may be ambiguous if the diagnosis is exclusively based on these criteria [6].

In contrast to MRI, CT, and angiography, that is, methods that provide structural data, proton magnetic resonance spectroscopy (^{1}H-MRS) provides nonanatomic information related to neuronal density and integrity, cell wall proliferation or degradation, energy metabolism [7], and necrotic transformation of brain and/or tumour tissues [8]. Hence, in conjunction with anatomic imaging modalities, ^{1}H-MRS is playing an increasingly important role in the discrimination of a number of common neurological disorders such as stroke, epilepsy, multiple sclerosis, HIV, dementia, head injury, and near drowning [6].

Conventional 1.5 T MRI is available at the Kenyatta National Hospital (which is Kenya's main public referral hospital), and a few of the major private diagnostic imaging establishments in Nairobi and Mombasa. This is a significant improvement from only a few years back when there were only two low strength MRI scanners in the whole country and no public hospital had access to these services [9, 10]. Today, MRS services in Kenya are only available at three private establishments, only one of them offering multivoxel MRS. All other MRI providers, including the national hospital, do not provide MRS facilities.

2. Materials and Methods

All patients were investigated under a constant single-volume ^{1}H-MRS protocol following structural MRI imaging. All imaging and spectroscopic studies were carried out with a 1.5 T Phillips Intera whole-body magnetic resonance scanner using a circularly polarized head coil.

Either T2 weighted or gadolinium enhanced T1 weighted axial images were used for voxel localization. Water-suppressed single-voxel spectra were acquired using a double spin-echo localization technique (PRESS, point-resolved excitation spin-echo sequence) with frequency-selective water suppression. ^{1}H-MRS was performed using automated spectroscopy sequences at short TE of 31msec, and intermediate TE of 144msec. A voxel of 2–8 mL, depending on the size of the lesion, was placed within the lesion.

All MRI and MRS examinations were reported by the attending radiologists. PACS archived images and reports were used to record and analyse the imaging and spectroscopy findings.

2.1. Ethical Considerations. This study was done after obtaining approval from KNH-UON ethical review commission. Patient autonomy was maintained throughout the study.

3. Results

A total of 68 patients presented to Plaza Imaging Solutions for Brain MR Spectroscopy between September 2012 and September 2013. Of these, 63 patients satisfied the study's selection criteria and were thus recruited for the study.

The average age (mean (±SD)) of patients with intracranial masses was 45.33 years (±20.14). The youngest patient was 5 years of age while the oldest was 90 years old. Of the 63 patients, 32 (50.8%) were male and 31 (49.2%) were female, representing an almost equal 1 : 1 male to female ratio.

3.1. MRI Diagnosis. All patients referred for brain MRS underwent conventional brain MRI scans before their spectroscopy examinations. All MRI and MRS studies were reported and reviewed with a consultant specialist neuroradiologist who has more than 10-year practice experience in neuroradiology based on clinical information and imaging features. These MRI examinations were initially reported independently of their corresponding MRS findings. When the reporting radiologist had more than one differential, even if there were two indisputable differentials, this was recorded as "no single diagnosis." The following diagnoses were made based on the clinical history provided and conventional MRI scans alone (Table 1).

It is clear that from all patients referred for brain MRS, a significant proportion (76.2%) (95% CI 63.8–86.0%) were unable to get a single definite diagnosis based on MRI alone.

3.2. Indication for MRS. Figure 1 lists the indications for which brain MR spectroscopies were performed during this study.

3.2.1. Spectroscopy. The largest proportion of brain MR spectroscopies (49.2%) ($p = 0.899$) were performed to help differentiate tumours from infections. Of these 31 indications, 30 (96.7%) ($p < 0.001$) were performed to differentiate tuberculoma, from glioblastoma multiforme (GBM). The remaining indication from this subgroup was to differentiate Primary CNS Lymphoma from toxoplasmosis in a patient with HIV infection. These statistics suggest that tuberculomas are statistically significantly the most common infectious intracranial mass lesions seen in this population. It is worth noting that no diagnosis of the pyogenic abscess was seen either based on MRI alone nor MRI + MRS during this study.

3.3. MRI + MRS Diagnosis. Figure 2 provides the diagnoses and their frequencies that were made after correlating the MRI findings to the findings of single-voxel MR spectroscopy performed on the intracranial mass lesions. It is important to note that only definitive imaging diagnoses were recorded as such. If there was more than one differential, this was recorded as "no single diagnosis." These diagnoses were made by combining MRI and MRS findings, not from MRS alone. The two most frequent diagnoses made using MRI

TABLE 1: Diagnoses using MRI alone.

MRI diagnosis	Frequency (%)
No single diagnosis	48 (76.2)
Low-grade glioma	4 (6.3)
High-grade glioma	3 (4.8)
Metastasis	1 (1.6)
Meningioma	1 (1.6)
Schwannoma	1 (1.6)
Cerebral infarct	1 (1.6)
Radiation necrosis	1 (1.6)
Pilocytic astrocytoma	1 (1.6)
Cavernoma	2 (3.2)

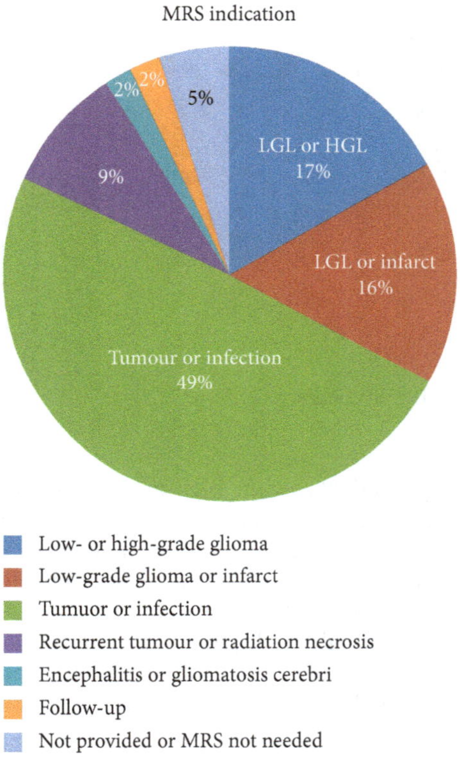

FIGURE 1: MRS indication.

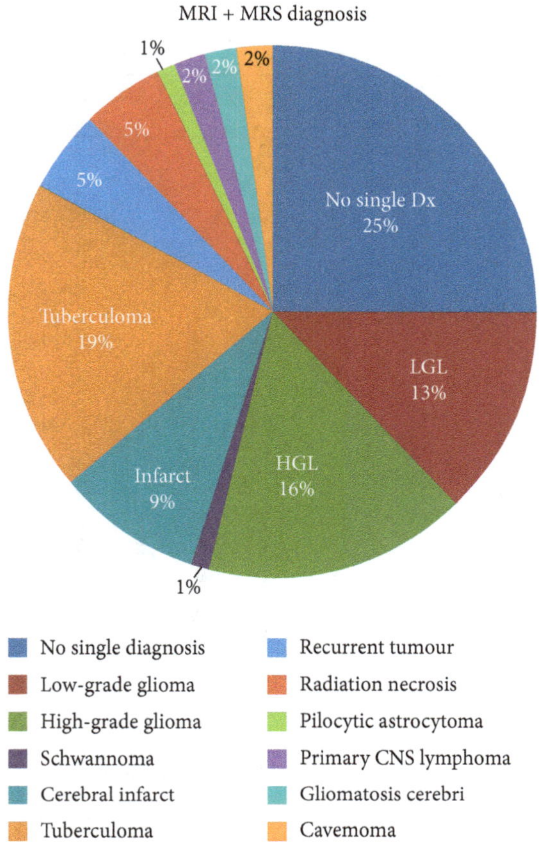

FIGURE 2: MRI + MRS diagnosis.

and MRS were high-grade gliomas (15.9%) (95% CI 7.9–27.3%) and tuberculomas (19%) (95% CI 10.3–30.9%).

3.3.1. Efficacy of MRI + MRS. Of all patients examined by MRI and MRS for intracranial mass lesions, the radiologists were able to offer a single definite imaging diagnosis based on MRI alone in only 23.8% of patients while when MRI imaging was combined with MR spectroscopy, a single imaging diagnosis was offered in 74.6% of patients. This was an overall statistically significant improvement of 313.4% (p value <0.001), a slightly more than 3-fold improvement in diagnostic performance (Table 2). It is important to note that the majority of this population was biased towards patients who had been referred for MRS because of inconclusive prior imaging.

When we combine all individual diagnoses made using MRI alone and MRI + MRS, from all 63 patients, the addition of MRS improved the imaging diagnosis in 35 of these patients (55.6%). This means that the radiologist was able to rule out some differentials and offer a single imaging diagnosis or was, in a few cases, able to change the single diagnosis that was offered based on MRI alone. In 28 patients (44.4%), the addition of MRS was either not able to rule out other differentials or it did not change the single diagnosis that was offered based on MRI alone. Although this is an improvement, it is not statistically significant ($p = 0.374$).

The combination of MRI with MRS significantly increased the radiologist's chances of confidently diagnosing high-grade gliomas, low-grade gliomas, cerebral infarcts, tuberculomas, recurrent tumours, and radiation necrosis, rather than with MRI alone ($p < 0.001$ based on Wilcoxon Rank test) as demonstrated in Figure 3.

3.4. MRS Spectral Changes Based on Diagnosis. The metabolite changes are as follows.

Creatine was depressed in 70% of lesions diagnosed as high-grade glioma, while it was unchanged in all but one lesion diagnosed as low-grade glioma ($p = 0.025$).

Decreased NAA, increased choline, lipid, and lactate were seen in both grades of tumours, with no significant difference in observed spectral changes. NAA was reduced and creatine was unchanged in both. Choline was increased in 75% of low-grade gliomas, while it was unchanged or decreased in 83.3% of cerebral infarcts. Although this trend is radiologically important for distinction between the two,

Table 2: Overall diagnostic performance between MRI diagnosis and MRI + MRS diagnosis.

Findings	MRI diagnosis n (%)	MRI + MRS diagnosis n (%)	P value
Single imaging diagnosis	15 (23.8)	47 (74.6)	<0.001
No single imaging diagnosis	48 (76.2)	16 (25.4)	

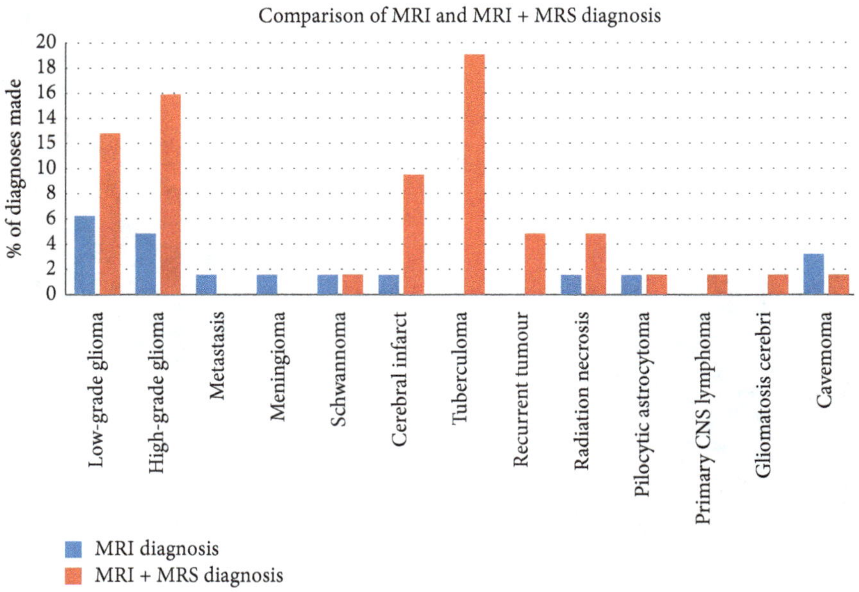

Figure 3: Comparison of MRI and MRI + MRS diagnosis.

the difference between the two groups was not statistically significant ($p = 0.149$).

This is most likely due to the small frequency of these lesions, and a larger frequency would likely show a statistically significant difference. Lipid and lactate were increased in both. Myo-inositol was increased in 75% of lesions diagnosed as low-grade gliomas while, in cerebral infarcts, it was either increased or decreased or no change was seen.

Metabolite spectral changes between recurrent tumour and radiation necrosis showed no statistically significant differences in metabolite changes between the two groups likely due to the very small frequencies encountered of these lesions. However, from a radiological perspective, choline was increased in all (100%) of the recurrent tumours, while it was not increased in any diagnosis of radiation necrosis ($p = 0.071$). Decreased NAA and increased lipid and lactate were seen in both groups.

Comparison of metabolite spectral changes between high-grade gliomas and tuberculomas showing that the only statistically significant difference between the two groups was increased myo-inositol in 50% of high-grade glioma diagnoses, while, in all tuberculomas, myo-inositol was either unchanged or decreased ($p = 0.007$). Decreased NAA, increased choline, lipid, and lactate were seen in both sets of diagnoses as shown in Figure 4.

Cho : Cr and Cho : NAA (at both TE 31 and 144 msec) were significantly higher in patients with high-grade glioma than in those with low-grade glioma. Conversely, NAA : Cho and NAA : Cr were significantly lower in patients with high-grade glioma than in those with low-grade glioma.

Similarly, patients with high-grade gliomas, tuberculomas, and recurrent tumours had significantly lower NAA : Cho ratios. NAA : Cr was increased in cerebral infarcts and radiation necrosis due to creatine depletion, while it was decreased in all other diagnoses. While NAA : Cr was decreased in both high-grade gliomas and tuberculomas, the decrease in high-grade gliomas was significantly more than in tuberculomas. Further analysis based on pairs of major diagnoses is provided below.

MRS was also useful in differentiating some tuberculomas from high-grade gliomas. Although increased choline was seen in both, Cho : Cr and Cho : NAA were significantly much higher in high-grade gliomas than in those confidently diagnosed as tuberculomas. NAA : Cr and NAA : Cho were reduced in both; however, only the reduction in NAA : Cr was statistically significantly more in high-grade gliomas than in tuberculomas (at TE 144 msec).

Brain MRS was also used to help differentiate low-grade gliomas from cerebral infarcts. The low frequency of cerebral infarcts diagnosed and the wide variation in ratios encountered meant that no statistically significant differences were seen between the two groups. However, NAA : Cr and NAA : Cho were much lower in low-grade gliomas compared to infarcts. The markedly reduced (almost zero) values of NAA and creatine, seen in several diagnosed cerebral infarcts (wide SD), caused deceptively elevated Cho : NAA (TE 31) and NAA : Cr and Cho : Cr ratios (TE 144).

A number of diagnoses of recurrent tumour versus radiation necrosis were made based on MRS findings. No statistically significant differences between the two groups

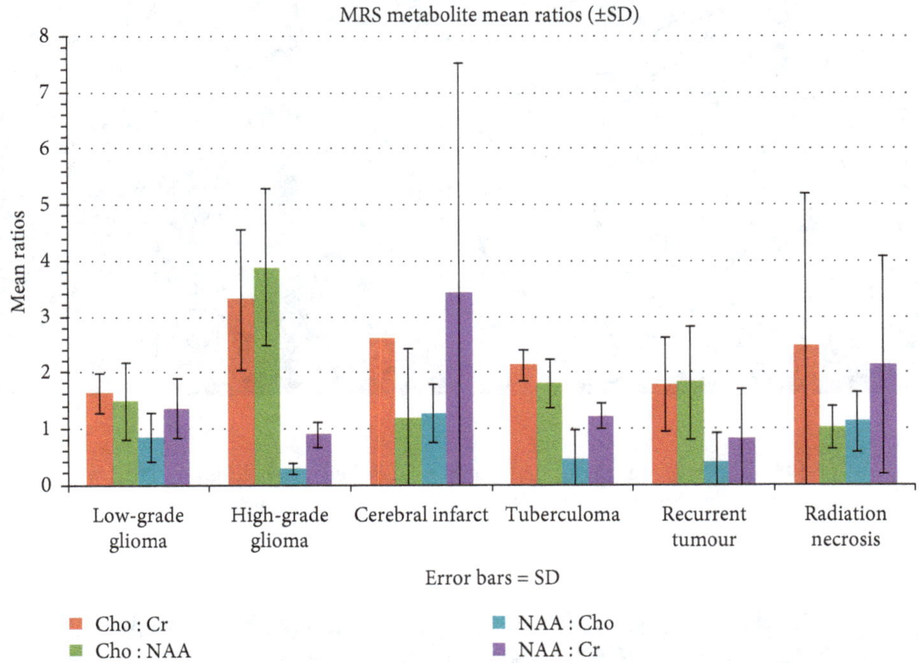

FIGURE 4: MRS ratios based on the diagnosis.

were seen due to the low frequency of the occurrences. However, of note is the trend that NAA : Cr and NAA : Cho were much lower in recurrent tumour than in radiation necrosis, and Cho : NAA was much higher in recurrent tumour than in radiation necrosis. The very low levels of creatine in radiation necrosis caused deceptively elevated Cho : Cr ratios.

3.5. Selected MRI/MRS Images from Study Sample. Images from selected cases representing the spectrum of findings encountered during the study are presented in Figures 5–9 below. All images shown are from actual cases of patients recruited in the study.

4. Discussion

Overall, the impact of combining MRI with MRS in improving the radiologist's ability to offer a single imaging diagnosis was significant. The number of "single diagnoses" increased by 3-fold (in 47/63) patients (74.6%) with MRI + MRS compared to MRI alone (15/63 patients (23.8%)). The most notable lesions, for which MRS aided the radiologist in offering a single diagnosis, were high and low-grade gliomas, tuberculomas, cerebral infarcts, recurrent tumours, and radiation necrosis. It is important to note that the majority of this sample population was biased towards patients who had been referred for MRS because of inconclusive prior imaging. This shows that, among the referring clinicians, there is awareness about the utility of and indications for brain MRS in the diagnosis of intracranial mass lesions.

Most patients presenting for brain MRS for intracranial mass lesions were in the age group of 41–50 years. By far the largest number of brain MR, spectroscopy examinations were performed to differentiate tuberculomas from high-grade gliomas, seeing that both may present as ring-enhancing mass lesions. We can infer that the age group of 41–50 years is like a watershed group which presents more of a challenge when differentiating tuberculomas from high-grade gliomas because epidemiologically high-grade gliomas tend to peak more in elderly patients, while tuberculomas tend to peak in younger patients [11–15].

Four major indications for brain MRS emerged from this study. These were to differentiate low- and high-grade gliomas; to differentiate tumours from infections (96.7% of these were to differentiate high-grade gliomas from tuberculomas); to differentiate low-grade gliomas from cerebral infarcts; and to differentiate recurrent tumour from radiation necrosis.

If we look at the efficacy of MRS added to MRI in improving the imaging diagnosis versus the four major indications described above, the addition of MRS to MRI did indeed improve the imaging diagnosis in all four indications. However, the improvement was not statistically significant ($p > 0.05$). It is possible that a larger sample size would probably show more statistically significant improvements.

When trying to differentiate between low-grade and high-grade gliomas, decreased NAA, increased Choline, lipid and lactate were seen in both grades of tumours, with no significant difference in observed spectral changes. Of statistical significance was the fact that creatine was depressed in a large proportion of diagnosed high-grade gliomas, while it remained unchanged in low-grade glioma diagnoses ($p = 0.025$).

Of important note is that myo-inositol was increased in 87.5% of lesions diagnosed as low-grade gliomas. However, in lesions diagnosed as high-grade glioma, myo-inositol was

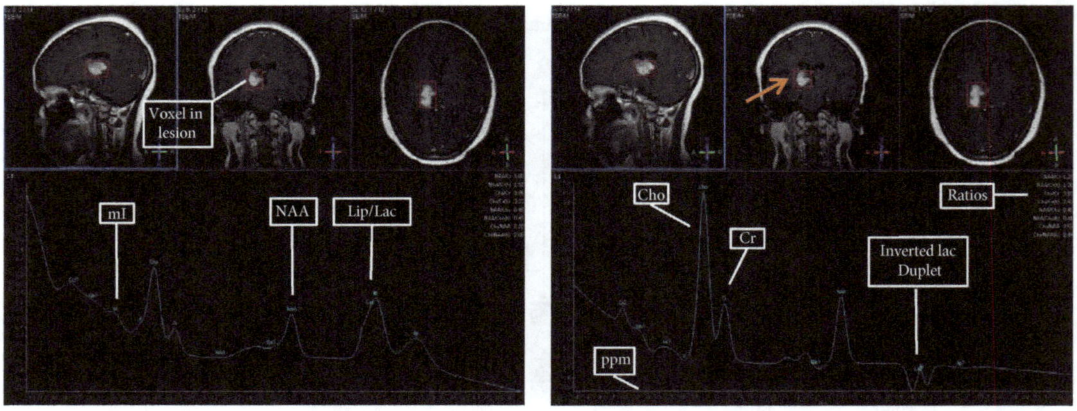

(a) (b)

Figure 5: (a) TE 31 msec. (b) TE 144 msec. MRS was performed to differentiate between high-grade and low-grade glioma. The lesion was diagnosed as a high-grade glioma. NAA is decreased. Lipid and lactate are increased. Choline is markedly elevated. Cho : Cr ratio is 2.93, and Cho : NAA ratio is 2.44. At TE31, myo-inositol is reduced. Myo-inositol decrease has been associated with high-grade gliomas (58).

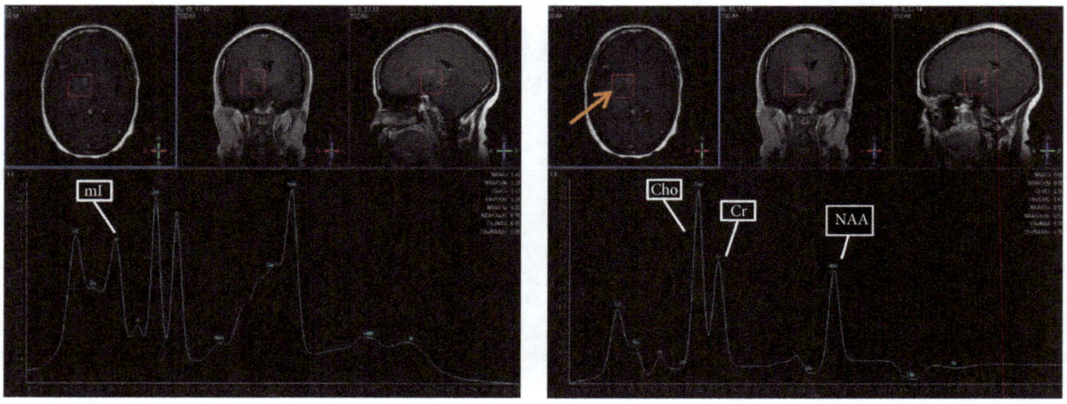

(a) (b)

Figure 6: (a) TE 31 msec. (b) TE 144 msec. MRS was performed to differentiate between high-grade and low-grade glioma. The lesion was diagnosed as a low-grade glioma. NAA is depressed. Choline is moderately elevated. Cho : Cr is 1.67, and Cho : NAA is 1.90. Increased myo-inositol is also seen at TE31.

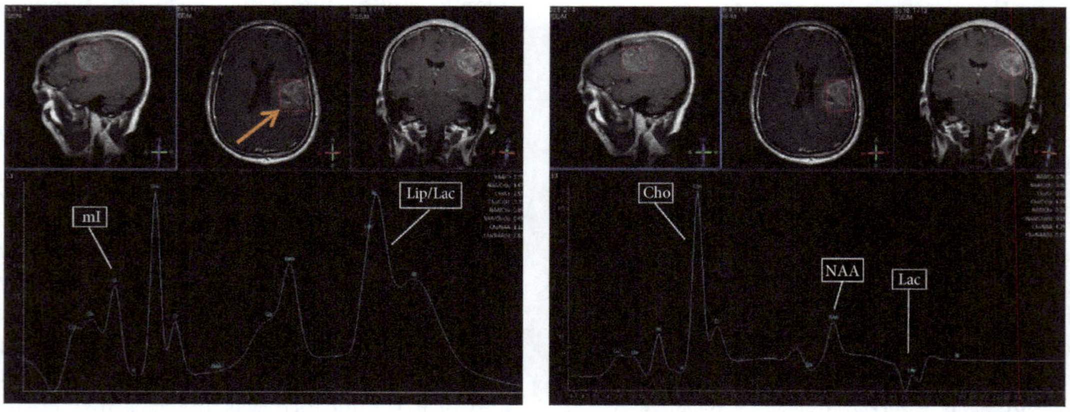

(a) (b)

Figure 7: (a) TE 31 msec. (b) TE 144 msec. MRS was performed to differentiate between high-grade and low-grade glioma. The lesion was diagnosed as a high-grade glioma. NAA is reduced. Lipid and lactate are elevated. Choline is markedly elevated. Cho : Cr is 4.74, and Cho : NAA is 5.19. However, at TE31, myo-inositol is slightly increased. Myo-inositol increase has been associated with low-grade gliomas (58).

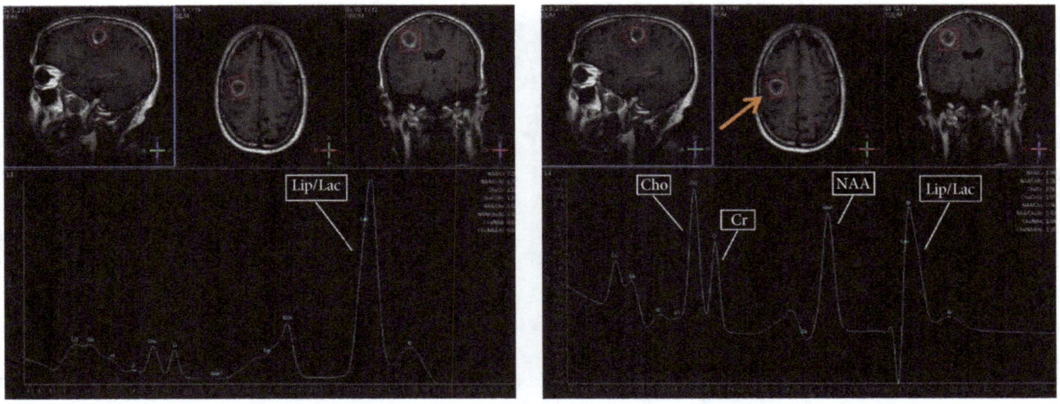

(a) (b)

FIGURE 8: (a) TE 31 msec. (b) TE 144 msec. MRS was performed to differentiate between high-grade glioma and tuberculoma. The lesion was diagnosed as a tuberculoma. At TE31 prominent, lipid peak is seen at 1.3 ppm. At TE144, choline is increased. However, Cho : Cr is 1.57 and Cho : NAA is 1.20.

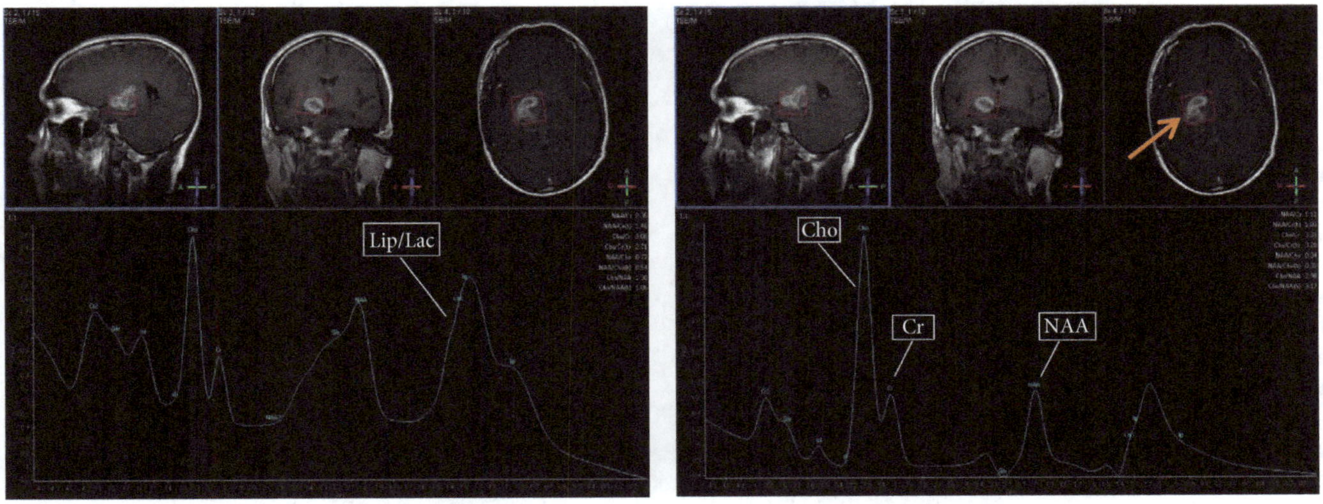

(a) (b)

FIGURE 9: (a) TE 31 msec. (b) TE 144 msec. MRS was performed to differentiate between high-grade glioma and tuberculoma. The lesion was diagnosed as a high-grade glioma. NAA is depressed. Lipid is elevated. Choline is markedly elevated. Cho : Cr is 3.28, and Cho : NAA is 3.17. Note that in this case diagnosed as high0grade glioma, myo-inositol at TE31 is not decreased.

decreased in only 30% of lesions, remained unchanged in 20%, and was increased in 50%. This contrasts the findings of Castillo et al. who reported a trend towards lower myo-inositol levels in high-grade gliomas compared to increased levels in those of low-grade gliomas [16].

More significant differences between low- and high-grade glioma diagnoses were seen when we look at metabolite ratios. Cho : Cr and Cho : NAA ratios were significantly higher in patients with high-grade glioma than in those with low-grade glioma. Conversely, NAA : Cho and NAA : Cr were significantly lower in patients with high-grade glioma than in those with low-grade glioma. Mean Cho : Cr and Cho : NAA ratios were <2.00 in low-grade gliomas [1.63 (±0.36)] and [1.48 (±0.68)] respectively, while they were >2.00 in high-grade gliomas [3.30 (±1.26)] and [3.88 (±1.40)], respectively. Mean NAA : Cr was <1.80 in low-grade gliomas [1.36 (±0.52)] and <1.00 in high-grade gliomas [0.89 (±0.23)], while mean NAA : Cho was <1.20 in low-grade gliomas [0.84 (±0.44)] and <0.50 in high-grade gliomas [±0.29 (0.10)]. Our findings compare favourably with those of Bertholdo et al. who report that at different institutions the threshold for Cho : Cr and Cho : NAA for differentiating low- and high-grade gliomas ranges between 2.0 and 2.5 [17].

The bulk of MRS examinations were performed to differentiate tuberculomas from high-grade gliomas. Based on MR spectrum appearance, decreased NAA, increased choline, lipid, and lactate were seen in both sets of diagnoses. Early work by Gupta et al. showed that tuberculomas tend to have prominent lipid peaks within the lesion, while all other metabolites are depressed [18]. However, our findings in tuberculomas compare to more recent work by Gupta et al.

and Gutch et al. which show that Choline increase is also seen in tuberculomas depending on the degree of cellular infiltrate and caseation [19, 20].

The only statistically significant difference between the two groups was that myo-inositol was increased in 50% of high-grade glioma diagnoses, while, in all tuberculomas, myo-inositol was either unchanged or decreased ($p = 0.007$).

Differentiating tuberculomas from high-grade gliomas can be particularly challenging based on the observed spectral changes of single-voxel MRS alone. Comparing metabolite ratios did assist in the differentiation. Although increased choline was seen in both, Cho : Cr and Cho : NAA were significantly much higher in high-grade gliomas, [3.30 (±1.26)] and [3.88 (±1.40)], respectively, than in those confidently diagnosed as tuberculomas [2.13 (±0.28)] and [1.80 (±0.43)]. NAA : Cr and NAA : Cho were reduced in both; however, only the reduction in NAA : Cr was statistically significantly more in high-grade gliomas [0.89 (±0.23)] than in tuberculomas [1.22 (±0.22)].

31(49.2%) of MR spectroscopies were performed to differentiate tumours from nontumours (infections). Of these, 30 (96.7%) were to differentiate tuberculomas from high-grade gliomas. The lowly diagnostic performance of MRS in this regard (51.6% improvement of imaging diagnosis) occurred mainly when elevated choline and lipids were seen in a lesion, and the Cho : NAA and Cho : Cr ratios were such that they could not be confidently diagnosed as one or the other. A large number (48.4%) of such MR spectroscopies led to "no single diagnosis," with both differentials still being considered. The age of the patients was also a factor in this diagnostic dilemma as explained above. It is in these situations where multivoxel MRS if available would have been particularly useful. Multivoxel MRS would allow different parts of the lesion; the central area of breakdown, the enhancing solid rim, and the peritumoural region to be interrogated separately. Increased choline in the peritumoural oedema would greatly increase the confidence of diagnosing a high-grade glioma. Differentiation of tumour from nonneoplastic lesions is possible using NAA/Cho and NAA/Cr ratios, with high choline levels seen in the neoplastic lesions [21].

When multiple ring-enhancing lesions were encountered, this would favour tuberculomas; however, when such lesions had markedly elevated Choline and Cho : NAA and Cho : Cr ratios, it would be difficult to confidently diagnose tuberculomas, as a multifocal aggressive tumour like metastasis would also need to be considered in the differential.

Only one MRS was performed to differentiate between primary CNS lymphoma and toxoplasmosis in an HIV patient. No pyogenic abscess diagnosis was encountered.

The third indication for which MRSs were performed was to differentiate low-grade gliomas from cerebral infarcts, in those whose prior imaging was inconclusive. Choline was increased in 75% of low-grade gliomas, while it was unchanged or decreased in 83.3% of cerebral infarcts. Although this trend is radiologically important for distinction between the two, the difference between the two groups was not statistically significant ($p = 0.149$). This is most likely due to the small frequency of these lesions encountered, and a larger frequency from a larger sample size would likely show a statistically significant difference. Another observation was that myo-inositol was increased in low-grade gliomas (75% of them), while in cerebral infarcts, no particular trend was seen although without any statistical significance.

MRS metabolite ratios showed no statistically significant differences between the two groups. However, mean NAA : Cr and NAA : Cho ratios were much lower in low-grade gliomas compared to infarcts. The markedly reduced (almost zero) values of NAA and creatine, seen in several diagnosed cerebral infarcts, caused deceptively elevated Cho : NAA (TE 31) and NAA : Cr and Cho : Cr ratios (TE 144). This suggests that the diagnosis of cerebral infarct versus low-grade glioma was more likely based on observed spectral changes of increased Choline in gliomas, rather than on metabolite ratios.

The indication for the fourth group of MRS examinations was to differentiate between recurrent tumour and radiation necrosis. Once again, due to the small frequencies encountered, no statistically significant differences in metabolite changes between the two groups were seen. However, from a radiological perspective, choline was increased in all (100%) of recurrent tumours, while it was not increased in any diagnosis of radiation necrosis ($p = 0.071$).

However, of note is the trend that NAA : Cr and NAA : Cho were much lower in recurrent tumour than in radiation necrosis, and Cho : NAA was much higher in recurrent tumour than in radiation necrosis. The very low levels of creatine in radiation necrosis caused deceptively elevated Cho : Cr ratios.

One MRS examination was performed to help differentiate between encephalitis and gliomatosis cerebri which has a varied MRI appearance. MRS was useful in this instance as it showed typical MRS features of gliomatosis cerebri, which include elevated myo-inositol together with features of aggressive tumour, that is, increased choline, increased Cho : Cr and Cho : NAA ratios, and decreased NAA : Cr and NAA : Cho ratios [22].

One MRS examination was performed for a child whose MRI imaging diagnosis was a pilocytic astrocytoma. MRS findings only confirmed the MRI findings by showing typical accepted paradoxical findings of an aggressive-appearing metabolite pattern and increased choline and lactate, which do not reflect the histologically benign nature of this tumour [23]. MRS in this case did not however improve the imaging diagnosis.

The main study limitation is that findings were not correlated with histology. The correlation of MRS and relative cerebral blood volume (rCBV) has been shown to increase diagnostic accuracy to 100% when compared with histopathology [23].

5. Conclusions

MRS combined with MRI is an important tool in the arsenal of a radiologist for diagnosing intracranial mass lesions and provides a noninvasive way of interrogating the biochemical make-up of lesions within the brain. Overall, when patients are selectively chosen who have more than one differential based on conventional MRI, in whom MRS has the potential to answer the diagnostic question, MRS combined with MRI showed a threefold increase in the number of single imaging diagnosis offered by the radiologist.

The most notable lesions, for which MRS aided the radiologist in offering a single diagnosis, were high- and low-grade gliomas, tuberculomas, cerebral infarcts, recurrent tumours, and radiation necrosis.

MRS combined with MRI "improved" the imaging diagnosis in more than half of all patients examined. MRS is also valuable in differentiating between recurrent tumour and radiation necrosis based on observing increased spectra of choline in recurrent tumours, along with increased Cho : NAA ratios and decreased NAA : Cr and NAA : Cho ratios.

6. Limitations

One of the limitations of this study was the fact that we were unable to compare the imaging diagnosis with the histopathological diagnosis; hence, the investigator has referred to his findings as "imaging diagnosis" and not definitive diagnosis. As a result, we were unable to provide local data on the sensitivity and specificity of MRS for the diagnosis of intracranial mass lesions.

Secondly, while MRS findings showed trends in metabolite spectral changes and ratios for particular diagnoses and indication groups in one way or another, the fact that the frequencies of several diagnoses encountered were small, it was difficult to determine the statistical significance of these trends. A larger sample size with a longer study duration, or a study designed to target particular diagnoses, would be required to resolve this.

An important factor to consider is that majority of patients recruited in this study may already have had prior imaging with an inconclusive diagnosis. Due to cost implications, the decision to refer a patient for MRS is often made by the clinicians, either on their own or upon the recommendation of the radiologist. This, coupled with the fact that a consecutive series sample selection method was used, may have introduced an element of selection bias.

References

[1] I. A. Chishty, M. Z. Rafique, M. Hussain et al., "MRI characterization and histopathological correlation of primary intra-axial brain glioma," *Journal of the Liaquat University of Medical and Health Sciences*, vol. 9, pp. 64–69, 2010.

[2] R. E. Latchaw, J. Kucharczyk, and M. E. Moseley, *Imaging of the Nervous System-Diagnostic and Therapeutic Applications*, Elsevier Mosby, Maryland, MI, USA, 2005.

[3] K. Sartor, "MR imaging of the brain: tumors," *European Radiology*, vol. 9, no. 6, pp. 1047–1054, 1999.

[4] S. J. Nelson, "Multivoxel magnetic resonance spectroscopy of brain tumors," *Molecular Cancer Therapeutics*, vol. 2, no. 5, pp. 497–507, 2003.

[5] P. B. Barker, "Fundamentals of MR spectroscopy," in *Clinical MR Neuroimaging*, J. H. W. A. Gillard and P. B. Barker, Eds., Cambridge University Press, Cambridge, UK, 2005.

[6] W. Möller-Hartmann, S. Herminghaus, T. Krings et al., "Clinical application of proton magnetic resonance spectroscopy in the diagnosis of intracranial mass lesions," *Neuroradiology*, vol. 44, no. 5, pp. 371–381, 2002.

[7] B. L. Miller, "A review of chemical issues in 1H NMR spectroscopy:N-acetyl-l-aspartate, creatine and choline," *NMR in Biomedicine*, vol. 4, no. 2, pp. 47–52, 1991.

[8] A. C. Kuesel, G. R. Sutherland, W. Halliday, and I. C. P. Smith, "1H MRS of high grade astrocytomas: mobile lipid accumulation in necrotic tissue," *NMR in Biomedicine*, vol. 7, no. 3, pp. 149–155, 1994.

[9] E. O. Amayo, "Kenya," *Practical Neurology*, vol. 6, no. 4, p. 261, 2006.

[10] G. Kenya, "Provision of vital equipment to government hospitals," Kenya National Assembly Official Report 2298, Hansard, London, UK, 2003.

[11] P. B. Barker, A. Bizzi, N. DeStefano et al., *Clinical MR Spectroscopy*, Cambridge University Press, Cambridge, UK, 2009.

[12] A. M. Mishra, R. K. Gupta, R. S. Jaggi et al., "Role of diffusion-weighted imaging and in vivo proton magnetic resonance spectroscopy in the differential diagnosis of ring-enhancing intracranial cystic mass lesions," *Journal of Computer Assisted Tomography*, vol. 28, no. 4, pp. 540–547, 2004.

[13] L. G. Astrakas, D. Zurakowski, A. A. Tzika et al., "Noninvasive magnetic resonance spectroscopic imaging biomarkers to predict the clinical grade of pediatric brain tumors," *Clinical Cancer Research*, vol. 10, no. 24, pp. 8220–8228, 2004.

[14] V. N. Kornienko and I. N. Pronin, *Diagnostic Neuroradiology*, Springer, Berlin, Germany, 2009.

[15] W. Dähnert, *Radiology Review Manual*, Lippincott Williams & Wilkins, Philadelphia, PA, USA, 2003.

[16] M. Castillo, J. K. Smith, and L. Kwock, "Correlation of myo-inositol levels and grading of cerebral astrocytomas," *AJNR. American Journal of Neuroradiology*, vol. 21, no. 9, pp. 1645–1649, 2000.

[17] D. Bertholdo, A. Watcharakorn, and M. Castillo, *Brain Proton Magnetic Resonance Spectroscopy: Introduction and Overview*, pp. 359–380, Neuroimaging Clinics, Gainesville, FL, USA, 2013.

[18] R. K. Gupta, H. Poptani, A. Kholi et al., "In vivo localized proton magnetic resonance spectroscopy of intracranial tuberculomas," *Indian Journal of Medical Research*, vol. 101, pp. 19–24, 1995.

[19] R. Trivedi, S. Saksena, and R. K. Gupta, "Magnetic resonance imaging in central nervous system tuberculosis," *Indian Journal of Radiology and Imaging*, vol. 19, pp. 256–265, 2009.

[20] M. Gutch, N. Jain, A. Agrawal et al., "MR spectroscopy in tuberculoma of brain," *BMJ Case Reports*, vol. 10, p. 1136, 2012.

[21] A. Jesrani, R. Ajmal, M. Asad, and S. N. Zehra, "Diagnostic accuracy of magnetic resonance spectroscopy in differentiating neoplastic from non-neoplastic enhancing brain lesions

taking histopathology as gold standard, experience at Liaquat National Hospital, Karachi, Pakistan," *Acta Scientific Cancer Biology*, vol. 3, no. 10, pp. 3–8, 2019.

[22] A. G. Osborn, K. L. Salzman, and A. J. Barkovich, *Diagnostic Imaging: Brain*, Amirsys, Salt Lake City, UT, USA, 2009.

[23] A. S. Hasan, A. K. Hasan, H. I. Megally et al., "The combined role of MR spectroscopy and perfusion imaging in preoperative differentiation between high- and low-grade gliomas," *Egyptian Journal of Radiology and Nuclear Medicine*, vol. 50, p. 72, 2019.

24

Comparison of Phase Estimation Methods for Quantitative Susceptibility Mapping Using a Rotating-Tube Phantom

Kathryn E. Keenan,[1] Ben P. Berman,[2] Slávka Rýger,[1] Stephen E. Russek,[1] Wen-Tung Wang,[3] John A. Butman,[4] Dzung L. Pham,[3] and Joseph Dagher[2]

[1]*National Institute of Standards and Technology, Physical Measurement Laboratory, 325 Broadway, Boulder, CO 80305, USA*
[2]*The MITRE Corporation, 7515 Colshire Dr, McLean, VA 22102, USA*
[3]*Henry M. Jackson Foundation, 10 Center Drive, Bethesda, MD 20892, USA*
[4]*Clinical Center, National Institutes of Health, 10 Center Drive, Bethesda, MD 20814, USA*

Correspondence should be addressed to Ben P. Berman; bberman@mitre.org

Academic Editor: André Luiz Ferreira Costa

Quantitative Susceptibility Mapping (QSM) is an MRI tool with the potential to reveal pathological changes from magnetic susceptibility measurements. Before phase data can be used to recover susceptibility ($\Delta\chi$), the QSM process begins with two steps: data acquisition and phase estimation. We assess the performance of these steps, when applied without user intervention, on several variations of a phantom imaging task. We used a rotating-tube phantom with five tubes ranging from $\Delta\chi = 0.05$ ppm to $\Delta\chi = 0.336$ ppm. MRI data was acquired at nine angles of rotation for four different pulse sequences. The images were processed by 10 phase estimation algorithms including Laplacian, region-growing, branch-cut, temporal unwrapping, and maximum-likelihood methods, resulting in approximately 90 different combinations of data acquisition and phase estimation methods. We analyzed errors between measured and expected phases using the probability mass function and Cumulative Distribution Function. Repeatable acquisition and estimation methods were identified based on the probability of relative phase errors. For single-echo GRE and segmented EPI sequences, a region-growing method was most reliable with Pr (relative error <0.1) = 0.95 and 0.90, respectively. For multiecho sequences, a maximum-likelihood method was most reliable with Pr (relative error <0.1) = 0.97. The most repeatable multiecho methods outperformed the most repeatable single-echo methods. We found a wide range of repeatability and reproducibility for off-the-shelf MRI acquisition and phase estimation approaches, and this variability may prevent the techniques from being widely integrated in clinical workflows. The error was dominated in many cases by spatially discontinuous phase unwrapping errors. Any postprocessing applied on erroneous phase estimates, such as QSM's background field removal and dipole inversion, would suffer from error propagation. Our paradigm identifies methods that yield consistent and accurate phase estimates that would ultimately yield consistent and accurate $\Delta\chi$ estimates.

1. Introduction

Quantitative Susceptibility Mapping (QSM)[1–3] is a method to estimate magnetic susceptibility of tissue from the phase of the magnetic resonance (MR) signal. QSM has potential clinical utility for characterizing neurological diseases [4–6], blood oxygen content [7], iron overload in the heart and liver [8], and quantitative tracking of contrast agent bolus perfusion [9, 10].

Repeatability and reproducibility of QSM have been assessed in phantoms and human subjects using different scanners, magnetic field strengths, and data processing methods. While some studies report high repeatability [11–18], both *in vivo* and in phantoms, recent *in vivo* studies report lower reproducibility across MRI scanners with the same data processing method [19] and across QSM algorithms using the same input data [20]. These conflicting results limit the clinical adoption of QSM.

A typical QSM process requires four steps: data acquisition (Step 1), phase estimation (Step 2), background field removal (Step 3), and magnetic susceptibility reconstruction (Step 4). Recently proposed methods combine Steps 2–4 into fewer steps [21].

In its standardization efforts, the QSM community has actively evaluated competing methods [17, 22, 23], in particular for methods in Steps 3 and 4 of the process [20]. However, the selection of the "best" QSM method is difficult for various reasons: (a) the appropriate definition of a quality metric, for example, accuracy versus repeatability; (b) competing quality metrics that favor different algorithms [20]; (c) the lack of a gold standard *in vivo*; (d) algorithm performance depending on imaging application (*in vivo* versus phantoms); and (e) the large number of methods for each QSM step, which would render any exhaustive validation effort to be combinatorial and quickly untenable.

We present an experimental setup that allows for an exhaustive quantitative analysis of all four QSM steps. This framework uses a rotating-tube phantom design introduced in the work of Erdevig et al. [24], which uses tubes that rotate, within a background solution, relative to the main magnetic field, B_0. The design enables the analysis of MRI data obtained in objects at any orientation, using common QSM techniques. The closed-form theoretical relationship between the magnetic field and magnetic susceptibility in the sample allows for mapping the magnetic field to magnetic susceptibility without having to solve the dipole inversion problem [25].

Our contributions include (a) a framework for evaluation of repeatability and reproducibility of QSM algorithms and (b) rigorous analysis of common methods in Steps 1 and 2 of the QSM process. We focus on the performance of QSM Steps 1 and 2 for the following reasons:

(a) There exist a large number of methods in each of the four QSM steps. We replicate here approximately 90 different combinations of Steps 1 and 2 methods. If we analyze all four steps simultaneously, the resulting data set would grow combinatorially and become difficult to interpret.

(b) Errors introduced early in the QSM process propagate downstream and have been overlooked in validation studies. For example, Olsson et al. used only one acquisition sequence and one phase estimation algorithm [22].

(c) It is well understood that phase unwrapping, a common algorithm used in Step 2, is a nondeterministic polynomial-time-hard problem (in two dimensions and higher) that often relies on user intervention and careful parameter tuning. Therefore, it is important to isolate the impact of such a problem in the QSM processing methods.

(d) Susceptibility weighted imaging [26, 27], electrical properties tomography [28], thermometry [29], flow [30], and elastography [31] use MR phase information, and this work can inform those applications.

We analyze Steps 1 and 2 of the QSM process to understand which are sufficiently robust to be executable without user intervention and independent of scanner, sequence, and other parameter variations.

2. Methods

We used a rotating-tube phantom (Figure 1(a)) to explore the reproducibility of phase estimates obtained after Steps 1 and 2. MRI data was acquired with different pulse sequences (Step 1), at nine angles, and the performance of a wide variety of phase estimation methods was compared to theory. The rotating-tube phantom was designed to take advantage of the analytical model for a long cylinder at an angle, θ, with respect to B_0. The internal z-axis field offset can be derived from Maxwell's equations and is shown to be [25]

$$\delta B_{\text{in}} = \frac{\Delta\chi B_0}{6}\left(3\cos^2\theta - 1\right), \tag{1}$$

where $\Delta\chi$ is the susceptibility difference between the inside and outside of the cylinder and χ^2 terms are ignored.

2.1. Experimental Setup.

The rotating-tube phantom consists of five cylindrical, polypropylene tubes (80 mm length and 10 mm outer diameter; Nalgene cryogenic storage vials) alternated orthogonally along the central axis of a larger cylinder (610 mm length and 140 mm outer diameter) containing water (Figure 1). Each tube contains one of the following: 0.5 mM $GdCl_3$, 1.0 mM $GdCl_3$, or 3.2 mM $CuSO_4$ (Figure 1(b)). This phantom is modifiable, and the range of susceptibility values can be focused on particular areas of interest. Here, the range of susceptibility values was selected to span those observed *in vivo* from venous blood (1.0 mM $GdCl_3$) to deep grey matter structures (0.5 mM $GdCl_3$) to the lower limits of MRI detection (3.2 mM $CuSO_4$) [32]. A rod extends from the internal rotation gears through the phantom and outside the MRI scanner, allowing the tubes to be manually rotated. Example MR images are shown for the three primary planes (Figure 1(c)) and in a 3D rendering of the tubes (Figure 1(d)). Temperature of the water was continuously monitored via a fiber optic probe (OpSens Medical, Québec, QC, Canada).

The paramagnetic salt solution $\Delta\chi$ values were estimated from susceptibility theory and corrected using Curie's law with the experimentally measured temperatures (21.0°C–22.0°C). $\Delta\chi$ values were 0.336 ppm and 0.168 ppm for the 1 mM $GdCl_3$ and 0.5 mM $GdCl_3$, respectively, and 0.0804 ppm for the 3.2 mM $CuSO_4$. Additional details on the calculation of $\Delta\chi$ are in the Supplementary Material.

2.2. Data Acquisition.

MR data was collected on a 3T Siemens Biograph mMR (MR-PET scanner, Syngo MR E11 software) with a 6-element torso array and 9-element spine array coil for a total of 15 elements. To assess the reproducibility of phase estimation across pulse sequences, we acquired data with four gradient echo (GRE) pulse sequences (details in Table 1):

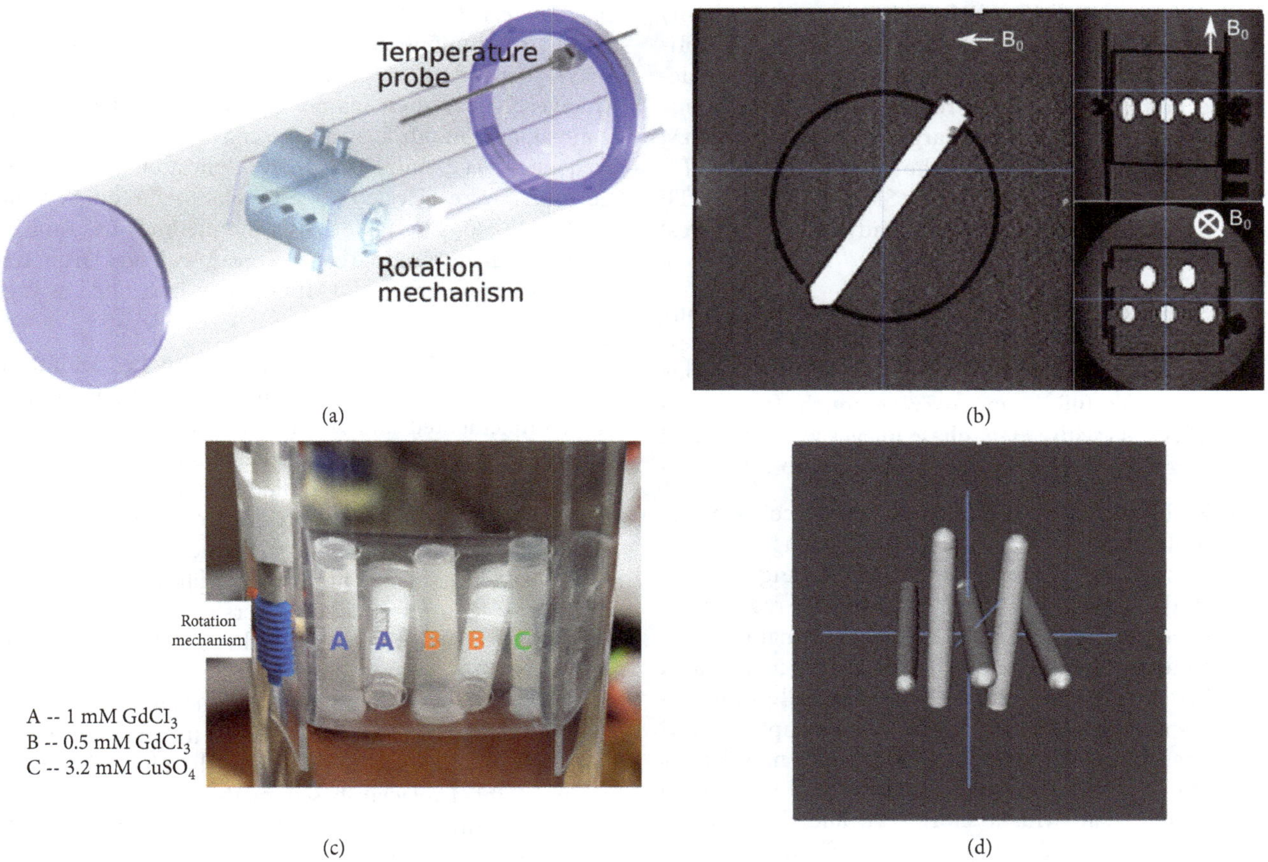

Figure 1: (a) 3D diagram of the rotating-tube phantom design with five smaller cylindrical samples along with temperature probe. (b) Magnitude images of the sagittal (one tube), axial, and coronal (multiple tube) views. (c) A photograph of the 5 tubes. (d) 3D rendering from MRI magnitude images.

Table 1: All data acquisition parameters.

Sequence	Scan ID	TR (ms)	Echo times (ms)	Bandwidth (Hz)	Alpha (deg)	Resolution (mm^3)	Acquisition time (min:s)
Single-echo GRE (SEGE)	1	25	16	80	15	1.0 × 1.0 × 2.0	1:59
	2	35	25.7	80	15	0.5 × 0.5 × 2.0	4:35
	3	45	30	80	15	1.0 × 1.0 × 2.0	3:35
Multiecho GRE (MEGE)	1	25	2.5, 6.2, 9.9, 13.6, 17.3, 21.0	500	15	1.0 × 1.0 × 2.0	1:59
	2	35	3, 7.8, 12.6, 17.4, 22.2, 27.0	530	15	0.5 × 0.5 × 2.0	4:35
	3	45	2.5, 6.2, 9.9, 13.6, 17.3, 21.0, 24.7, 28.4, 32.1, 35.7, 39.5	500	15	1.0 × 1.0 × 2.0	3:35
sEPI	1	72	27, ETL = 15	430	20	1.0 × 1.0 × 2.0	0:31
	2	72	27, ETL = 15	430	20	0.5 × 0.5 × 2.0	0:52
MAGPI	1	25	4.1, 8.9, 12.6, 16.3, 20.0	190	15	1.0 × 1.0 × 2.0	1:59
	2	35	7.6, 13.0, 17.3, 21.5, 25.7, 30.0	250	15	0.5 × 0.5 × 2.0	4:35
	3	45	6.6, 13.0, 18.5, 23.8, 29.0, 34.2, 39.4	200	15	1.0 × 1.0 × 2.0	3:35

(i) Single-echo GRE (SEGE): This is a commonly chosen protocol with QSM and other susceptibility-based techniques [33], wherein a single-echo time TE is measured as close to T_2^* of tissue of interest (here, the target is 60 ms for 1 mM $GdCl_3$). This maximizes the phase SNR at this T_2^*. To maximize the magnitude SNR at the chosen TE and TR, we set the readout bandwidth at its lowest possible value.

(ii) Segmented Echo Planar Imaging (sEPI): A recently proposed sEPI sequence was shown to possess similar quality phase images as SEGE [34], while acquiring full brain coverage much faster than SEGE. As with SEGE, phase images were generated at a single TE at the center of the echo train.

(iii) Multiecho GRE (MEGE): This protocol acquires multiple TEs in a single TR. The challenge with this technique is the choice of the echo spacing ΔTE and readout bandwidth BW. A short ΔTE reduces the likelihood of aliasing in the phase domain but introduces noise. A long ΔTE yields phase images with better SNR but suffers from potentially unrecoverable phase-aliasing errors. For example, to unwrap frequency offsets of ±150 Hz, ΔTE must be less than 3.33 ms. A common approach [33, 35] is to acquire data with a short ΔTE and, in order to recover SNR efficiency similar to SEGE sequences [36], acquire as many echoes as possible in a TR. However, due to hardware limitations, the readout bandwidth, BW, places a lower limit on ΔTE. We aimed to select the shortest ΔTE possible at the highest BW attainable with the MR system. This choice minimizes the likelihood of phase wrap errors, which may not be recoverable by all phase unwrapping algorithms. We elaborate on this choice further in the Discussion section.

(iv) MAGPI: This is an MEGE sequence that uses preoptimized echo times and bandwidths selection that, when paired with a corresponding phase estimation algorithm, yields maximum-likelihood optimal phase estimates in the presence of wrapping, noise, and phase-offset errors [37, 38].

All sequences were 3D excitations of a 128 mm × 128 mm × 128 mm slab (64 slices) with sagittal slab-selection and phase encode along the B_0 direction. We used anisotropic voxels to boost SNR, a common practice for QSM and Susceptibility-Weighted Imaging [26, 27, 39]. MAGPI and the sEPI sequences used alternating gradient polarity, while the other sequences did not. Autoshimming was completed prior to the first data acquisition, and then the same shim parameters were used over time, over all sequences and methods.

We assessed the effect of in-plane resolution and TR on phase estimate reproducibility with each protocol (Table 1). We also examined the reproducibility of phase estimates across nine different angles by advancing the apparatus approximately 18 degrees per turn.

2.3. Phase Estimation. Images generated in Steps 2–3 of QSM are commonly referred to as frequency, phase, or field maps, depending on the units of the data. We interchangeably use these names in this work depending on context, and, in our analysis, we convert all phase images to frequency via a simple scalar multiplication. Ten phase algorithms were selected to estimate the frequency offset image [37, 40–47]. Table 2 lists the methods used for each pulse sequence; multiple codes were downloaded from freely available resources (e.g., MEDI) and integrated with the pipeline.

All phase estimation methods were applied with default parameters in 3D over the entire acquisition volume and were implemented and run blinded to the theoretical solution. Apart from the MAGPI algorithm, which operates on raw k-space channel-uncombined data, all methods (including MAGPI-unopt) operated on unprocessed phase data obtained using the vendor-provided adaptive-coil-combine method. While this is "unprocessed phase data," different vendors may apply different filters, phase corrections, or other adjustments that could influence the phase quality. Here, adaptive-coil-combine describes the algorithm used by this vendor to combine multichannel coil data [48]. Each unwrapping method used the SNR in the magnitude image to guide unwrapping orientation in the phase domain: for example, the Laplacian-based methods used this SNR to mask the entire image, while others (region-growing, GBC) masked the phase values in regions with poor SNR. SNR was measured as approximately 30 dB in water, similar to *in vivo* values ranging from 25 to 30 dB.

For MEGE sequences, the multiecho data is processed using the five following categories of algorithms:

(1) Spatial phase unwrapping at each echo, followed by temporal combination of the resulting images using a weighted averaging method, that is, phase SNR-optimal [49].

(2) Spatial phase unwrapping at each echo with weighted averaging (as in 1), but a 1D phase unwrapping step is used just before weighted averaging. This is meant to correct any remaining aliasing that spatial unwrapping failed to correct.

(3) Direct temporal phase estimation (Slope, Division) applied in complex domain. These methods correctly unwrap the phase over time, provided the inherent frequency is less than the Nyquist frequency associated with the echo spacing.

(4) Temporal phase combination (as in 3), followed by 3D spatial phase unwrapping to correct errors encountered with temporal phase estimation.

(5) Maximum-likelihood-based combination of multi-echo and multichannel data (MAGPI) [37]. This method solves the phase estimation problem on a voxel-by-voxel basis, without resorting to spatial averaging techniques.

All phase images are eventually converted to frequency offset (Hz) by dividing by $2\pi\ x$ phase evolution time.

TABLE 2: All phase estimation methods. The first six methods were combined with other common phase processing techniques to process the multiecho data, as described in the Methods section.

Sequence	Method	Summary
SEGE, MEGE, sEPI	Unprocessed	Default channel combined output phase image produced by the scanner
	Phun	Region-based algorithm [46]
	GBC	Goldstein's branch cut method [42]
	MEDI.RG	Region growing algorithm from MEDI Toolbox [45, 47]
	MEDI.LP	Laplacian algorithm from MEDI Toolbox [44, 45]
	Laplace	Laplacian algorithm [40]
MEGE	Slope	Computes the frequency offset from the slope of the complex data across echoes [41]
	Division	Computes the frequency offset from the complex division of the data at successive echoes [43]
	MAGPI-unopt	Applies the MAGPI postprocessing algorithm using a random (unoptimized) subset of echoes from the MEGE sequence. Since MAGPI requires uneven echo spacing, only four unequally spaced echoes were selected [37]
MAGPI	MAGPI	Maximum-likelihood estimate of phase from optimal echo spacing [37]

2.4. Adjusting for Field due to Rotation of Apparatus. To accurately estimate $\Delta\chi$ from the phase images, we need to remove the global field effects resulting from the tubes rotating in the magnetic field, as well as field effects from the apparatus itself. We call this process "frequency referencing" (FR).

The scalar magnitude of the complete field inside a voxel can be written as follows:

$$\delta B(r,\theta) = \delta B_{\Delta\chi}(r,\theta) + \delta B_0(r,\theta), \quad (2)$$

where r is the spatial coordinate of the voxel and θ is the rotation angle of the tube relative to B, $\delta B_{\Delta\chi}(r,\theta)$ is the field caused by magnetic susceptibility variations (such as the one due to a homogeneous cylindrical object immersed in a homogeneous sphere), and $\delta B_0(r,\theta)$ is an unknown field offset component. We separate $\delta B_0(r,\theta)$ into a component that varies only spatially and a component that varies only with the rotation of the apparatus:

$$\delta B_0(r,\theta) = \delta B_0^{bkg}(r) + \delta B_0^{rot}(\theta). \quad (3)$$

At a given angle of rotation, sources of spatially varying global offsets $\delta B_0^{bkg}(r)$ are field inhomogeneity (imperfections of magnetic field/coils), bulk magnetic susceptibility of the apparatus [50, 51], and coil phase offset [52]. As the apparatus is rotated, in the absence of "shimming" at the console, the center frequency will be shifted due to the bulk magnetic susceptibility of the entire apparatus [53, 54]. Our goal is to extract $\Delta\chi$ by fitting $\delta B(r,\theta)$ to the angle of rotation θ, inside the tube. $\delta B_0^{bkg}(r)$ is a nuisance parameter that can be easily accounted for during the fitting process by allowing for a constant shift to the cosine.

First, we compute an estimate of $\delta B_0^{rot}(\theta)$ using the average frequency in a static region outside the "Tube + - Sphere" system (Figure2(a)). The average (indicated by < >) is taken over pixels in a region r_{out} distant from local susceptibility effects:

$$\langle \delta B(r,\theta)\rangle_{r\in r_{out}} = \langle \delta B_0^{bkg}(r)\rangle_{r\in r_{out}} + \delta B_0^{rot}(\theta) = C_{r_{out}} + \delta B_0^{rot}(\theta), \quad (4)$$

where we define $C_{r_{out}}$ to be a variable that is only a function of the referencing region. Then, the referencing step consists of

$$\delta B_{ref}(r,\theta) \equiv \delta B(r,\theta) - \langle \delta B(r,\theta)\rangle_{r\in r_{out}} = \delta B_{\Delta\chi}(r,\theta) + \left(\delta B_0^{bkg}(r) - C_{r_{out}}\right), \quad (5)$$

thus removing $\delta B_0^{rot}(\theta)$. Our goal is to use the referenced field, $\delta B_{ref}(r,\theta)$, at every pixel in the tube center, $r = r_{in}$, to fit the field variation to the angle of rotation θ. The only component that varies with θ is the first term on right side of equation (5). The estimation step is a simple fit with respect to θ, along with an arbitrary shift for the constant: $c = \delta B_0^{bkg}(r) - C_{r_{out}}$. For the case of a cylinder (equation (1)), the estimate can be obtained by solving

$$\left(\widehat{\Delta\chi}(r_{in}), c^*\right) = \arg\min_{\Delta\chi,c} \left\| \widehat{\delta B}_{ref}(r_{in},\theta) - \left(\frac{\Delta\chi}{6}\left(3\cos^2\theta - 1\right)B_0 + c\right)\right\|_2. \quad (6)$$

Fitting c effectively amounts to shifting the midline of the data to match the model (across all angles). We used a bisquare-weighting method to fit this midline. We include a few examples of $\widehat{\Delta\chi}$ estimation using equation (6) in Table S.1.

We apply this frequency referencing method after each phase estimation algorithm. To investigate repeatability with respect to the location of frequency reference estimate, we apply this process in 13 different regions selected across static areas of the phantom (Figure 2(a)).

2.5. Error Analysis. We use the theoretically determined values of $\Delta\chi$ to predict the field values at each angle that would have been measured with ideal methods in Steps 1 and 2. We then compute the error (Hz) between measured frequency $\widehat{\delta B}_{ref}(r_{in},\theta)$ and expected frequency offset:

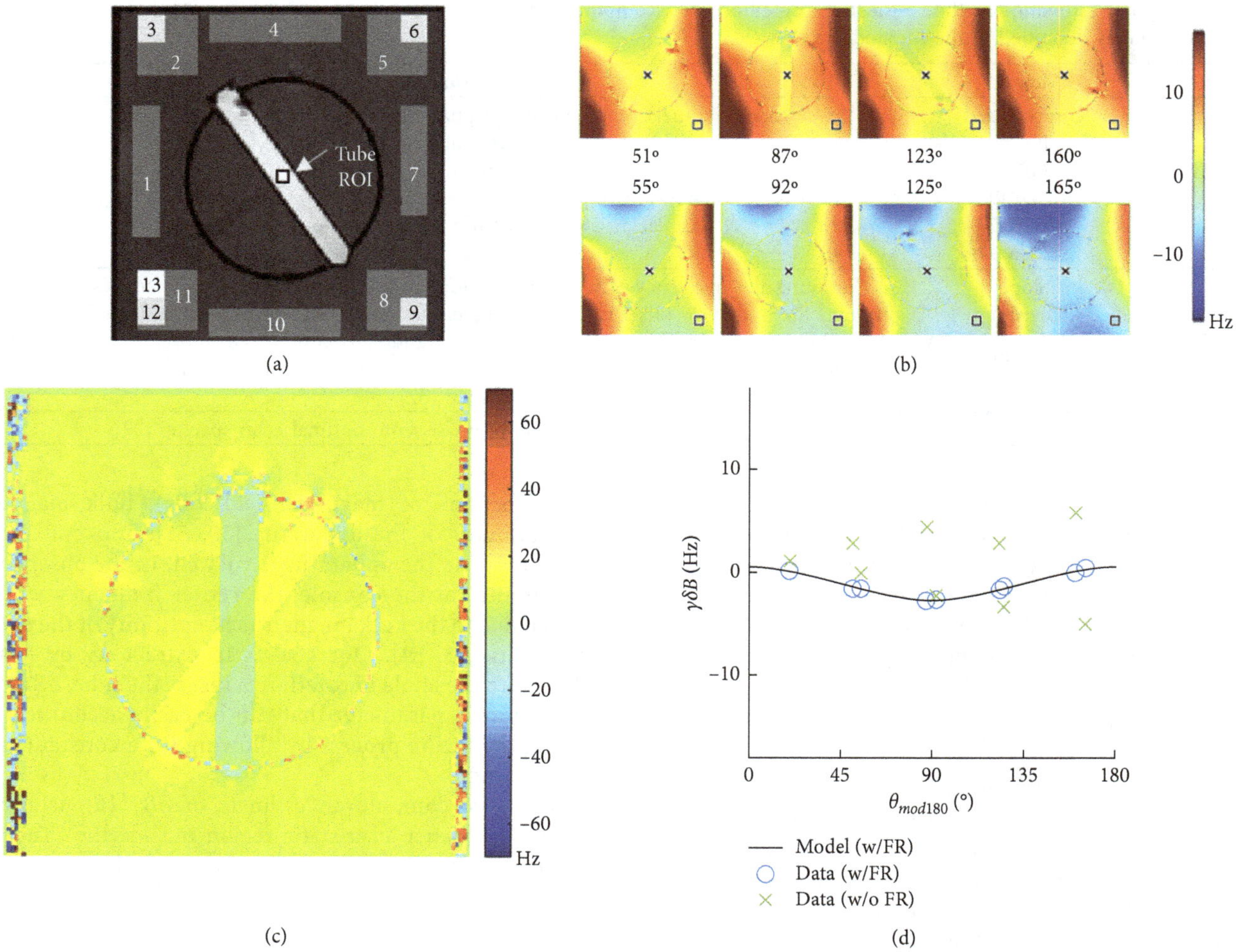

FIGURE 2: (a) An example magnitude GRE image showing both the tube ROI (small black box in center) used for the analysis and the placement of the 13 background ROIs. (b) Example frequency images in tube 3 (0.5 mM GdCl3) obtained with the single GRE sequence (1 mm, TR 45 ms) and reconstructed with MEDI.RG phase estimation method. (c) Also using SEGE + MEDI.RG, the field difference between two angles ($\delta\mathbf{B}_{\mathbf{total}}(\mathbf{r}, \theta_2) - \delta\mathbf{B}_{\mathbf{total}}(\mathbf{r}, \theta_1)$) showing that this difference is attributable to the spatially invariant component (in homogeneous areas) and a spatially variant component (in areas close to material boundaries). The spatially invariant component of the field difference is removed with frequency referencing (FR). (d) A plot of the frequency against the angle of rotation (modulo 180°) is shown for each of the data without frequency referencing (in green (x), data after frequency referencing using the frequency reference ROI #9 (blue circles), and the model's prediction of the frequency (solid red line).

$$\varepsilon(r_{\text{in}}, \theta) = \widehat{\delta B}_{\text{ref}}(r_{\text{in}}, \theta) - \left(\frac{\Delta\chi_{\text{true}}}{6}\left(3\cos^2\theta - 1\right)B_0 + c^*\right), \tag{7}$$

where $c^*$is obtained by solving equation (6) with $\Delta\chi$ set to $\Delta\chi_{\text{true}}$.

To account for any dependence on tube content, we compute the absolute relative error:

$$\epsilon_{\mathbf{r}}(\mathbf{r}_{\mathbf{in}}, \boldsymbol{\theta}) = \frac{|\epsilon(\mathbf{r}_{\mathbf{in}}, \boldsymbol{\theta})|}{\mathbf{B}_0\Delta\boldsymbol{\chi}}, \tag{8}$$

where the absolute value is used instead of the signed error due to the irrelevance of sign in this context.

Error statistics were computed for each voxel in the tube ROI (mean tube ROI sizes were 17 pixels at 1 mm resolution and 57 pixels at 0.5 mm resolution), for each slice (2 slices per tube), each tube (5 total), each angle (9 total rotations), using each applicable phase estimation method (from a possible 10), each background phase removal ROI (13 total), and each sequence with its respective resolution and TR variations (11 total). Cumulatively, 2.36 million frequency values were analyzed in this experiment.

The large number of data points allows us to extract statistics about ε and ε_r including their probability mass function, $\Pr(\varepsilon)$ and $\Pr(\varepsilon_r)$. The probability of ε can exhibit a multimodal distribution and therefore is not a Gaussian. While we can report the absolute bias and standard deviations from such a distribution, it would not be descriptive of $\Pr(\varepsilon)$. A more practical measure is the likelihood of observing absolute relative errors less than or equal to a threshold, τ. This is obtained by integrating $\Pr(\varepsilon_r)$ between 0 and τ a measure known as the Cumulative Distribution Function (CDF),

$$F_{\varepsilon_r}(\tau) = \Pr(\varepsilon_r \le \tau). \quad (9)$$

The CDF can be used to capture phase errors that are dominated by outliers, as well as phase errors that result from generally poor/unreliable model fitting. The ideal CDF is a step function, and any presence of outliers/large errors yields a CDF with slow convergence to 1. The frequency of large errors is seen from the magnitude of the deviation of the CDF from 1.0 at any given threshold.

3. Results

Figure 2(a) shows a magnitude GRE image of tube 3 (0.5 mM $GdCl_3$) in one orientation. Figure 2(b) shows frequency offset images corresponding to different rotations. Figure 2(c) shows a typical field difference between two angles ($\delta B(r,\theta_2) - \delta B(r,\theta_1)$). According to equation (3), this difference is equal to $\delta B_{\Delta\chi}(r,\theta_2) - \delta B_{\Delta\chi}(r,\theta_1) + \delta B_0^{rot}(\theta_2) - \delta B_0^{rot}(\theta_1)$, predicting spatial variations only in locations close to areas with susceptibility changes and a constant field in homogeneous locations. This is precisely what we observe in Figure 2(c). Figure 2(d) shows a plot of the frequency values for a voxel inside the tube prior to frequency referencing (symbol "x"). The resulting plot does not follow the expected sinusoid (solid line). After applying the frequency referencing step, we observe the expected sinusoidal shape (symbol "o").

Figure 3 shows the resulting histogram of frequency errors and resulting CDF. From Figures 3(a) and 3(b), we note the probability of ε for this example exhibits a multimodal distribution. We can see from the CDF in Figure 3(c) that the probability of observing errors less than 10% ($F_{\varepsilon_r}(0.1)$) is about 66%.

Table 3 summarizes the error statistics for all combination of sequences and algorithms. The first column lists the sequence type, and the second and third columns indicate the name and category of each postprocessing algorithm, respectively. We report the mean and standard deviations of both ε and ε_r. We also report $F_{\varepsilon_r}(0.1)$ pooled over all background ROIs, as well as the range (minimum, $F_{\varepsilon_{rW}}(0.1)$, and maximum, $F_{\varepsilon_{rB}}(0.1)$) of $F_{\varepsilon_r}(0.1)$ encountered in those ROIs. These quantities are computed from data that includes all tubes and angles. A representative subset of these results is selected for more detailed analysis and illustration in Figures 4–6.

Figure 4 shows a subset of frequency-offset images for different sequence + algorithm pairs, at 3 of the 9 angles of rotation. This figure illustrates typical challenges with phase estimation methods. For example, in Figure 4(a), we observe phase unwrapping errors in SEGE + GBC, with abrupt jumps across contiguous regions. The corresponding frequency versus angle plot (last column in Figure 4(a)) shows that incorrect frequency referencing in these areas (square in figure) yields occasional mismatch between measurement and predictions at certain angles. SEGE + Laplace demonstrates a smoothly varying frequency map across the FOV; however, the resulting data deviates from the expected theoretical values at almost every angle (Figure 4(b)). MEGE + Slope, a direct temporal phase estimation method (MEGE category 3), exhibits phase wrapping errors when the underlying frequency value is larger than the bandwidth allowable by ΔTE(Figure 4(c)). Placing a frequency referencing ROI in these areas yields incorrect values at the respective angles. Note that the example frequency reference ROI (#9 in Figure 2) is meant to highlight the phase errors or artifacts observed. Figures 4(d) and 4(e) show that the results from MAGPI-unopt and MAGPI are consistent with those predicted from theory.

The CDF of ε_r collects the errors, such as those observed in Figure 4, over a variety of acquisition and processing parameters. Figure 5 shows $F_{\varepsilon_r}(\tau)$ for all algorithms when ε_r is pooled over all voxels, background ROIs, slices, tubes, and sequence variations. This represents an overall summary of algorithm behavior, irrespective of which parameter was used in acquisition and postprocessing. We see that MAGPI attains a nearly ideal CDF, with 0.91 probability of relative errors, ε_r, less than 0.1 ($F_{\varepsilon_r}(0.1) = 0.91$) and rapidly converges to 1 (Figure 5). MAGPI and MAGPI-unopt achieve similar CDFs, with MAGPI performing slightly better, as expected. MEDI.RG and GBC phase unwrapping methods, both based on region growing, have similar CDFs, with $F_{\varepsilon_r}(0.1) = 0.69$ and $F_{\varepsilon_r}(0.1) = 0.70$, respectively. The unprocessed phase images have the most artifacts and, thus, the lowest CDF across all ε_r. Figure 5 focuses on the CDF for ε_r in [0, 1.0] to highlight the different convergence pattern (distribution/frequency of errors) in that domain. The CDF extends beyond $\varepsilon_r = 1.0$ for any occurrence of relative errors greater than 100%.

Next, we explore the behavior of $F_{\varepsilon_r}(\tau)$ as a function of data acquisition strategy. In Figures 6(a)–6(c), we group results by three sequence types: SEGE, sEPI, and MEGE. Since MAGPI is a multiecho sequence, we include MAGPI in the MEGE category. For each CDF curve $F_{\varepsilon_r}(\tau)$, ε_r is pooled across all pixels, background ROIs, slices, tubes, and variations of TR and resolution within that sequence type. We also explore variability of $F_{\varepsilon_r}(\tau)$ with the frequency referencing method. For each sequence, we show CDFs in the ROI with the maximum $F_{\varepsilon_r}(\tau = 0.1)$ ($F_{\varepsilon_{rB}}$, Figures 6(d)–6(f)) and the ROI with the minimum $F_{\varepsilon_r}(\tau = 0.1)$ ($F_{\varepsilon_{rW}}$, Figures 6(g)–6(i)) for a given data set. The separation between $F_{\varepsilon_{rB}}$ and $F_{\varepsilon_{rW}}$ demonstrates the robustness (or lack thereof) of a method to frequency reference ROI selection.

Table 4 shows the dependence of the CDF on scan variability and tube contents. Because the performance of some methods is dominated by frequency reference ROI (seen in Table 3 and Figure 6), Table 4 shows results for the largest $\mathbf{F}_{\varepsilon_r}(10\%)$ for a given sequence + method pair observed over all frequency reference ROIs, for every method, sequence, scan variation, tube, and slice.

4. Discussion

A reliable pulse sequence protocol, with repeatable and reproducible phase estimation, is a necessary step to develop robust QSM methods for clinical use. Previous work examined the reproducibility of certain QSM methods using phantoms [22, 25, 55], simulation [22, 25, 56], and human subjects [19, 56]. We used a rotating-tube phantom to

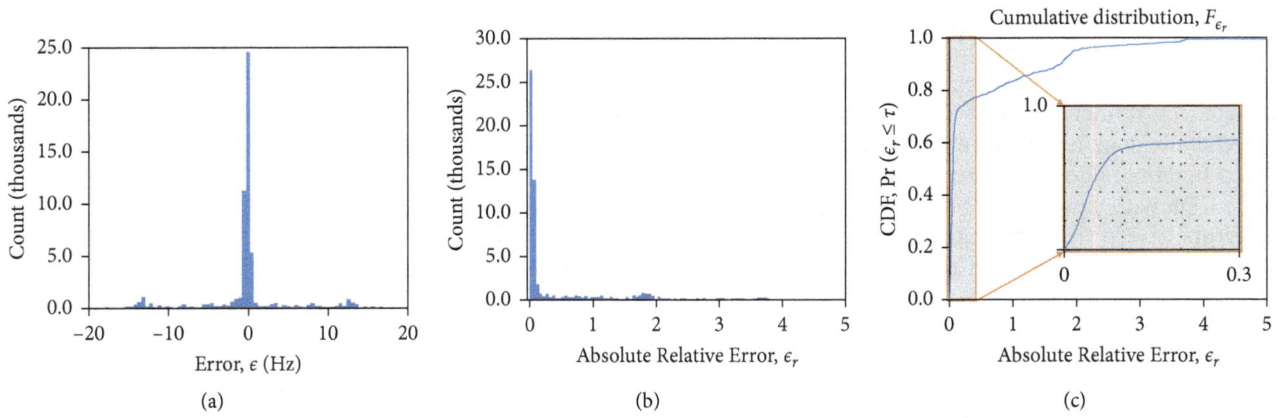

FIGURE 3: (a) The histogram of the error ε (in Hz) when the measurement is obtained with the SEGE + GBC phase estimation method. The error data is pooled over all ROI voxels, all backgrounds, rotations, and tubes. (b) The histogram of the absolute relative error ε_r seen with the same measurement. (c) The corresponding Cumulative Distribution Function $\mathbf{F}_{\epsilon_r}$ of the error in (b). The inset figure shows a portion of this CDF within [0, 0.3] to better illustrate the distributions within reasonable error range. In this case, the CDF shows that the probability of obtaining ε_r less than 0.1 is around 0.66 with the SEGE + GBC pair. The maximum observed ϵ was 27.0 Hz, and the maximum observed ε_r was 6.85, illustrating the occasional large errors that may result with SEGE + GBC.

TABLE 3: Error statistics for each of the estimation methods and acquisition protocols. The mean and standard deviation of error measurements ε (Hz), as well as the absolute relative errors ε_r, are provided in columns 4–7. Columns 8-9 show $F_{\epsilon_r}(0.1)$ of the overall data, as well as the range (min and max) of $F_{\epsilon_r}(0.1)$ across reference backgrounds.

Protocol	Postprocessing	Method	μ_ϵ(Hz)	σ_ϵ (Hz)	μ_{ϵ_r}	σ_{ϵ_r}	$\mathbf{F}_{\epsilon_r}(0.1)$	$[\mathbf{F}_{\epsilon_{rW}}(0.1), \mathbf{F}_{\epsilon_{rB}}(0.1)]$
SEGE	Spatial 3D unwrap	Unprocessed	0.29	3.85	0.52	0.92	0.48	[0.24, 0.76]
		Phun	0.21	5.12	0.35	1.38	0.67	[0.49, 0.89]
		GBC	−0.22	4.83	0.53	1.08	0.66	[0.47, 0.82]
		MEDI.RG	−0.19	1.60	0.08	0.22	0.90	[0.84, 0.96]
		MEDI.LP	−0.01	1.07	0.14	0.12	0.50	[0.38, 0.62]
		Laplace	0.00	1.01	0.14	0.15	0.54	[0.40, 0.66]
sEPI	Spatial 3D unwrap	Unprocessed	−0.34	4.19	0.58	0.76	0.43	[0.32, 0.52]
		Phun	−0.10	5.23	0.73	1.30	0.45	[0.31, 0.56]
		GBC	−0.32	3.80	0.42	0.97	0.66	[0.31, 0.91]
		MEDI.RG	1.03	4.14	0.32	1.15	0.85	[0.79, 0.91]
		MEDI.LP	0.00	1.14	0.12	0.12	0.57	[0.51, 0.65]
		Laplace	0.00	0.95	0.12	0.11	0.58	[0.47, 0.68]
Multiecho	1. Spatial 3D unwrap ⟶ temporal average	(i) Unprocessed	0.01	2.60	0.48	0.41	0.16	[0.08, 0.23]
		(ii) Phun	0.39	4.75	0.30	1.23	0.57	[0.48, 0.69]
		(iii) GBC	0.31	2.21	0.15	0.36	0.78	[0.59, 0.91]
		(iv) MEDI.RG	−0.37	3.47	0.66	0.95	0.35	[0.09, 0.63]
		(v) MEDI.LP	−0.01	0.89	0.11	0.09	0.58	[0.49, 0.67]
		(vi) Laplace	0.00	0.82	0.12	0.12	0.58	[0.44, 0.68]
	2. Spatial 3D unwrap ⟶ temporal 1D unwrap ⟶ temporal average	(i) Phun	0.19	7.66	0.94	2.23	0.55	[0.12, 0.96]
		(ii) GBC	0.20	7.78	0.96	2.25	0.55	[0.12, 0.96]
		(iii) MEDI.RG	0.13	7.95	0.97	2.29	0.55	[0.12, 0.96]
		(iv) MEDI.LP	−0.01	0.89	0.11	0.09	0.58	[0.49, 0.67]
		(v) Laplace	0.00	0.82	0.12	0.13	0.58	[0.45, 0.68]
	3. Temporal estimation	(i) Slope	0.26	9.28	1.15	2.79	0.55	[0.13, 0.96]
		(ii) Division	0.26	9.27	1.15	2.78	0.55	[0.13, 0.95]
	4. Temporal estimation ⟶ spatial 3D unwrap	(i) Phun	0.04	11.04	1.17	3.02	0.53	[0.06, 0.95]
		(ii) GBC	0.17	9.18	1.10	2.69	0.54	[0.09, 0.95]
		(iii) MEDI.RG	0.47	62.07	10.11	16.54	0.21	[0.00, 0.76]
		(iv) MEDI.LP	0.16	3.87	0.54	1.16	0.43	[0.20, 0.70]
		(v) Laplace	0.22	6.89	0.89	2.05	0.36	[0.10, 0.66]
	5. MAGPI	(i) MAGPI unopt	0.00	0.30	0.05	0.05	0.90	[0.78, 0.97]
		(ii) MAGPI	0.00	0.27	0.05	0.04	0.91	[0.84, 0.98]

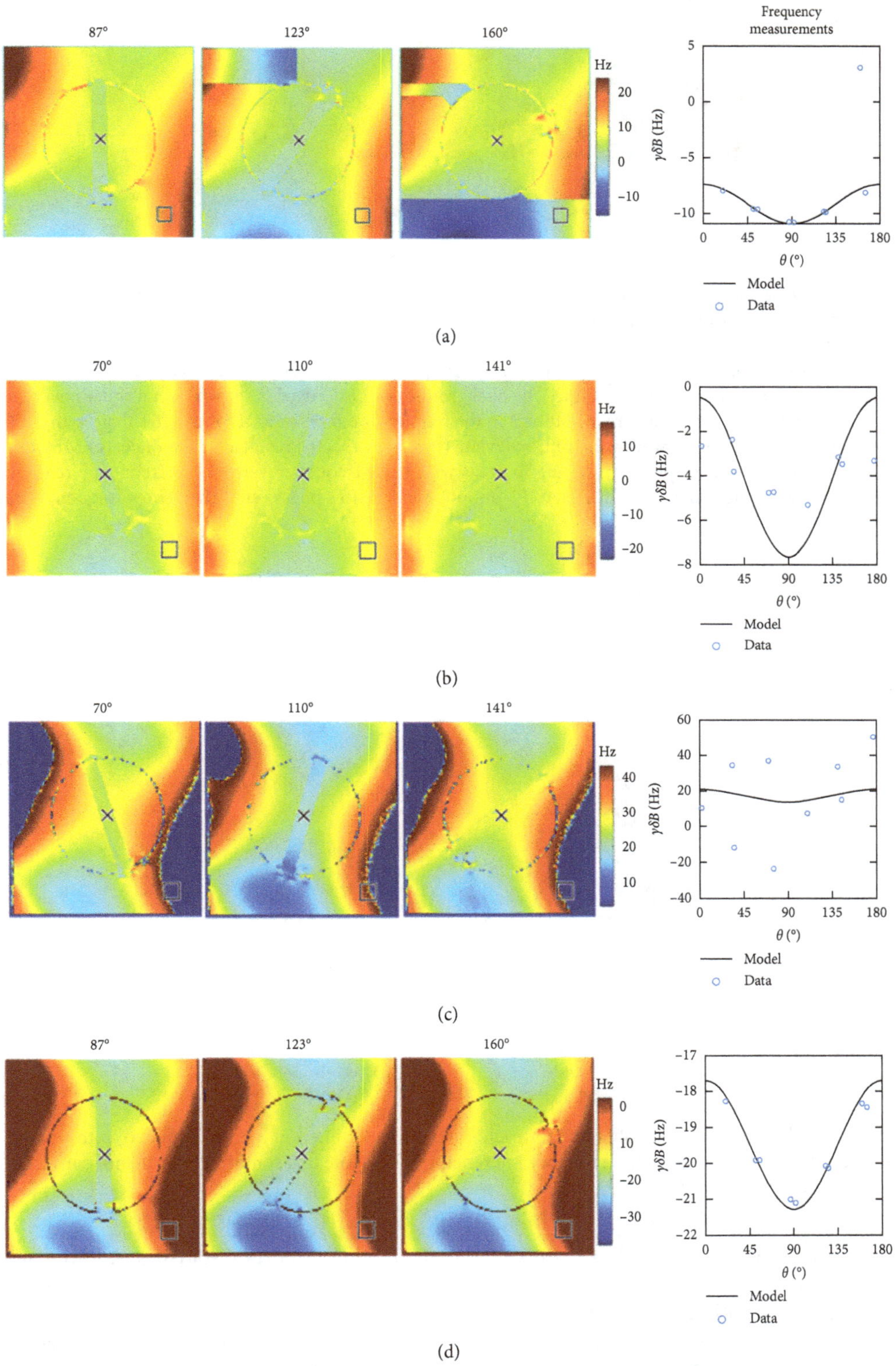

Figure 4: Continued.

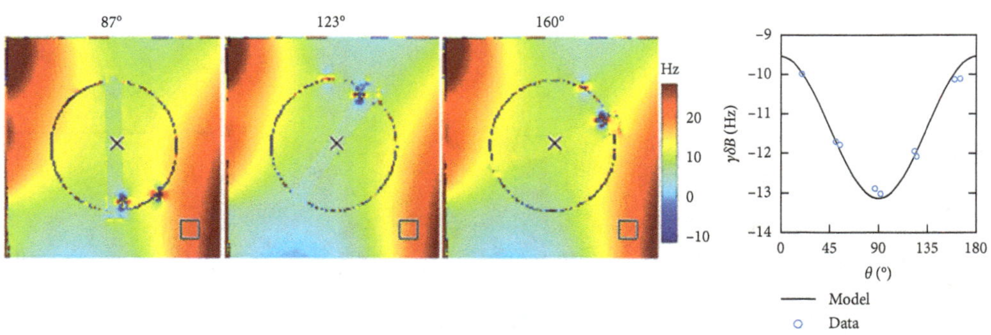

(e)

FIGURE 4: Each row in this figure shows five different examples of sequence (at 1 mm resolution, TR = 45 ms) and phase estimation method pairs for three different angles of rotation in different tubes. These examples were selected to illustrate the spatial nature of different phase estimations errors and artifacts. The corresponding plots in the last column show the resulting frequency measurements as a function of angle of rotation (modulo 180°), for a voxel inside the tube, after frequency referencing (blue circle). The predicted frequency offset as obtained from equation (1) is also shown in solid red line. The background ROI (#9) used is shown with a square overlaid on the frequency maps. (a) SEGE + GBC shows a phase wrapping error in tube 3 in the frequency reference ROI for the 160-degree angle. (b) SEGE + Laplace shows smoothly varying frequency maps; however, the values deviate from the expected result at every angle. (c) MEGE + Slope, without 3D phase unwrapping, shows the presence of phase wrapping in areas with large frequency values. The frequency reference ROI is within a phase wrapped region across all angles. (d, e) MEGE + MAGPI-unopt and MAGPI's phase estimation show frequency maps consistent with values predicted from the model.

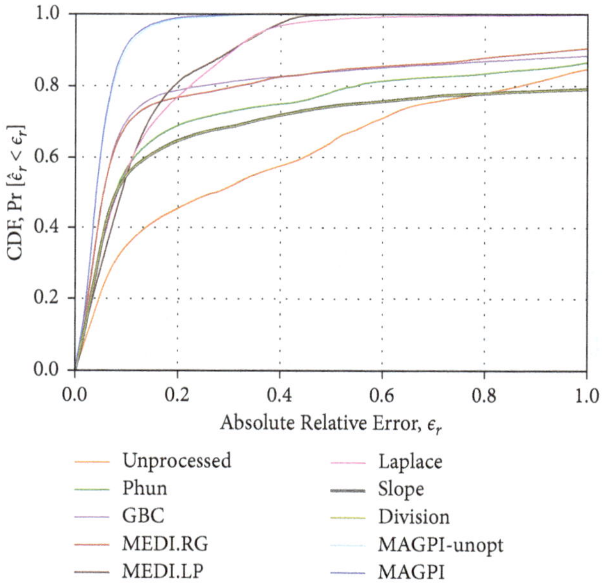

FIGURE 5: CDF $\mathbf{F}_{\epsilon_r}$ of the absolute relative error obtained for each of the phase estimation methods studied in this work, when the error is pooled over all sequences, slices, tubes, angles, and frequency referencing ROIs. Note that some methods do not converge to probability of 1, due to the presence of errors greater than 100%.

quantitatively evaluate methods used for data acquisition and phase estimation. This is not the first study using long tubes nor is it the first to position tubes relative to B_0; however, compared to previous work [22, 24, 25, 55, 57–59], more acquisition and phase estimation methods were considered. Specifically, we used ~90 different combinations of pulse sequences and phase estimation methods to analyze millions of measurements from different ROIs, tube contents, rotations, and sequence parameters. This vast amount of data ultimately allowed us to estimate the probability distribution of phase error with every QSM method, along with other important statistics. Additional phase estimation methods could be retrospectively used on the data set, which we aim to make publicly available.

Our results showed varying degrees of accuracy and precision over all tested methods. For example, while the majority of methods resulted in μ_ϵ less than 1 Hz (note the particularly small μ_ϵ with MEDI.LP, Laplace, MEGE + MAGPI-unopt, and MAGPI), the only methods with μ_{ϵ_r} <10% are SEGE + MEDI.RG (7.6%), MEGE + MAGPI-unopt (5.3%), and MAGPI (5.0%). We observed a similar trend with precision, whereby methods

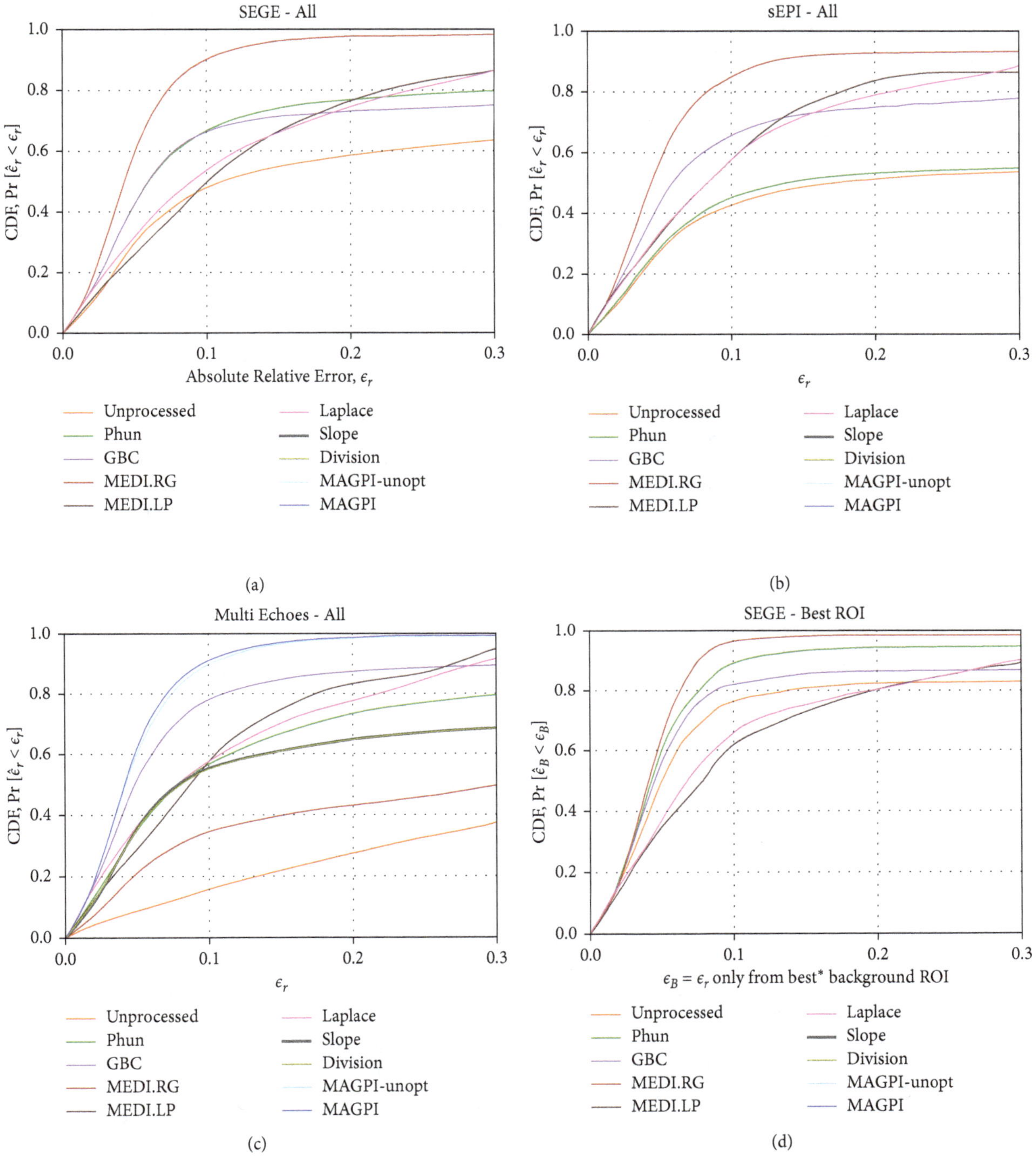

Figure 6: Continued.

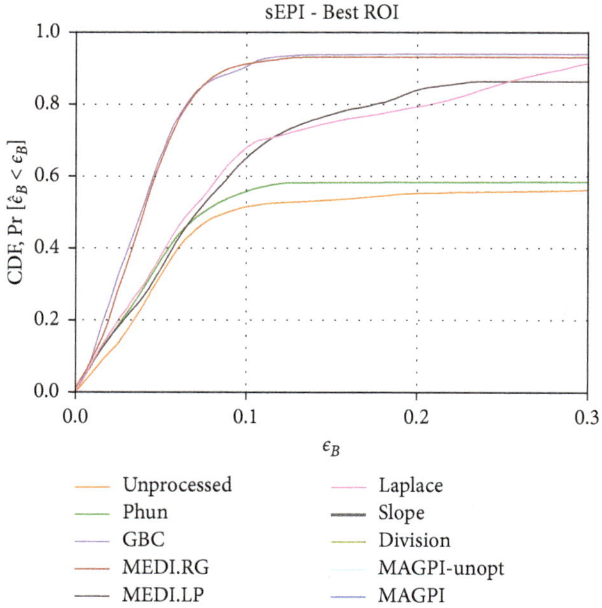

(e)

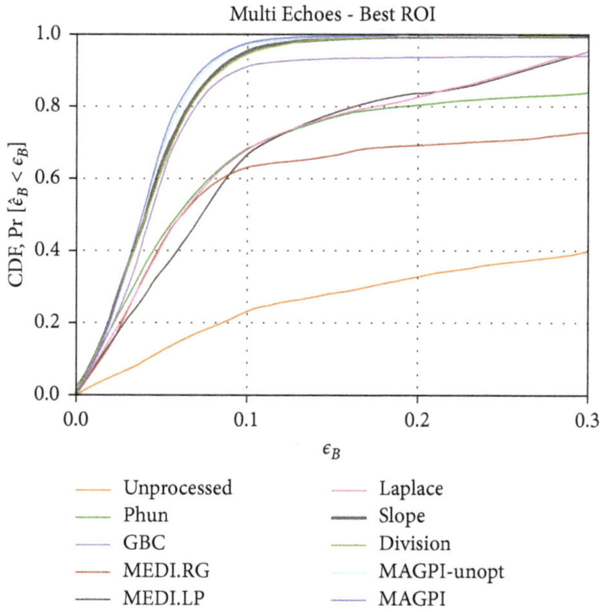

(f)

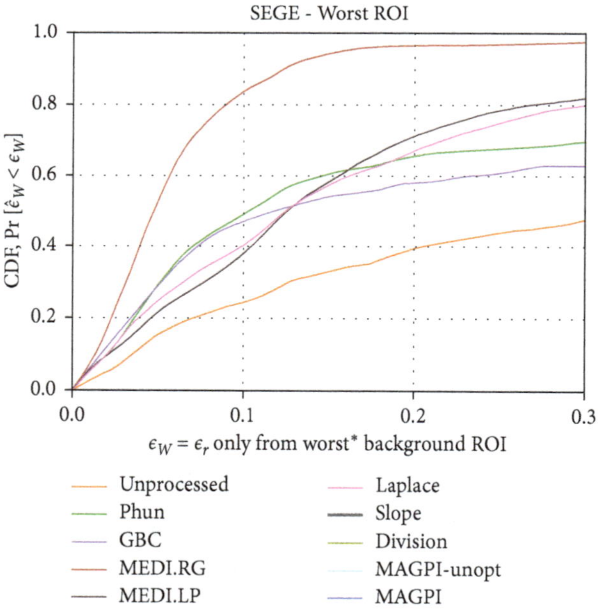

(g)

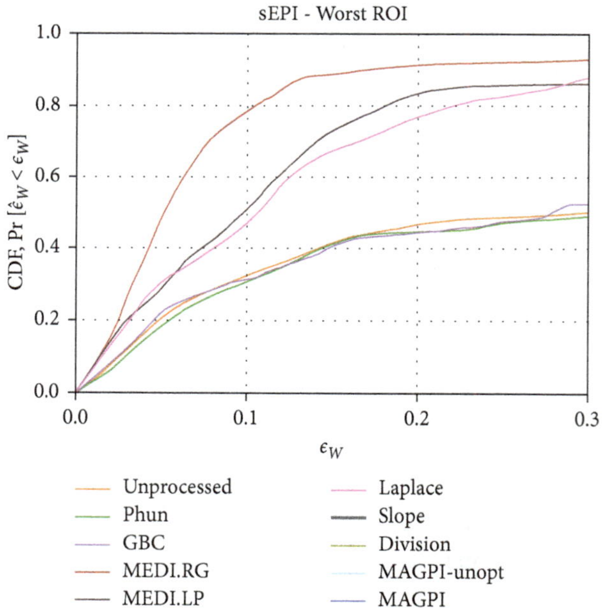

(h)

Figure 6: Continued.

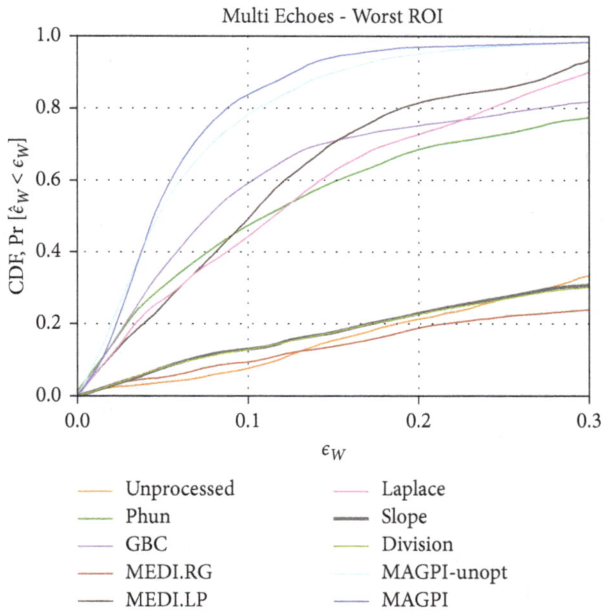

(i)

FIGURE 6: The CDFs for each acquisition and phase estimation method pair. Each column corresponds to a different type of acquisition: single-echo acquisitions (SEGE) are shown in the first column, accelerated acquisitions with sEPI in the second, and multiecho acquisitions (MEGE and MAGPI) in the third. The first row (a–c) shows the CDF when all the error data is pooled, over all voxels, slices, tubes, and background ROIs. Given the large variability in performance for different background ROIs, we show in the second (d–f) and third (g–i) rows the CDFs obtained in the ROIs with the maximum and minimum $\mathbf{F}_{\epsilon_r}(0.1)$, respectively. A highly reproducible method will have a similar curve shape across all plots.

TABLE 4: Probability of relative errors <0.1 in the background ROI that maximizes $\mathbf{F}_{\epsilon_r}(0.1)$ across sequences, scan variability (ID is as listed in Table 1), and phantom tube components. The tube contents are 1.0 mM $GdCl_3$ in tubes 1 and 2, 0.5 mM $GdCl_3$ in tubes 3 and 4, and 3.2 mM $CuSO_4$ in tube 5. The last column is the standard deviation of all $F_{\epsilon_{rB}}(0.1)$ for the given method.

Method	Sequence	Scan ID 1	Scan ID 2	Scan ID 3	Tube 1	Tube 2	Tube 3	Tube 4	Tube 5	Std $\mathbf{F}_{\epsilon_{rB}}(0.1)$
	SEGE	0.79	0.86	0.47	0.59	0.88	0.83	0.89	0.68	
Unprocessed	MEGE	0.25	0.21	0.27	0.25	0.23	0.25	0.26	0.18	0.32
	sEPI	0.51	0.55	—	1.00	0.00	0.86	0.06	0.77	
	SEGE	0.91	0.96	0.68	0.98	0.88	0.83	0.87	0.88	
Phun	MEGE	0.67	0.73	0.64	0.89	0.51	0.54	0.66	0.80	0.24
	sEPI	0.56	0.58	—	0.92	0.00	0.87	0.37	0.79	
	SEGE	0.96	0.73	0.96	0.75	0.79	0.97	0.93	0.73	
GBC	MEGE	0.95	0.88	0.96	0.89	0.93	0.97	1.00	0.80	0.08
	sEPI	0.89	0.97	—	0.95	0.89	0.90	1.00	0.82	
	SEGE	0.97	0.96	0.97	1.00	0.94	1.00	1.00	0.89	
MEDI.RG	MEGE	0.24	0.76	0.65	0.63	0.61	0.64	0.67	0.63	0.20
	sEPI	0.91	0.92	—	1.00	0.84	0.94	0.97	0.84	
	SEGE	0.63	0.63	0.59	0.36	0.58	0.53	0.96	0.70	
MEDI.LP	MEGE	0.68	0.67	0.64	0.36	0.75	0.53	0.95	0.76	0.18
	sEPI	0.65	0.66	—	0.36	0.63	0.53	1.00	0.78	
	SEGE	0.57	0.68	0.68	0.36	0.97	0.52	0.85	0.56	
Laplace	MEGE	0.62	0.72	0.64	0.36	1.00	0.69	0.90	0.46	0.19
	sEPI	0.66	0.74	—	0.40	0.93	0.58	0.89	0.60	
Slope	MEGE	0.96	0.95	0.97	0.99	1.00	0.95	0.99	0.82	0.06
Division	MEGE	0.95	0.94	0.96	0.99	1.00	0.95	0.99	0.78	0.07
MAGPI-unopt	MEGE	0.97	0.97	0.97	1.00	1.00	0.98	1.00	0.87	0.04
MAGPI	MAGPI	0.97	0.98	0.97	1.00	1.00	0.98	1.00	0.91	0.03

with the lowest relative standard deviation σ_{ϵ_r} were MEGE + MEDI.LP (8.9%), MEGE + MAGPI-unopt (4.8%), and MAGPI (4.1%). The detailed behavior of the error is captured by the CDF (or PDF) of the data (Figure 5). A summary of the CDF is in the second-to-last column of Table 3 where we show the probability of observing relative errors <10%, $F_{\epsilon_r}(10\%)$, which captures the frequency by which *relatively* acceptable errors occur. An advantage of the Laplace-based methods is that they had smooth phase maps with qualitatively no apparent phase jumps. However, analysis showed that Laplace phase images result in quantitatively larger errors (a low $F_{\epsilon_r}(10\%)$) than other methods, suggesting incorrect phase unwrapping results, similar to the work of Chen et al. [60]. Other methods with low $F_{\epsilon_r}(10\%)$ were the unprocessed phase data, MEGE + Slope/Div, and MEGE + MEDI.RG, which had large phase unwrapping errors in a significant proportion of the data. $F_{\epsilon_r}(10\%)$ is an arbitrary point at which we highlight the behavior of F_{ϵ_r} and does not represent the entirety of the distribution of error (or CDF). For example, $F_{\epsilon_r}(10\%)$ of SEGE + MEDI.RG was comparable to MEGE + MAGPI-unopt and MAGPI, despite the comparatively poorer (larger) μ_{ϵ_r} and σ_{ϵ_r} of SEGE + MEDI.RG. This is due to relative errors falling mostly within the chosen 10% threshold for these methods.

We explored the dependence of errors on frequency reference ROI location (Figure 6). Since phase estimation errors (particularly large errors) are undesirable anywhere in the FOV, any spatial variation of the CDF highlights the potential dependence of the method on user intervention and/or its automated processing. We show the range of $F_{\epsilon_r}(10\%)$ observed across the 13 different frequency reference ROIs in the last column of Table 3. The results suggest that the most repeatable methods across background ROIs are SEGE + MEDI.RG, sEPI + MEDI.RG, MEGE + MAGPI-unopt, and MAGPI.

The MEGE data was processed using four broad classes of postprocessing algorithms. We note the following about these algorithms:

(i) The results obtained with methods in Categories 1 and 2 were fundamentally similar. That is, additional 1D-temporal processing does not alter the performance of 3D spatial unwrapping methods (with the exception of Laplacian-based methods, which we discuss below). This redundancy is due to the inherent Nyquist limitation associated with the echo spacing. As a result, we focus on the distinctive results of Category 1: spatial phase unwrapping + weighted averaging of echoes (Table 3).

(ii) Some postprocessing methods used in MEGE Categories 1 and 2 performed more poorly with MEGE than with SEGE (e.g., MEDI.RG). We believe this is due to the relatively larger bandwidth used with MEGE acquisitions, resulting in noisier images at each echo. Higher BW acquisitions were needed with MEGE to accommodate temporal methods (MEGE Categories 3 and 4), which require short echo spacing. It is possible that MEGE + MEDI.RG would perform better with lower BW (wider echo spacing). Due to time/complexity constraints, we were unable to explore every possible MEGE variation that favors specific algorithms. This is a limitation of this study.

(iii) MEGE Category 3 methods (Division/Slope) were straightforward to apply but resulted in a wide range of errors. This is due to large errors observed in frequency reference ROIs where the underlying frequency-offset value is larger than what is allowable by the smallest echo spacing. While such errors are avoidable with shorter echo spacing, this is not always possible (as was the case here) due to hardware constraints on readout bandwidth, resolution, FOV, and so forth. While Slope and Division are straightforward to apply, they result in a suboptimal combination of echoes, with noisy phase estimates.

(iv) MEGE Category 4 methods have a similar performance to that of Category 3 methods. That is, spatial phase unwrapping did not seem to markedly improve the performance of temporal phase unwrapping. This is potentially due to the hard-to-unwrap noisy boundary lines observed with Category 3 methods, as shown in MEGE + Slope example in Figure 4, which are still present with Category 4 methods.

Finally, we explored the dependence of the CDF on scan variability and tube contents (Table 4), and we note the following:

(1) Not all sequence + method pairs were invariant to scan and/or tube content. sEPI + Phun and sEPI + Unprocessed had greatest variability, followed by all of the Laplace-based methods (LP, MEDI.LP), indicating that some methods produced inconsistent phase even in their best-case scenario. Laplace-based techniques generated smoothly varying, though numerically inaccurate phase maps, irrespective of sequence, and sEPI + Phun suffered from sequence-dependent errors.

(2) Considering the best-case ROI scenario, we did not observe consistent performance differences between pairing methods with either SEGE or sEPI. The sEPI sequence provides a significant acceleration over SEGE via its segmented GRE approach and performed better with some methods (GBC) and worse with others (Phun).

(3) Table 4 compares Sequence + Method pair performance as a function of variability of scan parameters. For example, MEGE + Slope performed consistently well ($F_{\epsilon_{rB}}(10\%) > 0.95$) irrespective of the scan type used, while SEGE + Laplace was not always able to estimate the correct phase, irrespective of scan. SEGE + GBC, though, only struggled with Scan 2, which had a shorter TR than Scan 1.

(4) The same analysis can be applied to tube contents. MAGPI achieved $F_{\epsilon_{rB}}(10\%)$ close to 1.0 for all tubes and $F_{\epsilon_{rB}}(10\%) = 0.91$ in Tube 5. sEPI + Phun had inconsistent performance across tubes of similar

content (Tubes 1, 2, 3, and 4). Among the methods that maximized $F_{\epsilon_r}(0.1)$, Tube 5 exhibited lower $F_{\epsilon_{rB}}(10\%)$ compared to other tubes, which could be due to challenges defining $\Delta\chi_{th}$ and the complexity of $CuSO_4$ compared to $GdCl_3$.

Overall, the consistently good performance across tube content, scan, and rotation angle in the absence of phase estimation errors validates the $\Delta\chi$ model (equation (1)) and demonstrates that the rotating-tube phantom itself did not introduce unexpected detrimental effects to the phase measurements. In previous work, QSM performance improved with higher isotropic spatial resolution and higher coverage [56, 61]. Here, slice thickness was 2.0 mm for all scans, which may explain why performance did not drastically change with resolution. Additionally, Zhou et al. [61] and Karsa et al. [56] examined the entire QSM process, including inversion, which was not addressed here. Olsson et al. [22] used a phantom with tubes of Gd in comparable concentrations, though only one tube was used when varying angle with respect to B_0 (five angles). That study used one method to estimate QSM [62–64] over multiple spatial resolutions, volumes, and inversion parameters. Similar to the work of Karsa et al. [56], Olsson et al.'s results improved with increasing resolution and volume coverage, and, similar to our results, Olsson et al. observed errors in phase estimation using [47], compared to the theoretical result.

A limitation of this work is that the geometric structure of the phantom was not identical to that encountered *in vivo*. *In vivo* imaging may present different sources of phase errors not included here (e.g., eddy currents, susceptibility-induced signal drops), and the phantom could present some challenges that are not encountered or are less prominent in the brain. This is a common problem with nearly all phantom studies, and it is counterbalanced by the advantage of having a known truth, which is not possible *in vivo*. Errors observed in phantoms are frequently observed *in vivo*, even when the geometry of the phantom is a gross simplification of human anatomy. For example, in T_1 estimation, while phantoms can be used to refine a method, errors are amplified when methods are applied *in vivo* [65]. The many parameters, sequences, and processing steps considered here are useful to evaluate the robustness of phase estimation techniques, and this work can be viewed as a complement to other efforts seeking to evaluate the accuracy of QSM techniques, such as the use of simulated data [66, 67].

We introduced a wide range of variability to test repeatability and reproducibility of many data acquisition scenarios. While the performance of each method could be improved with additional "intervention" and potentially adapting the acquisition parameters to the intended post-processing methods to be used later, our intent was to assess the ability of existing techniques in diverse imaging scenarios encountered in reality. The degree to which Steps 3 and 4 of QSM are sensitive to the errors introduced in Steps 1 and 2 requires further investigation. This phantom validation study allowed us to set a quantitative limit on the performance of various Steps 1 and 2 methods. Ongoing work focuses on evaluating the performance of a subset of these methods, paired with Steps 3 and 4 methods.

5. Conclusion

In this work, we used a rotating-tube phantom to explore sources of error in QSM data acquisition and phase estimation. To assess the robustness and repeatability of methods, we did not manually intervene. The two most impactful parameters on reproducibility of measurements were (a) acquisition protocol (e.g., single echo or multiple echoes) and (b) phase errors. The most repeatable and reproducible approaches were MAGPI and MAGPI-unopt, both methods based on the maximum-likelihood approach in phase estimation. For the remaining methods, performance varied greatly, even when systematically applied to the same underlying data from the same sequence or with the same method across different sequences. This assessment of which methods are repeatable and reproducible without manual intervention is an important step towards using QSM pipelines in clinical settings without experienced users.

Abbreviations

BW: Bandwidth
CDF: Cumulative Distribution Function
FOV: Field of view
FR: Frequency referencing
GBC: Goldstein's branch cut
GRE: Gradient echo
LP: Laplace
MAGPI: Maximum AmbiGuity distance for Phase Imaging
MEDI: Morphology enabled dipole inversion
MEGE: Multiecho gradient echo
QSM: Quantitative Susceptibility Mapping
RG: Region growing
ROI: Region of interest
SEGE: Single-echo gradient echo
sEPI: Segmented Echo Planar Imaging.

Disclosure

A preprint has previously been published [68]. Certain commercial instruments and software are identified to specify the experimental study adequately. This does not imply endorsement by NIST or that the instruments and software are the best available for the purpose.

Acknowledgments

The authors W.-T.W., J. A.B., and D. L.P. would like to acknowledge funding from the Department of Defense in the Center for Neuroscience and Regenerative Medicine and the intramural research program of the National Institutes of Health. The authors K. E.K, S. C., and S. E.R. acknowledge funding from their employer, the National Institute of Standards and Technology. The authors B. P.B. and J. D. acknowledge funding from their employer, the MITRE Corporation.

References

[1] Y. Wang and T. Liu, "Quantitative susceptibility mapping (QSM): decoding MRI data for a tissue magnetic biomarker," *Magnetic Resonance in Medicine*, vol. 73, no. 1, pp. 82–101, 2015.

[2] E. M. Haacke, N. Y. C. Cheng, M. J. House et al., "Imaging iron stores in the brain using magnetic resonance imaging," *Magnetic Resonance Imaging*, vol. 23, no. 1, pp. 1–25, 2005.

[3] I. R. Young, S. Khenia, D. G. T. Thomas et al., "Clinical magnetic susceptibility mapping of the brain," *Journal of Computer Assisted Tomography*, vol. 11, no. 1, pp. 2–6, 1987.

[4] J. H. Jensen, K. Szulc, C. Hu et al., "Magnetic field correlation as a measure of iron-generated magnetic field in homogeneities in the brain," *Magnetic Resonance in Medicine*, vol. 61, no. 2, pp. 481–485, 2009.

[5] K. Shmueli, J. A. de Zwart, P. van Gelderen, T.-Q. Li, S. J. Dodd, and J. H. Duyn, "Magnetic susceptibility mapping of brain tissue in vivo using MRI phase data," *Magnetic Resonance in Medicine*, vol. 62, no. 6, pp. 1510–1522, 2009.

[6] H. Tan, T. Liu, Y. Wu et al., "Evaluation of iron content in human cerebral cavernous malformation using quantitative susceptibility mapping," *Investigative Radiology*, vol. 49, no. 7, pp. 498–504, 2014.

[7] E. M. Haacke, K. Prabhakaran, I. R. Elangovan, Z. Wu, and J. Neelavalli, "Oxygen saturation: quantification, susceptibility weighted imaging in MRI," in *MRI: Basic Concepts and Clinical Applications*, M. Haacke and J. Reichenbach, Eds., John Wiley & Sons, Inc, Hoboken, NJ, USA, pp. 517–528, 2011.

[8] S. D. Sharma, D. Hernando, D. E. Horng, and S. B. Reeder, "Quantitative susceptibility mapping in the abdomen as an imaging biomarker of hepatic iron overload," *Magnetic Resonance in Medicine*, vol. 74, no. 3, pp. 673–683, 2015.

[9] D. Bonekamp, P. B. Barker, R. Leigh, P. C. M. van Zijl, and X. Li, "Susceptibility-based analysis of dynamic gadolinium bolus perfusion MRI," *Magnetic Resonance in Medicine*, vol. 73, no. 2, pp. 544–554, 2015.

[10] E. Lind, L. Knutsson, R. Kämpe, F. Ståhlberg, and R. Wirestam, "Assessment of MRI contrast agent concentration by quantitative susceptibility mapping (QSM): application to estimation of cerebral blood volume during steady state," *Magnetic Resonance Materials in Physics, Biology and Medicine*, vol. 30, no. 6, pp. 555–566, 2017.

[11] K. Deh, T. D. Nguyen, S. Eskreis-Winkler et al., "Reproducibility of quantitative susceptibility mapping in the brain at two field strengths from two vendors," *Journal of Magnetic Resonance Imaging*, vol. 42, no. 6, pp. 1592–1600, 2015.

[12] K. Deh, K. Kawaji, M. Bulk et al., "Multicenter reproducibility of quantitative susceptibility mapping in a gadolinium phantom using MEDI+0 automatic zero referencing," *Magnetic Resonance in Medicine*, vol. 81, no. 2, pp. 1229–1236, 2019.

[13] X. Feng, A. Deistung, and J. R. Reichenbach, "Quantitative susceptibility mapping (QSM) and R 2 ∗ in the human brain at 3 T," *Zeitschrift für Medizinische Physik*, vol. 28, no. 1, pp. 36–48, 2018.

[14] T. Hinoda, Y. Fushimi, T. Okada et al., "Quantitative susceptibility mapping at 3 T and 1.5 T," *Investigative Radiology*, vol. 50, no. 8, pp. 522–530, 2015.

[15] P.-Y. Lin, T.-C. Chao, and M.-L. Wu, "Quantitative susceptibility mapping of human brain at 3T: a multisite reproducibility study," *American Journal of Neuroradiology*, vol. 36, no. 3, pp. 467–474, 2015.

[16] M. D. Santin, M. Didier, R. Valabrègue et al., "Reproducibility of R2∗ and quantitative susceptibility mapping (QSM) reconstruction methods in the basal ganglia of healthy subjects," *NMR in Biomedicine*, vol. 30, no. 4, Article ID e3491, 2017.

[17] S. D. Robinson, K. Bredies, D. Khabipova, B. Dymerska, J. P. Marques, and F. Schweser, "An illustrated comparison of processing methods for MR phase imaging and QSM: combining array coil signals and phase unwrapping," *NMR in Biomedicine*, vol. 30, no. 4, Article ID e3601, 2017.

[18] R. Wang, G. Xie, M. Zhai et al., "Stability of R2∗ and quantitative susceptibility mapping of the brain tissue in a large scale multi-center study," *Scientific Reports*, vol. 28, no. 1, Article ID 45261, 2017.

[19] M. Lancione, G. Donatelli, P. Cecchi, M. Cosottini, M. Tosetti, and M. Costagli, "Echo-time dependency of quantitative susceptibility mapping reproducibility at different magnetic field strengths," *NeuroImage*, vol. 197, pp. 557–564, 2019.

[20] C. Langkammer, F. Schweser, K. Shmueli et al., "Quantitative susceptibility mapping: report from the 2016 reconstruction challenge," *Magnetic Resonance in Medicine*, vol. 79, no. 3, pp. 1661–1673, 2018.

[21] Z. Liu, Y. Kee, D. Zhou, Y. Wang, and P. Spincemaille, "Preconditioned total field inversion (TFI) method for quantitative susceptibility mapping," *Magnetic Resonance in Medicine*, vol. 78, no. 1, pp. 303–315, 2017.

[22] E. Olsson, R. Wirestam, and E. Lind, "MRI-based quantification of magnetic susceptibility in gel phantoms: assessment of measurement and calculation accuracy," *Radiology Research and Practice*, vol. 2018, Article ID 6709525, 13 pages, 2018.

[23] V. Fortier and I. R. Levesque, "Phase processing for quantitative susceptibility mapping of regions with large susceptibility and lack of signal," *Magnetic Resonance in Medicine*, vol. 79, no. 6, pp. 3103–3113, 2018.

[24] H. E. Erdevig, S. E. Russek, S. Carnicka, K. F. Stupic, and K. E. Keenan, "Accuracy of magnetic resonance based susceptibility measurements," *AIP Advances*, vol. 7, no. 5, Article ID 056718, 2017.

[25] Y.-C. N Cheng, C.-Y. Hsieh, J. Neelavalli, and E. M. Haacke, "Quantifying effective magnetic moments of narrow cylindrical objects in MRI," *Physics in Medicine and Biology*, vol. 54, no. 22, pp. 7025–7044, 2009.

[26] C. Liu, W. Li, K. A. Tong, K. W. Yeom, and S. Kuzminski, "Susceptibility-weighted imaging and quantitative susceptibility mapping in the brain," *Journal of Magnetic Resonance Imaging*, vol. 42, no. 1, pp. 23–41, 2015.

[27] S. Liu, S. Buch, Y. Chen et al., "Susceptibility-weighted imaging: current status and future directions," *NMR in Biomedicine*, vol. 30, no. 4, Article ID e3552, 2017.

[28] U. Katscher, T. Voigt, and C. Findeklee, "Electrical conductivity imaging using magnetic resonance tomography," in *Proceedings of the 2009 Annual International Conference of the IEEE Engineering in Medicine and Biology Society*, pp. 3162–3164, Munich, Germany, September 2009.

[29] V. Rieke and K. Butts Pauly, "MR thermometry," *Journal of Magnetic Resonance Imaging*, vol. 27, no. 2, pp. 376–390, 2008.

[30] S. Ley, D. Mereles, M. Puderbach et al., "Value of MR phase-contrast flow measurements for functional assessment of pulmonary arterial hypertension," *European Radiology*, vol. 17, no. 7, pp. 1892–1897, 2007.

[31] R. Muthupillai, D. J. Lomas, P. J. Rossman, J. F. Greenleaf, A. Manduca, and R. L. Ehman, "Magnetic resonance elastography by direct visualization of propagating acoustic strain waves," *Science*, vol. 269, no. 5232, pp. 1854–1857, 1995.

[32] A. Deistung, A. Schäfer, F. Schweser, U. Biedermann, R. Turner, and J. R. Reichenbach, "Toward in vivo histology: a comparison of quantitative susceptibility mapping (QSM) with magnitude-, phase-, and R2-imaging at ultra-high magnetic field strength," *NeuroImage*, vol. 65, pp. 299–314, 2013.

[33] E. M. Haacke, S. Liu, S. Buch, W. Zheng, D. Wu, and Y. Ye, "Quantitative susceptibility mapping: current status and future directions," *Magnetic Resonance Imaging*, vol. 33, no. 1, pp. 1–25, 2015.

[34] P. Sati, D. Thomasson, N. Li et al., "Rapid, high-resolution, whole-brain, susceptibility-based MRI of multiple sclerosis," *Multiple Sclerosis Journal*, vol. 20, no. 11, pp. 1464–1470, 2014.

[35] W. Feng, J. Neelavalli, and E. M. Haacke, "Catalytic multiecho phase unwrapping scheme (CAMPUS) in multiecho gradient echo imaging: removing phase wraps on a voxel-by-voxel basis," *Magnetic Resonance in Medicine*, vol. 70, no. 1, pp. 117–126, 2013.

[36] G. Helms and P. Dechent, "Increased SNR and reduced distortions by averaging multiple gradient echo signals in 3D FLASH imaging of the human brain at 3T," *Journal of Magnetic Resonance Imaging*, vol. 29, no. 1, pp. 198–204, 2009.

[37] J. Dagher and K. Nael, "MAGPI: a framework for maximum likelihood MR phase imaging using multiple receive coils," *Magnetic Resonance in Medicine*, vol. 75, no. 3, pp. 1218–1231, 2016.

[38] J. Dagher and K. Nael, "MR phase imaging with bipolar acquisition," *NMR in Biomedicine*, vol. 30, no. 4, Article ID e3523, 2017.

[39] A. M. Halefoglu and D. M. Yousem, "Susceptibility weighted imaging: clinical applications and future directions," *World Journal of Radiology*, vol. 10, no. 4, pp. 30–45, 2018.

[40] C. J. G. Bakker, H. de Leeuw, and P. R. Seevinck, "Selective depiction of susceptibility transitions using Laplace-filtered phase maps," *Magnetic Resonance Imaging*, vol. 30, no. 5, pp. 601–609, 2012.

[41] N.-k. Chen and A. M. Wyrwicz, "Correction for EPI distortions using multi-echo gradient-echo imaging," *Magnetic Resonance in Medicine*, vol. 41, no. 6, pp. 1206–1213, 1999.

[42] R. M. Goldstein, H. A. Zebker, and C. L. Werner, "Satellite radar interferometry: two-dimensional phase unwrapping," *Radio Science*, vol. 23, no. 4, pp. 713–720, 1988.

[43] K. Lu, T. T. Liu, and M. Bydder, "Optimal phase difference reconstruction: comparison of two methods," *Magnetic Resonance Imaging*, vol. 26, no. 1, pp. 142–145, 2008.

[44] M. A. Schofield and Y. Zhu, "Fast phase unwrapping algorithm for interferometric applications," *Optics Letters*, vol. 28, no. 14, pp. 1194–1196, 2003.

[45] Y. Wang, "Cornell MEDI Toolbox," http://pre.weill.cornell.edu/mri/pages/qsm.html.

[46] S. Witoszynskyj, A. Rauscher, J. R. Reichenbach, and M. Barth, "Phase unwrapping of MR images using ΦUN-a fast and robust region growing algorithm," *Medical Image Analysis*, vol. 13, no. 2, pp. 257–268, 2009.

[47] R. Cusack and N. Papadakis, "New robust 3-D phase unwrapping algorithms: application to magnetic field mapping and undistorting echoplanar images," *NeuroImage*, vol. 16, no. 3 Pt 1, pp. 754–764, 2002.

[48] D. L. Parker, A. Payne, N. Todd, and J. R. Hadley, "Phase reconstruction from multiple coil data using a virtual reference coil," *Magnetic Resonance in Medicine*, vol. 72, no. 2, pp. 563–569, 2014.

[49] B. Wu, W. Li, A. V. Avram, S.-M. Gho, and C. Liu, "Fast and tissue-optimized mapping of magnetic susceptibility and T2 with multi-echo and multi-shot spirals," *NeuroImage*, vol. 59, no. 1, pp. 297–305, 2012.

[50] J. L. R. Andersson, M. S. Graham, I. Drobnjak, H. Zhang, and J. Campbell, "Susceptibility-induced distortion that varies due to motion: correction in diffusion MR without acquiring additional data," *NeuroImage*, vol. 171, pp. 277–295, 2018.

[51] J. A. Lundman, M. Bylund, A. Garpebring, C. Thellenberg Karlsson, and T. Nyholm, "Patient-induced susceptibility effects simulation in magnetic resonance imaging," *Physics and Imaging in Radiation Oncology*, vol. 1, pp. 41–45, 2017.

[52] P. B. Roemer, W. A. Edelstein, C. E. Hayes, S. P. Souza, and O. M. Mueller, "The NMR phased array," *Magnetic Resonance in Medicine*, vol. 16, no. 2, pp. 192–225, 1990.

[53] B. Gruber, M. Froeling, T. Leiner, and D. W. J. Klomp, "RF coils: a practical guide for nonphysicists," *Journal of Magnetic Resonance Imaging*, vol. 48, no. 3, pp. 590–604, 2018.

[54] K. C. Chu, Y. Xu, J. A. Balschi, and C. S. Springer Jr, "Bulk magnetic susceptibility shifts in NMR studies of compartmentalized samples: use of paramagnetic reagents," *Magnetic Resonance in Medicine*, vol. 13, no. 2, pp. 239–262, 1990.

[55] C.-Y. Hsieh, Y.-C. N. Cheng, J. Neelavalli, E. M. Haacke, and R. J. Stafford, "An improved method for susceptibility and radius quantification of cylindrical objects from MRI," *Magnetic Resonance Imaging*, vol. 33, no. 4, pp. 420–436, 2015.

[56] A. Karsa, S. Punwani, and K. Shmueli, "The effect of low resolution and coverage on the accuracy of susceptibility mapping," *Magnetic Resonance in Medicine*, vol. 81, no. 3, pp. 1833–1848, 2019.

[57] M. J. Cronin, N. Wang, K. S. Decker, H. Wei, W.-Z. Zhu, and C. Liu, "Exploring the origins of echo-time-dependent quantitative susceptibility mapping (QSM) measurements in healthy tissue and cerebral microbleeds," *NeuroImage*, vol. 149, pp. 98–113, 2017.

[58] Y. Kanazawa, Y. Matsumoto, M. Harada, H. Hayashi, T. Matsuda, and H. Otsuka, "Appropriate echo time selection for quantitative susceptibility mapping," *Radiological Physics and Technology*, vol. 12, no. 2, pp. 185–193, 2019.

[59] W. Zheng, H. Nichol, S. Liu, Y.-C. N. Cheng, and E. M. Haacke, "Measuring iron in the brain using quantitative susceptibility mapping and X-ray fluorescence imaging," *NeuroImage*, vol. 78, pp. 68–74, 2013.

[60] M.-C. Hsieh, C.-Y. Tsai, M.-C. Liao, J.-L. Yang, C.-H. Su, and J.-H. Chen, "Quantitative susceptibility mapping-based microscopy of magnetic resonance venography (QSM-mMRV) for in vivo morphologically and functionally assessing cerebromicrovasculature in rat stroke model," *PLoS One*, vol. 11, no. 3, Article ID e0149602, 2016.

[61] D. Zhou, J. Cho, J. Zhang, P. Spincemaille, and Y. Wang, "Susceptibility underestimation in a high-susceptibility phantom: dependence on imaging resolution, magnitude contrast, and other parameters," *Magnetic Resonance in Medicine*, vol. 78, no. 3, pp. 1080–1086, 2017.

[62] L. de Rochefort, T. Liu, B. Kressler et al., "Quantitative susceptibility map reconstruction from MR phase data using bayesian regularization: validation and application to brain imaging," *Magnetic Resonance in Medicine*, vol. 63, no. 1, pp. 194–206, 2010.

[63] J. Liu, T. Liu, L. de Rochefort et al., "Morphology enabled dipole inversion for quantitative susceptibility mapping using

structural consistency between the magnitude image and the susceptibility map," *NeuroImage*, vol. 59, no. 3, pp. 2560–2568, 2012.

[64] T. Liu, C. Wisnieff, M. Lou, W. Chen, P. Spincemaille, and Y. Wang, "Nonlinear formulation of the magnetic field to source relationship for robust quantitative susceptibility mapping," *Magnetic Resonance in Medicine*, vol. 69, no. 2, pp. 467–476, 2013.

[65] N. Stikov, M. Boudreau, I. R. Levesque, C. L. Tardif, J. K. Barral, and G. B. Pike, "On the accuracy of T1mapping: searching for common ground," *Magnetic Resonance in Medicine*, vol. 73, no. 2, pp. 514–522, 2015.

[66] Q. S. M. C. O. Committee, B. Bilgic, C. Langkammer et al., "QSM reconstruction challenge 2.0: design and report of results," *Magnetic Resonance in Medicine*, vol. 86, no. 3, pp. 1241–1255, 2021.

[67] J. P. Marques, J. Meineke, C. Milovic et al., "QSM reconstruction challenge 2.0: a realistic in silico head phantom for MRI data simulation and evaluation of susceptibility mapping procedures," *Magnetic Resonance in Medicine*, vol. 86, no. 1, pp. 526–542, 2021.

[68] K. E. Keenan, B. P. Berman, and S. C. Carnicka, "Validation of data acquisition and phase estimation for quantitative susceptibility mapping with a rotating-tube phantom," *bioRxiv*, 2021, preprint.

25

Comparative Study on the Outcomes of Elective-Start versus Urgent-Start Peritoneal Dialysis Catheter Placement

Ahmed Kamel Abdel Aal,[1] Khalid Mahmoud,[2] Amr Soliman Moustafa,[3,4] Noha Alaaeldin Aboueldahab,[2] Anas Souid,[2] Andrew Gunn,[2] Yufeng Li,[5] Zhixin Wang,[5] and Ammar Almehmi[6]

[1]*Department of Diagnostic and Interventional Imaging, University of Texas Health Science Center at Houston, Houston, TX 77030, USA*
[2]*Department of Radiology, University of Alabama at Birmingham, Birmingham, AL 35233, USA*
[3]*Department of Radiology, University of Arkansas for Medical Sciences, Little Rock, AR 72205, USA*
[4]*Department of Radiology, Zagazig University, Zagazig, Egypt*
[5]*Department of Medicine, Division of Preventive Medicine, University of Alabama at Birmingham, Birmingham, AL 35233, USA*
[6]*Department of Medicine, Division of Nephrology, University of Alabama at Birmingham, Birmingham, AL 35233, USA*

Correspondence should be addressed to Ahmed Kamel Abdel Aal; ahmed.k.abdelaal@uth.tmc.edu

Academic Editor: Paul Sijens

The aim of this study is to compare the outcomes of the elective-start versus urgent-start use of peritoneal dialysis (PD) catheters using percutaneous radiologic or laparoscopic techniques. Patients having their first peritoneal dialysis catheter placed and used between January 2005 and January 2018 were identified, and their medical records were retrospectively reviewed. Two groups were identified: elective-start ($n = 211$) and urgent-start ($n = 29$). Patient's demographics were similar between the two groups with the exception of age, which was higher in the elective-start group. The catheter complication rates and catheter removal rates at 3 and 12 months, mean days-to-first complication, mean days-to-catheter removal, and overall patient survival at 12 months were analyzed. Catheter complication rates at 3 and 12 months were similar between the two groups (27.8% and 48.9%, respectively, in the elective-start group versus 35.9% and 54.2%, respectively, in the urgent-start group, $p = 0.415$). The catheter removal rates at 3 and 12 months were also similar between the two groups ($p = 0.088$). Catheter leak was higher in the urgent-start group (13.8% versus 3.3%, respectively, $p = 0.011$). There was no difference between the elective-start and the urgent-start groups in the mean days-to-first complication (95 vs 69, $p = 0.086$), mean days-to-catheter removal (145 vs 127, $p = 0.757$), and overall patient survival at 12 months (100% vs 97%, $p = 0.41$). In conclusion, apart from catheter leak, there were similar rates of catheter complication and removal for PD catheter used for the elective-start compared to the urgent-start PD. Furthermore, the technique of placement did not affect the outcomes.

1. Introduction

Chronic kidney disease (CKD) as well as end-stage renal disease (ESRD) is prevalent throughout the world with an incidence of 13.6% and 0.14%, respectively [1]. More than 25,000 patients in the United States receive dialysis via peritoneal dialysis (PD) [2]. PD is a patient-centered cost-effective modality compared to hemodialysis (HD) [3]. This is because PD can be carried out at home, affording unique lifestyle benefits for patients, and allowing for lower dialysis costs [4]. PD also provides preservation of kidney function [5] and improved mortality [6] when compared to HD.

It is expected that PD will be utilized at a higher rate in the United States as recent modifications by the Centers for Medicare and Medicaid Services (CMS) resulted in higher reimbursement for PD services [7]. The distinct advantages of PD have led to the "PD First" position by some clinicians and to consider PD for urgent dialysis commencement and not only for the elective-start dialysis settings [8–10]. The urgent-start dialysis is a term used to describe patients needing immediate dialysis initiation with no preestablished vascular or PD access, where initiation of the PD occurs within 2 weeks after catheter insertion [8]. Therefore, the urgent-start PD is an attractive option for patients presenting with ESRD without prior access preparation [11].

Nevertheless, PD in the urgent-start setting is frequently underutilized for several reasons. First, patients may have difficulty making a decision regarding a dialysis modality. Second, there may be limited experience with PD or a lack of resources at multiple levels, leading to reluctance in using PD especially in patients with severe uremic symptoms and volume overload. Third, the urgent-start PD requires prompt PD catheter placement (typically within 24 to 48 hours of presentation), which might not be available in all institutions and medical facilities [12, 13]. While PD catheters are better in terms of overall morbidity and mortality, they are not entirely without risk. Abdominal wall complications, most commonly hernia and leak, may occur owing to the increased intra-abdominal pressure from high dialysate volume infused in the peritoneal cavity [14]. Technical failure from malpositioned catheters may also occur [15]. Data regarding the outcomes of the elective-start compared to the urgent-start PD is limited, with few published studies available in the literature [16–18].

The purpose of this study was to compare the outcomes of PD catheter placement in the elective-start versus urgent-start settings.

2. Methods

2.1. Study Population. This study was approved by the local institutional review board, and informed consent was waived. A total of two hundred and sixty patients who underwent PD catheter placement between January 2005 and January 2018 were retrospectively reviewed. Two groups were identified: the elective-start group, which comprised of patients who had PD catheters inserted as part of patient preparation for dialysis access, and, the urgent-start group, which included patients who presented with no preestablished access and had their PD catheters placed for the immediate initiation of dialysis. PD catheter insertion was performed either by an interventional radiologists and nephrologists using percutaneous, image-guided technique (fluoroscopy and ultrasound guidance) using conscious sedation, or by surgeons using laparoscopic technique using general anesthesia. The decision to perform percutaneous image-guided versus laparoscopic placement of the catheters was mainly based on physician discretion taking into consideration the age and comorbidity of the patients, and the ability to perform general anesthesia. Older patients with comorbid conditions who were not eligible to obtain general anesthesia were referred for percutaneous catheter placement.

Some of the study subjects may overlap with another study titled "Outcomes of fluoroscopic and ultrasound-guided placement versus laparoscopic placement of peritoneal dialysis catheters," which was published in the Clinical Kidney Journal [19]. The objective of that study was to compare the fluoroscopy and ultrasound guidance technique with the laparoscopic technique. This study focuses on comparing the outcomes of PD catheter placement in the elective-start versus urgent-start settings regardless of the technique.

Patients with stage-5 CKD or with ESRD, age ≥19 years, and with PD catheter placed during the study period were the inclusion criteria. Exclusion criteria were patients with no documentation of follow-up at our institution or those with a PD catheter buried under the skin and not used during the study period due to the patients who did not meet the criteria for dialysis (embedded catheters). Patients who underwent laparoscopic adhesiolysis, hernia repair, or omentopexy, patients who had previous abdominal surgery, or patients with severe obesity, defined as BMI of 30 or higher, were included in both groups. Figure 1 illustrates the algorithm of including and excluding patients. Two hundred and forty patients were included in the study.

The demographics and comorbidities of the patients were obtained from the medical records. BMI was classified into 3 categories: Class-1 is BMI of 30 to <35, Class-2 is BMI of 35 to <40, and class-3 is BMI of 40 or higher. We also recorded the prior surgeries of the patients.

There were 211 patients in the elective-start group as well as 29 patients in the urgent-start group. Patients in both groups had similar demographics and medical comorbidities except for age, which was higher in the elective-start group (55.8 years, SD = 15.6) compared to the urgent-start group (47.2 years, SD = 15.9) (p = 0.0094) (Table 1). The elective-start group consisted of 121 (57.3%) females and 90 (42.7%) males, while the urgent-start group included 16 (55.2%) males and 13 (44.8%) females. Obesity was similar in the elective-start and urgent-start groups and was seen in 73 patients (34.6%) and 12 patients (41.3%), respectively (p = 0.47). The mean BMI was also similar between the elective-start group (29.2) and the urgent-start group (28.4) (p = 0.855). In the elective-start group, 32 patients (15.2%), 26 patients (12.3%), and 15 (7.1 %) were class-1, class-2, and class-3 obesity, respectively. In the urgent-start group, 8 patients (27.6%), 3 patients (10.3%), and 1 patient (3.4%) were class-1, class-2, and class-3 obesity, respectively. Prior surgical procedures were performed more commonly in the elective-start group (117 patients, 55.5%) compared to the urgent-start group (10 patients, 34.5%) (p = 0.034) (Table 2).

2.2. Study Outcomes. Following PD catheter placement, the patients were followed up regularly by their nephrologists. Information on catheter complication and removal was obtained from the nephrology clinic notes in the patients' medical records.

The occurrence of PD catheter-related complications at 3 and 12 months was a composite endpoint that included infectious, mechanical, and technical complications. The infectious complications included the following: exit-site infection and tunnel infection as well as peritonitis. Peritonitis was defined as an infectious process that starts at the exit site, migrates along the subcutaneous tunnel, and ends in peritonitis. The

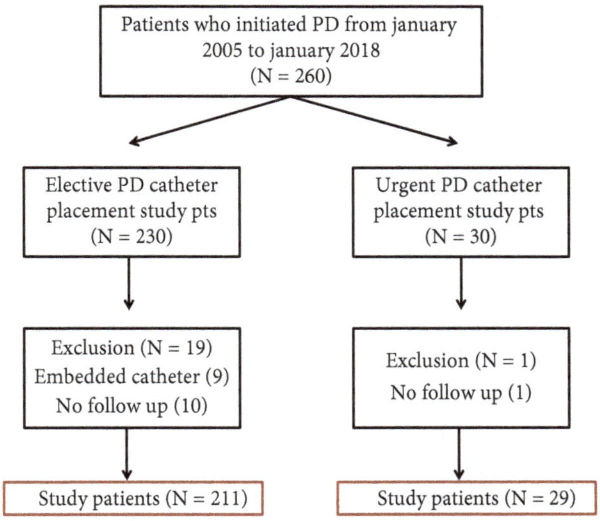

FIGURE 1: Algorithm for patients' inclusion and exclusion.

TABLE 1: Demographics and comorbidities of the elective-start and urgent-start groups.

Characteristics	Elective-start group, $N = 211$ (%)	Urgent-start group, $N = 29$ (%)	p value
Age*	55.8 (15.6)	47.2 (15.9)	0.009
Sex			0.203
Female	121 (57.3)	13 (44.8)	
Male	90 (42.7)	16 (55.2)	
Body Mass index (BMI)*	29.2 (7.4)	28.4 (6.8)	0.855
Diabetes	100 (47.4)	15 (51.8)	0.662
Hypertension	193 (91.5)	29 (100)	0.102
Coronary artery disease	53 (25.1)	6 (20.7)	0.604
Congestive heart failure	52 (24.6)	5 (17.2)	0.380
Peripheral vascular disease	26 (12.3)	3 (10.3)	0.759
Cerebrovascular disease	13 (6.2)	1 (3.5)	0.559

*Mean (Standard deviation).

mechanical complications included the following: catheter leakage through the exit-site, catheter malfunction caused by insufficient catheter drainage, and the development of abdominal hernia. The technical complications included the following: bowel perforation, muscle hematoma, intraperitoneal bleeding, and insertion failure resulting from either failing to insert the catheter or inability to use it after successful insertion. Comparison between radiologic and laparoscopic techniques in each of the two groups was performed.

Catheter removal at 3 and 12 months (catheter removal), mean days-to-first complication, mean days-to-catheter removal, and overall patient survival were calculated. All information regarding the catheter's placement, complications, and removal were acquired from the patients' electronic medical records.

2.3. Radiologic and Laparoscopic Technique of PD Catheter Placement. Percutaneous PD catheter insertion utilizing image-guided technique (fluoroscopy and ultrasound) has been described in the literature [4, 20, 21]. The laparoscopic technique has likewise been described in the literature [22]. In the urgent-start group, dialysis was started within 48 hours of catheter insertion with low-volume dialysis until wound healing occurred. In the elective-start group, dialysis was started with large volume after complete wound healing, which typically occurs within 21 days.

2.4. Statistical Analysis. Descriptive analysis was presented for patient demographics, clinical history, imaging, and laboratory data, including mean, standard deviation, count, and percentage. To compare continuous variables between the two groups, two sample t-tests were conducted. Careful attention was given to the normality assumption, which was examined by normal probability plots and histograms. To compare categorical variables, Fisher's exact test was conducted. Time to complication and time to catheter removal were analyzed using the Kaplan–Meier (KM) method. The 3 and 12 months complication-free and catheter removal rates were estimated from KM curves. Time to complication and time to catheter removal were calculated from the date of procedure to the date of complication and the date of catheter removed within 12 months. Right censor was considered if patients lost at the end of the study or if the event did not occur within the study duration. For all

TABLE 2: Prior surgical procedures in the elective-start and urgent-start groups.

Type of surgery	Elective-start group, $N = 211$ (%)	Urgent-start group, $N = 29$ (%)	p value
Total no. of surgeries	117 (55.5)	10 (34.5)	
Abdominal exploration	4 (1.9)	0 (0)	
Appendectomy	10 (4.7)	1 (3.4)	
Caesarean section	26 (12.3)	2 (6.9)	
Cholecystectomy	29 (13.7)	0 (0)	
Colon surgery	3 (1.4)	0 (0)	
Fundoplication	1 (0.5)	0 (0)	
Gastric bypass	4 (1.9)	0 (0)	0.034
Hernia repair	21 (10)	2 (6.9)	
Hysterectomy	40 (19)	1 (3.4)	
Kidney transplantation	18 (8.5)	3 (10.3)	
Myomectomy	1 (0.5)	0 (0)	
Nephrectomy	13 (6.2)	1 (3.4)	
Salpingo-oophorectomy	7 (3.3)	1 (3.4)	
Tubal ligation	13 (6.2)	0 (0)	

inferences, the significant level was set to $p \leq 0.05$. All analyses were conducted using SAS v.9.4 (SAS Inc., USA).

3. Results

Catheter complication rates are shown in Table 3. In both groups, the most common complications were catheter malfunction and peritonitis accounting for 28.4% and 15.1%, respectively, in the elective-start group compared to 17.2% and 27.6%, respectively, in the urgent-start group but without a significant difference ($p = 0.203$ and $p = 0.092$, respectively). Catheter leakage was more frequent in the urgent-start group when compared to the elective-start group (13.8% versus 3.3%, respectively, $p = 0.011$). Bowel injury resulting in perforation was documented in one of the patients in the elective-start group and was placed using the image-guided technique. This patient was treated conservatively using prophylactic antibiotic administration.

Kaplan–Meier analysis revealed nonsignificant difference in the rates of catheter complications when comparing the two groups ($p = 0.415$) (Figure 2). The estimated catheter complication rates at 3 and 12 months from the KM analysis were 27.8% and 48.9%, respectively, in the elective-start group versus 35.9% and 54.2%, respectively, in the urgent-start group (Table 4). When patients were compared based on the technique of catheter placement (radiologic versus laparoscopic) in each group separately, there was no difference in the rate of catheter complications between the two techniques ($p = 0.834$ and $p = 0.264$ for the elective-start and urgent-start groups, respectively) (Figures 3(a) and 3(b)). No difference was noted in the mean days-to-first complication which was 95 days (SD = 88, range 0–350 days) in the elective-start group compared to 69 days (SD = 97, range 1–300 days) in the urgent-start group ($p = 0.086$).

Kaplan–Meier analysis demonstrated no difference in the overall catheter removal rates when comparing the two groups ($p = 0.088$) (Figure 4). The estimated catheter removal rates from the KM analysis are shown in Table 4. The overall catheter removal at 3 and 12 months were 7.3% and 26.9%, respectively, in the elective-start group versus 7.7% and 34.8%, respectively, in the urgent-start group. There was no difference in the mean days-to-catheter removal, which was 145 days (SD = 95, range 0–338 days) in the elective-start group compared to 127 days (SD = 79, range 14–235 days) in the urgent-start group ($p = 0.757$).

Kaplan–Meier survival analysis revealed no difference in the overall survival of the patients when comparing the two groups ($p = 0.41$) (Figure 5), although the mean age was higher in the elective-start group. The urgent-start group had no estimated deaths at 3 and 12 months compared to 1.0% and 3.33%, respectively, in the elective-start group. Four patients died in the first year in the elective-start group, and the causes of death were not related to the procedure or catheter complications, but were due to septic shock from pneumonia in one patient, multiorgan failure in one patient, and cardiopulmonary arrest in two patients.

4. Discussion

PD has several advantages over HD including an improved lifestyle for patients and enhanced outcomes [23, 24]. Survival superiority of PD over HD in the first two-years of therapy has been shown, with similar outcomes up to five years [25–29]. Typically, the late-referred patients who are good candidates for PD are usually started on HD using a temporary central venous catheter due to the inability to place PD catheter in a timely manner [16]. However, temporary central venous catheters are usually associated with increased risk of complications including but not limited to sepsis and bacteremia requiring hospitalization and catheter malfunction requiring catheter replacement [30].

PD catheter placement utilizing image-guided percutaneous methods is essential for rapid commencement of PD in late-presenting patients [31]. Various centers have established pathways for surgical and image-guided percutaneous PD catheter placements to provide rapid initiation of PD, in which assisted PD treatments are provided by dedicated PD nursing staff in the outpatient setting until clinical improvement, and then, the patient is trained on self-care at home [31–33].

TABLE 3: Catheter complication rates for the elective-start and urgent-start groups.

	Elective-start group, $N = 211$ (%)	Urgent-start group, $N = 29$ (%)	p value
Exit site infections	11 (5.2)	1 (3.5)	0.683
Peritonitis	32 (15.1)	8 (27.6)	0.092
Catheter malfunction	60 (28.4)	5 (17.2)	0.203
Catheter leak	7 (3.3)	4 (13.8)	0.011
Primary leak	2 (1)	1 (3.5)	0.256
Hernia	9 (4.3)	3 (10.3)	0.159
Muscle hematoma or bleeding	6 (2.8)	0 (0)	0.358
Bowel perforation	1 (0.5)	0 (0)	0.710

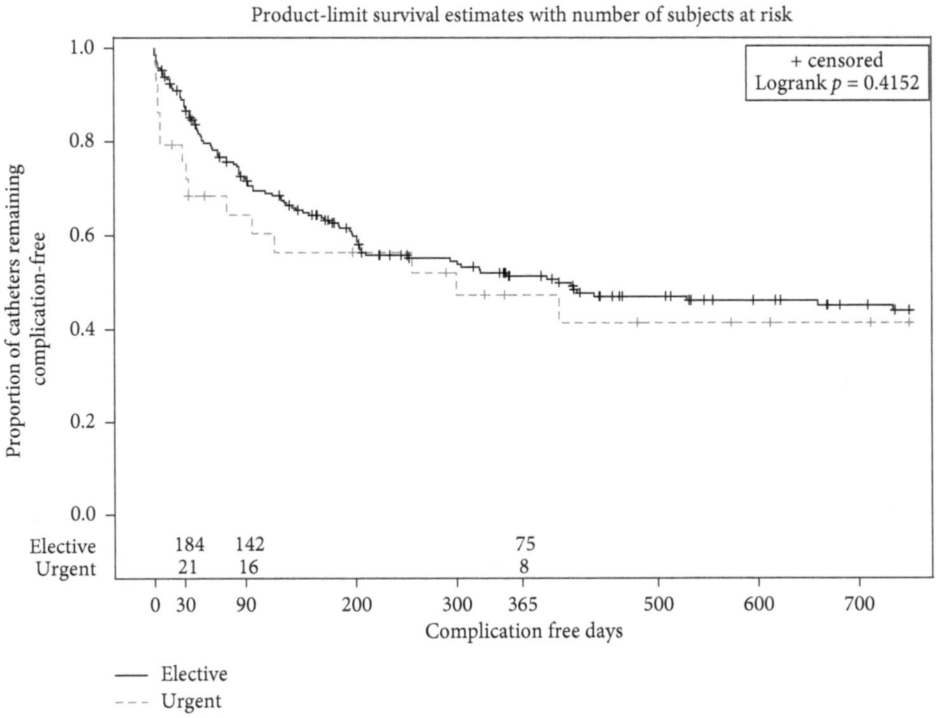

FIGURE 2: Kaplan–Meier curves for catheter complication rates in the elective-start and urgent-start groups, showing no difference between both groups.

TABLE 4: Estimated catheter complications and removal rates for the elective-start and urgent-start groups from the Kaplan–Meier curves.

	Elective-start group, $N = 211$ (%)	Urgent-start group, $N = 29$ (%)	p value*
Catheter complication rate at 3 months	27.8	35.9	0.415
Catheter complication rate at 12 months	48.9	54.2	
Catheter removal at 3 months	7.3	7.7	0.088
Catheter removal at 12 months	26.9	34.8	

*Logrank test.

Rapid placement of PD catheters with rapid initiation of dialysis allows for a single procedure to provide both short-term and long-term access. However, these patients frequently find themselves faced with the risk of dialysate leak by earlier use of the PD catheter [9, 16]. In the urgent-start setting, catheter leak is one of the most commonly encountered complications ranging 0–33.3% [9, 33–39]. Our study is consistent with the published literature showing a similar risk of leak with a rate of 13.8% for the urgent-start group, which was higher than that of the elective-start group. Several maneuvers have been described to minimize the risk of dialysate leak associated with PD catheter placement in the urgent-start setting. These include recumbent dialysis only with lower dwell volumes and avoidance of dialysate dwells while the patient is upright [9]. In the elective-start setting, patients typically initiate PD after 2–3 weeks to allow

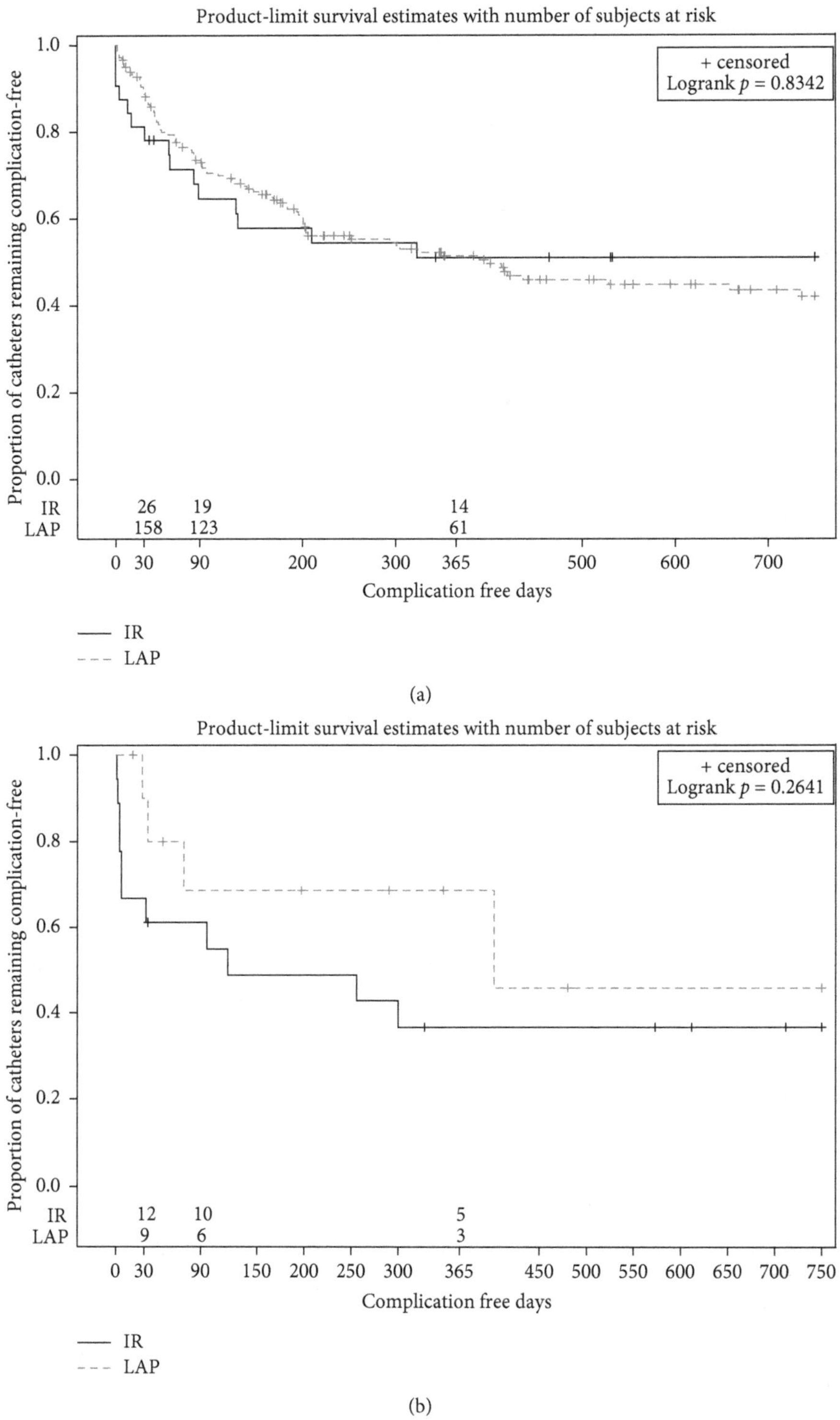

FIGURE 3: Kaplan–Meier curves for catheter complication rates based on radiologic and laparoscopic techniques in the (a) elective-start group and (b) urgent-start group. There was no difference in the complication rates based on the technique used for catheter placement.

for tissue ingrowth of the deeper Dacron cuff, which significantly minimize the risk of dialysate leak into the subcutaneous tissue [9].

The complication-free catheter survival or catheter removal rates in each group did not differ based on the technique of PD catheter placement used. Nayak et al. [16] conducted a prospective case-controlled study on 56 patients comparing the outcomes of patients who underwent conventional PD fourteen days after catheter insertion with those who underwent the urgent-start automated PD within 48 hours of catheter placement. Exit-site leak, catheter blockage, and peritonitis at 90 days were similar in both

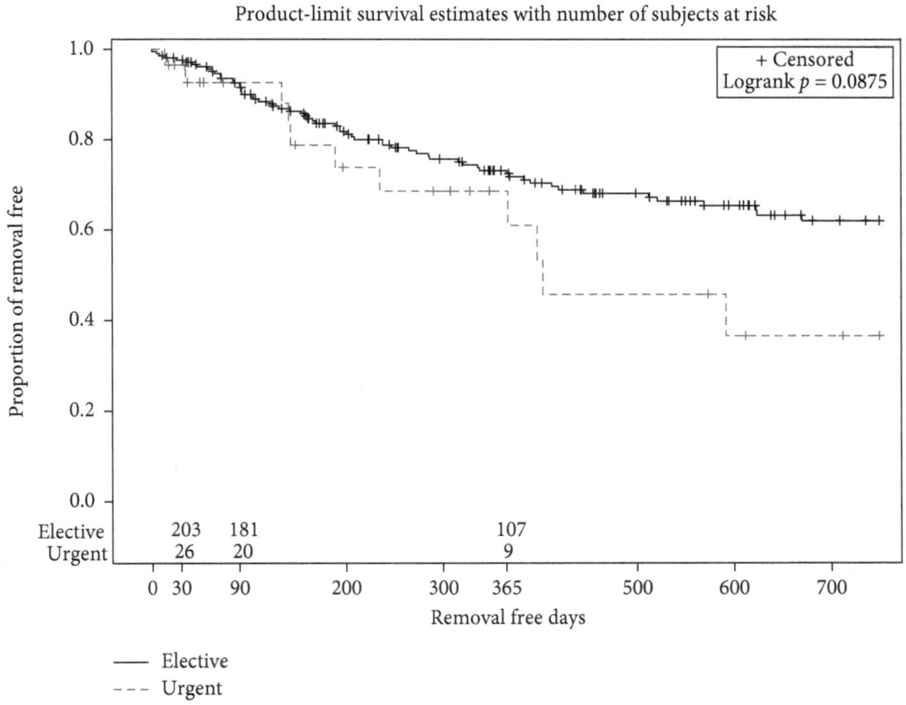

FIGURE 4: Kaplan–Meier curves for overall catheter removal in the elective-start and urgent-start groups showing no difference between the two groups.

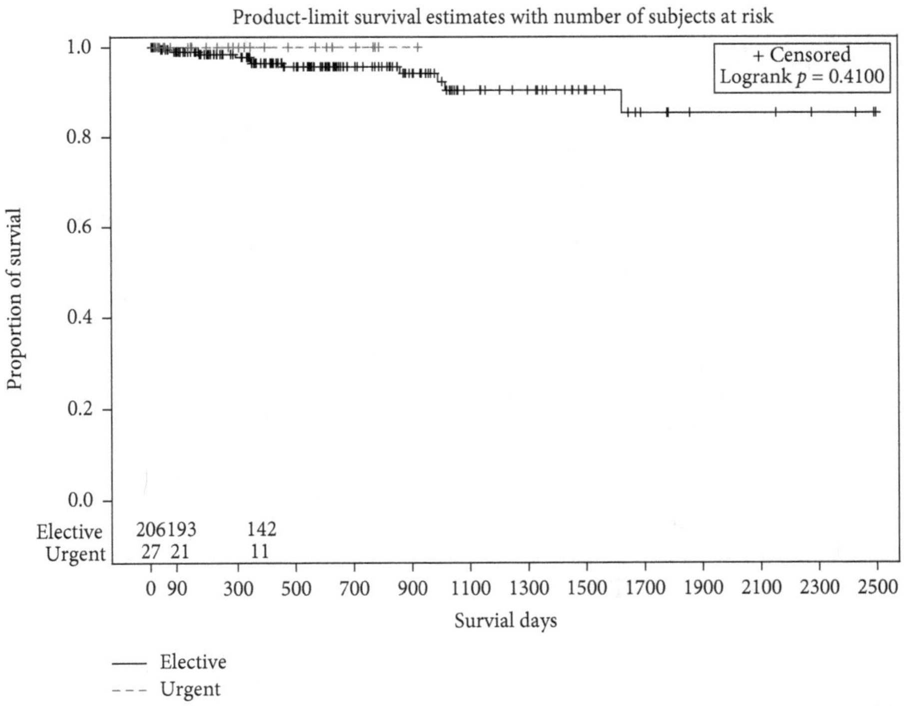

FIGURE 5: Kaplan–Meier curves for overall patient survival in the elective-start and urgent-start groups showing no difference in survival at 12 months.

groups, and the study concluded that urgent-start automated PD in the unplanned patient is an appropriate approach. Another recent study evaluated the safest and shortest interval to commence PD after catheter insertion [17]. Patients were randomized to 3 groups in which PD was started at 1 week, 2 weeks, and 4 weeks. Catheter leak was significantly higher in patients who initiated PD at 1 and 2 weeks compared to 4 weeks. The usage of manual exchanges in that study could have been responsible for the increased incidence of leaks.

A single-center study assessed 30 patients who started on urgent PD, which was initiated within 2 weeks of catheter insertion (range: 0–13 days, median = 6 days), with 66.7% of the PD catheters inserted percutaneously versus 33.3% inserted laparoscopically. Minor pericatheter leak developed in 10% of the patients during the first week of training was treated conservatively. Catheter migration resulting in dysfunction was seen in 20% of patients and was treated by repositioning, without any need for catheter exchange or change in dialysis modality. The study concluded that urgent-start PD is safe and a reasonable alternative option to hemodialysis for patients who need to start PD urgently with no preexisting dialysis access [34]. Several other retrospective studies supported the concept that shorter break-in periods are not associated with more catheter-related complications [9, 35, 36].

Comparison between radiologic and laparoscopic techniques for placement of peritoneal dialysis catheters has been previously published in the literature [19], with no significant difference in the safety and outcomes between the two techniques. This study adds to the evolving literature signifying that PD catheter placement in the urgent-start setting, regardless of the technique used for catheter placement whether radiologic or laparoscopic, is not inferior compared to placement in the elective-start settings and therefore may offer late-referred ESRD patients an alternative patient-centered dialysis option, while avoiding the side effects of placing a CVC.

Future directions will probably focus on continued improvement in the insertion techniques to prevent leaks, implementing protocols that address the urgent-start PD needs to facilitate patient transition to outpatient home dialysis training, and increasing the awareness of the urgent-start PD program to combat the deficits seen among the ER physicians, nephrologists, hospitalists, nursing staff, and discharge planners. The success of an urgent-start program depends on the institution of a multidisciplinary approach to ensure rapid initiation and proper monitoring of PD therapy and smooth transition to long-term PD therapy. This requires teamwork of dedicated interventional radiologists and surgeons, PD nurses, renal nutritionists, and the ancillary hospital resource staff including pharmacy [16].

Limitations of this current study include its retrospective design with selection-bias being an inherent disadvantage. In addition, the study describes a single-center experience, and the results cannot be generalized. Clinical outcomes such as duration of hospital stay and mortality were not included in the analysis.

In conclusion, apart from the higher incidence of catheter leak, the outcomes of PD catheters in the urgent-start setting are not inferior to the elective-start setting with similar complication-free catheter survival and catheter removal rates at 3 and 12 months regardless of the technique used for catheter placement. These findings suggest that urgent-start PD is as safe as elective-start PD and has the advantage of avoiding the side effects and complications associated with CVC placement in late-referred ESRD patients who are considered for PD.

Abbreviations and acronyms

CKD: Chronic kidney disease
ESRD: End-stage renal disease
PD: Peritoneal dialysis
HD: Hemodialysis
CMS: Centers for Medicare and Medicaid Services
KM: Kaplan–Meier.

References

[1] United States Renal Data System, "USRDS 2014 annual data report: atlas of chronic kidney disease and end-stage renal disease in the United States," in *Ch. 1: CKD in the general population*, National Institutes of Health, National Institute of Diabetes and Digestive and Kidney Diseases, Bethesda, MD, USA, 2014.

[2] United States, Department of Health and Human Services, National Institutes of Health, *USRDS 2010 Annual Data Report: Atlas of Chronic Kidney Disease and End-Stage Renal Disease in the United States*, National institute of diabetes and digestive and kidney diseases, US renal data system (USRDS), Bethesda, MD, USA, 2010.

[3] S. W. Klarenbach, M. Tonelli, B. Chui, and B. J. Manns, "Economic evaluation of dialysis therapies," *Nature Reviews Nephrology*, vol. 10, no. 11, pp. 644–652, 2014.

[4] A. K. Abdel-aal, P. Dybbro, P. Hathaway, S. Guest, M. Neuwirth, and V. Krishnamurthy, "Best practices consensus protocol for peritoneal dialysis catheter placement by interventional radiologists," *Peritoneal Dialysis International: Journal of the International Society for Peritoneal Dialysis*, vol. 34, pp. 481–493, 2014.

[5] C. R. Blagg, "Dialysis composite rate bundling: potential effects on the utilization of home hemodialysis, daily and nocturnal hemodialysis, and peritoneal dialysis," *Seminars in Dialysis*, vol. 24, no. 6, pp. 674–677, 2011.

[6] K. Yeates, N. Zhu, E. Vonesh, L. Trpeski, P. Blake, and S. Fenton, "Hemodialysis and peritoneal dialysis are associated with similar outcomes for end-stage renal disease treatment in Canada," *Nephrology Dialysis Transplantation*, vol. 27, no. 9, pp. 3568–3575, 2012.

[7] T. A. Golper, S. Guest, J. D. Glickman, J. Turk, and J. P. Pulliam, "Home dialysis in the new USA bundled payment plan: implications and impact," *Peritoneal Dialysis International: Journal of the International Society for Peritoneal Dialysis*, vol. 31, no. 1, pp. 12–16, 2011.

[8] K. Chaudhary, H. Sangha, and R. Khanna, "Peritoneal dialysis first: rationale," *Clinical Journal of the American Society of Nephrology*, vol. 6, no. 2, pp. 447–456, 2011.

[9] A. Ghaffari, "Urgent-start peritoneal dialysis: a quality improvement report," *American Journal of Kidney Diseases*, vol. 59, no. 3, pp. 400–408, 2012.

[10] R. Arramreddy, S. Zheng, A. B. Saxena, S. E. Liebman, and L. Wong, "Urgent-start peritoneal dialysis: a chance for a new beginning," *American Journal of Kidney Diseases*, vol. 63, no. 3, pp. 390–395, 2014.

[11] M. J. Schreiber Jr., "Changing landscape for peritoneal dialysis: optimizing utilization," *Seminars in Dialysis*, vol. 30, no. 2, pp. 149–157, 2017.

[12] L. M. Moist and C. E. Lok, "Incident dialysis access in patients with end-stage kidney disease: what needs to Be improved," *Seminars in Nephrology*, vol. 37, no. 2, pp. 151–158, 2017.

[13] A. Ghaffari, V. Kumar, and S. Guest, "Infrastructure requirements for an urgent-start peritoneal dialysis program," *Peritoneal Dialysis International: Journal of the International Society for Peritoneal Dialysis*, vol. 33, no. 6, pp. 611–617, 2013.

[14] J. M. Bargman, "Complications of peritoneal dialysis related to increased intraabdominal pressure," *Kidney International Supplements*, vol. 40, pp. S75–S80, 1993.

[15] B. B. McCormick and J. M. Bargman, "Noninfectious complications of peritoneal dialysis: implications for patient and technique survival: table 1," *Journal of the American Society of Nephrology*, vol. 18, no. 12, pp. 3023–3025, 2007.

[16] K. S. Nayak, S. V. Subhramanyam, N. Pavankumar, S. Antony, and M. A. Sarfaraz Khan, "Emergent start peritoneal dialysis for end-stage renal disease: outcomes and advantages," *Blood Purification*, vol. 45, no. 4, pp. 313–319, 2018.

[17] D. Ranganathan, G. T. John, E. Yeoh et al., "A randomized controlled trial to determine the appropriate time to initiate peritoneal dialysis after insertion of catheter (Timely PD study)," *Peritoneal Dialysis International: Journal of the International Society for Peritoneal Dialysis*, vol. 37, no. 4, pp. 420–428, 2017.

[18] E. J. See, Y. Cho, C. M. Hawley, L. R. Jaffrey, and D. W. Johnson, "Early and late patient outcomes in urgent-start peritoneal dialysis," *Peritoneal Dialysis International: Journal of the International Society for Peritoneal Dialysis*, vol. 37, no. 4, pp. 414–419, 2017.

[19] A. K. Abdel Aal, S. S. Guest, S. Moawad et al., "Outcomes of fluoroscopic and ultrasound-guided placement versus laparoscopic placement of peritoneal dialysis catheters," *Clinical Kidney Journal*, vol. 11, no. 4, pp. 549–554, 2018.

[20] A. K. Abdel Aal, S. Gaddikeri, and S. Saddekni, "Technique of peritoneal catheter placement under fluoroscopic guidance," *Radiology Research and Practice*, vol. 2011, Article ID 141707, 4 pages, 2011.

[21] A. K. Abdel-Aal, A. K. Joshi, S. Saddekni, and I. D. Maya, "Fluoroscopic and sonographic guidance to place peritoneal catheters: how we do it," *American Journal of Roentgenology*, vol. 192, no. 4, pp. 1085–1089, 2009.

[22] E. Maher, M. J. Wolley, S. A. Abbas, S. P. Hawkins, and M. R. Marshall, "Fluoroscopic versus laparoscopic implantation of peritoneal dialysis catheters: a retrospective cohort study," *Journal of Vascular and Interventional Radiology*, vol. 25, no. 6, pp. 895–903, 2014.

[23] A. W. Yu, K. F. Chau, Y. W. Ho, and P. K. Li, "Development of the "peritoneal dialysis first" model in Hong Kong," *Peritoneal Dialysis International*, vol. 27, no. 2, pp. S53–S55, 2007.

[24] P. K.-T. Li and C.-C. Szeto, "Success of the peritoneal dialysis programme in Hong Kong," *Nephrology Dialysis Transplantation*, vol. 23, no. 5, pp. 1475–1478, 2008.

[25] E. F. Vonesh, J. J. Snyder, R. N. Foley, and A. J. Collins, "The differential impact of risk factors on mortality in hemodialysis and peritoneal dialysis," *Kidney International*, vol. 66, pp. 2398–2401, 2004.

[26] J. G. Heaf, H. Løkkegaard, and M. Madsen, "Initial survival advantage of peritoneal dialysis relative to haemodialysis," *Nephrology Dialysis Transplantation*, vol. 17, no. 1, pp. 112–117, 2002.

[27] S. S. A. Fenton, D. E. Schaubel, M. Desmeules et al., "Hemodialysis versus peritoneal dialysis: a comparison of adjusted mortality rates," *American Journal of Kidney Diseases*, vol. 30, no. 3, pp. 334–342, 1997.

[28] B. G. Jaar, J. Coresh, L. C. Plantinga et al., "Comparing the risk for death with peritoneal dialysis and hemodialysis in a national cohort of patients with chronic kidney disease," *Annals of Internal Medicine*, vol. 143, no. 3, pp. 174–183, 2005.

[29] E. D. Weinhandl, R. N. Foley, D. T. Gilbertson, T. J. Arneson, J. J. Snyder, and A. J. Collins, "Propensity-matched mortality comparison of incident hemodialysis and peritoneal dialysis patients," *Journal of the American Society of Nephrology*, vol. 21, no. 3, pp. 499–506, 2010.

[30] H. S. Vats, "Complications of catheters: tunneled and non-tunneled," *Advances in Chronic Kidney Disease*, vol. 19, no. 3, pp. 188–194, 2012.

[31] F. X. Liu, A. Ghaffari, H. Dhatt et al., "Economic evaluation of urgent-start peritoneal dialysis versus urgent-start hemodialysis in the United States," *Medicine*, vol. 93, no. 28, p. e293, 2014.

[32] A. Masseur, S. Guest, and V. Kumar, "Early technique success after initiation of treatment with urgent-start peritoneal dialysis," *Advances in Peritoneal Dialysis*, vol. 30, no. 30, pp. 36–39, 2014.

[33] A. Casaretto, R. Rosario, W. R. Kotzker, Y Pagan-Rosario, C Groenhoff, and S Guest, "Urgent-start peritoneal dialysis: report from a U.S. private nephrology practice," *Advances in Peritoneal Dialysis*, vol. 28, no. 28, pp. 102–105, 2012.

[34] A. M. A. Alkatheeri, P. G. Blake, D. Gray, and A. K. Jain, "Success of urgent-start peritoneal dialysis in a large Canadian renal program," *Peritoneal Dialysis International: Journal of the International Society for Peritoneal Dialysis*, vol. 36, no. 2, pp. 171–176, 2016.

[35] Y.-F. Yang, H.-J. Wang, C.-C. Yeh, H.-H. Lin, and C.-C. Huang, "Early initiation of continuous ambulatory peritoneal dialysis in patients undergoing surgical implantation of tenckhoff catheters," *Peritoneal Dialysis International: Journal of the International Society for Peritoneal Dialysis*, vol. 31, no. 5, pp. 551–557, 2011.

[36] J. V. Povlsen and P. Ivarsen, "How to start the late referred ESRD patient urgently on chronic APD," *Nephrology Dialysis Transplantation*, vol. 21, no. 2, pp. ii56–ii59, 2006.

[37] J. H. Song, G. A. Kim, S. W. Lee, and M.-J. Kim, "Clinical outcomes of immediate full-volume exchange one year after peritoneal catheter implantation for CAPD," *Peritoneal Dialysis International: Journal of the International Society for Peritoneal Dialysis*, vol. 20, no. 2, pp. 194–199, 2000.

[38] O. Banli, H. Altun, and A. Oztemel, "Early start of CAPD with the Seldinger technique," *Peritoneal Dialysis International: Journal of the International Society for Peritoneal Dialysis*, vol. 25, no. 6, pp. 556–559, 2005.

[39] Y. Jo, S. K. Shin, J. Lee, J. Song, and J. Park, "Immediate initiation of CAPD following percutaneous catheter placement without break-in procedure," *Peritoneal Dialysis International: Journal of the International Society for Peritoneal Dialysis*, vol. 27, no. 11, pp. 179–183, 2007.

26

Not All Embolizations Are Created Equally in the Management of Posterior Epistaxis: Discussion of Safety Measures Avoiding Neurological Complications

Mareike Franke[1,2] **Jasper Franke,**[3] **Christian Saager,**[1] **Sven Barthel,**[1] **Randolf Riemann,**[4] **and Kersten Mueckner**[1]

[1]*Diagnostic and Interventional Radiology, Dr. Hancken Clinic, 21680 Stade, Germany*
[2]*Department of Radiology, Wesling Hospital Minden, University Hospital of the Ruhr University Bochum, 32429 Minden, Germany*
[3]*53 N Studios, 21682 Stade, Germany*
[4]*Otorhinolaryngology, Head and Neck Surgery, Elbe Hospitals, 21680 Stade, Germany*

Correspondence should be addressed to Mareike Franke; mfr@hancken.de

Academic Editor: Paul Sijens

Today, there are still no uniform guidelines for the treatment of epistaxis. Furthermore, it is widely debated whether embolization or surgical approaches should be the first choice of treatment for intractable posterior epistaxis after conservative measures have failed. In several meta-analyses, it is reported that endoscopic sphenopalatine artery ligation and embolization have similar success rates, but embolization was associated with more severe neurological complications. Regarding existing literature, there are many comparative analyses of surgical methods but none for embolization protocols. Against this backdrop of a lack of uniform standards in embolization techniques, we present a retrospective evaluation of what has emerged to be best procedural practice for endovascular treatment of epistaxis in our department using microsphere particles and microcoils, in particular regarding precaution measures to avoid neurological complications. In our retrospective data analysis of 141 procedures in 123 patients, performed between 2008 and 2019, we find success rates very similar to those reported in other studies (95.1% immediate-stop-of-bleeding success and 90.2% overall embolization success) but did not encounter any major neurological complication opposed to other reports. We suggest some aspects of our protocol as precaution measure to avoid neurological complications. More generally and perhaps even more importantly, we make a strong case for standardization for embolization techniques to the level of details in surgical procedure standardization to enable an apples to apples comparison of embolization techniques to each other and of intervention vs. surgery.

1. Introduction

Epistaxis is a common medical condition but is rarely a direct cause for hospital admission. Up to 60% of adult population experience nasal bleeding at some stage of their lives, but only 6% need medical help [1].

In most cases, the bleeding starts from the anterior septal area (Little area), which is vascularized by Kiesselbach's plexus. As the Little area is readily accessible, hemorrhage from this region can usually be managed by applying pressure to the nostrils, chemical or electrocautery, topical hemostatic or vasoconstricting agents, cryotherapy, or anterior nasal packing. However, severe, intractable bleeding usually arises from a posterior source, causing conservative measures to fail [2].

In general, for sufficient therapeutic management of anterior or posterior epistaxis, a profound anatomical knowledge of the branches of the external carotid artery and arterial blood supply of the nasal cavity is absolutely necessary (Figure 1).

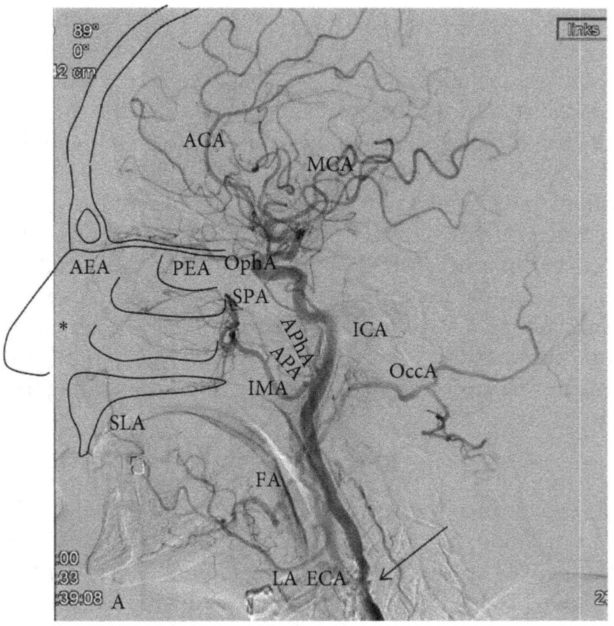

FIGURE 1: Arterial supply of nasal cavity. Digital subtraction angiography via the common carotid artery shows branches of the external and internal carotid artery (ECA and ICA; 90° LAO). For better understanding of the anatomy some anatomical structures like the nasal conchae, the floor of nasal cavity, nose, and frontobasis are drawn schematically. The major part of blood supply for the nasal cavity is provided via branches of the ECA. Especially the sphenopalatine artery (SPA), and end-branch of the internal maxillary artery (IMA), is the main blood supply for the nasal cavity and for Kiesselbach's plexus (asterisk). The roof of the nasal cavity is supplied by the anterior ethmoidal artery (AEA) and posterior ethmoidal artery (PEA), which are branches of the ophthalmic artery (OphA), i.e., branches of the internal carotid artery (ICA). The blood supply to the floor of the nasal cavity originates from ascending palatine arteries (APA) from the facial artery (FA) and descending palatine artery (DPA) from IMA. Little supply to Kiesselbach's plexus comes from the superior labial artery (SLA), an end-branch of the FA. And, finally minor supply to the posterior area of the nasal cavity is provided by the ascending pharyngeal artery (APhA), which originates from the ECA. Note the calcification of proximal ICA (arrow). Also shown are occipital artery (OccA), ophthalmic artery (OPhA), and intracranial arteries like anterior and middle cerebral artery (ACA and MCA). As ICA and ECA both contribute to the blood supply of the nasal cavity sometimes, there are some "dangerous" anastomoses, which can cause blindness or stroke when accidentally embolized during the procedure. These potentially "dangerous" anastomoses include the artery of the foramen rotundum, the middle meningeal artery, the accessory meningeal artery, the ethmoidal arteries, the APhA, and of course the communications between the FA and OPhA[3].

An option to control such posterior bleeding is the application of anterior and posterior packs (AP packs). These packs have been reported to have a success rate between 48% and 83% [4–6]. As they can lead to nasal trauma, vagal response, aspiration, infection, allergic reactions, and airway obstruction they should be applied with care and under patient monitoring [7, 8].

If conservative measures fail, reducing the blood supply to the sinonasal area is an option. This can be achieved either with a surgical or endovascular approach. Different surgical methods have been described: there is a wide range from transantral artery ligation, submoucous resection, external carotid artery (ECA) ligation, and anterior ethmoidal artery ligation to endoscopic sphenopalatine artery ligation [9]. So far, endoscopic sphenopalatine artery ligation has the most favorable adverse effect profile and success rate compared with other surgical approaches [9–13].

Endovascular treatment of epistaxis was first presented in 1974 as an alternative to surgery by Sokoloff et al. [14] and consisted of particle embolization of the ipsilateral internal maxillary artery (IMA). Later, Lasjaunias et al. [15] refined the technique stressing the need for a standardized angiographic and therapeutic protocol. Due to dangerous anastomoses between the external and internal carotid arteries with the risk of embolic material entering the internal carotid artery or ophthalmic artery, the procedure comes with the risk of severe neurologic complication, such as hemiplegia, ophthalmoplegia, facial paralysis/paresthesia, or blindness [16, 17]. Cases of facial necrosis are published as well [18–20].

As with surgery, there are many different protocols and techniques for embolization described (reviewed in [9] and [21]). Despite this multitude of techniques and protocols, no comparing study exists. The following methods have been individually described in literature [19, 21, 22]:

(a) Embolization of the ipsilateral IMA and sphenopalatine artery (SPA) or
(b) Embolization the ipsi- and contralateral IMA/SP or
(c) Embolization of the ipsilateral or both ipsi- and contralateral IMA/SPA in combination with embolization of the ipsilateral or both ipsi- and contralateral facial artery.

There are also many different embolization materials used (polyvinyl alcohol, coils, microspheres, gelfoam, etc. [21]). In general, the success rates of endovascular therapy have been reported between 75 and 92% [9, 21].

Today, the possible treatment options for intractable epistaxis are widely debated. While endovascular treatment is arguably easier on the patient requiring no general anesthesia and has a shorter hospital stay [23], the presence of "dangerous anastomoses" and the associated risk of cerebrovascular accident (CVA) is feared [3, 16].

We believe the main contribution of this paper to be twofold: (1) we retrospectively evaluated 141 mostly microsphere-based procedures performed on 123 patients at our hospital, thus contributing to a still very thin report base. (2) We find that—besides an encouragingly high success rate and a tolerable rate of rebleedings—not a single CVA occurred in our sample. We believe this to be due to the precautionary measures developed as part of our interventional protocol using calibrated microspheres and coils.

2. Materials and Methods

Between 2008 and 2019, 141 percutaneous endovascular embolization procedures for epistaxis were performed on

123 patients (80 male, 43 female, mean age 66, ranging from 18 to 90 years). Patients were referred to us by the hospital's otorhinolaryngologist after failed conventional treatment, involving anterior and posterior nasal packing and/or cauterization. Preinterventional imaging was not mandatorily performed. Patients suffered from severe epistaxis (as classified in [24]). Approximately 20% of patients required blood transfusion due to chronic blood loss over a time period of several days with a drop in hemoglobin levels. Interventions were performed with AP packs in situ. None of the patients which underwent intervention were in hemorrhagic shock.

All interventions were performed on an emergency basis in the angiographic facility of our department (until 2008 using a Siemens Axiom Artis angiography unit; from 2008 until today using a Philips Allura XP angiography unit). Patients received a mild sedation (1–2.5 mg Midazolam i.v.). Monitoring of blood pressure and pulse oximetry was performed during the procedure. Patient assessment was performed according to Table 1.

Pathologic coagulation parameters had to be balanced by the referring department (INR < 1.5, platelets > 60,000 per μl). The embolization procedure was performed according to Table 2 (Figure 2).

For synergistic effects, AP packs were left overnight and removed the next day. 6 Patients had an embolization only with coils, without particles due to re-embolization of contralateral side during the first five days or an embolization of other arteries than SPA/distal IMA (Figures 3 and 4).

Data were analyzed in terms of etiologies of epistaxis, duration of procedure (i.e., duration of vulnerable time with catheters in the carotid arteries), overall embolization success, immediate-stop-of-bleeding success, and complications. Overall embolization success of endovascular treatment was defined as successful one- or double-sided embolization of IMA/SPA avoiding surgery during a follow-up period of at least 6 months. Note that this definition of success also includes cases of patients which had to be re-embolized as the first embolization did in some cases not stop the bleeding immediately, but in all cases of embolization success, the patient avoided the more invasive treatment of surgery. Immediate-stop-of-bleeding success was classified as stopping the bleeding immediately for the next five days. While in some cases, the patients had to be re-embolized or required subsequent surgery; we considered it a success because the patient had at least five days during which they did not lose blood and did not require blood transfusion and could recover without AP packs. These two types of success are individually important but represent two distinct dimensions of benefit to the patient and are thus evaluated separately. Adverse effects were classified in major and minor complications according to [25].

3. Results and Discussion

3.1. Results. As described in the literature, many cases of epistaxis were idiopathic (Table 3).

Due to noncompliance, 4 patients needed general anesthesia. In terms of overall embolization success, one-sided or double-sided embolization safely controlled hemorrhage in 111 of 123 patients, which needed no further surgery (Table 4). Technical success rate was 99.3% with one technical failure. In this case, a catheterization of the IMA was not possible. Immediate-stop-of-bleeding success could be achieved in 117 of 123 patients (95.1%). Early rebleeding within the first five days after first embolization could be observed in six patients (4.8%). In 16 cases, rebleeding occurred more than five days after embolization (13.0%).

No life-threatening adverse event occurred (Table 4). Especially no CVA could be observed. The average procedure duration (i.e., duration of vulnerable period with catheters in carotid arteries) was 17.4 minutes, ranging from 4 to 31 minutes.

3.2. Discussion. There are some meta-analyses stating that there are more neurological complications for endovascular treatment of epistaxis compared to surgery [3] (in contrary to other [26]) and case series/reports showing neurological and facial complications of endovascular treatment [16, 18]. This leads to the opinion that endoscopic ligation of the sphenopalatine artery should be the method of choice and embolization should be performed in cases where surgical treatment fails or the patient has a high anesthetic risk. In our center, however, the endovascular treatment after failure of conservative measure is routine, which emerged also from the discussion with our otorhinolaryngologists. It has been investigated that there is a high risk of contamination of medical staff with patient`s blood during surgery [27, 28]. Since we are frequently asked to treat epistaxis, we developed a protocol with high safety standards to avoid CVA. All patients were hemodynamically stable with nasal packs in situ. The INR/platelet count had to be normalized before therapy (INR < 1.5 and platelets >60,000 μl). Despite being admitted with diagnosis of intractable epistaxis, all patients received a dose of 5,000 I.E. heparin at the procedure's beginning to avoid clot formation in catheters or adherent to the wires [29]. As complication rate increases with arteriosclerotic vessel changes and procedure time [30–32], we try to keep the time of carotid catheterization as low as possible. Therefore, we prefer a "no-touch of ICA" strategy: In contrary to other publications (e.g., [15, 33]), we do not perform a selective angiogram of the ICA because of calcifications in the passing region with the risk of thrombus release and in addition increasing time of procedure. Only an angiogram of the carotid bifurcation is performed in every patient to identify ICA stenosis or occlusion which could lead to recruitment of ECA/ICA collateral pathways requiring special attention. To detect the dangerous ICA/ECA-anastomoses, we perform an accurate angiogram of ECA and of the pterygopalatinal segment of IMA.

Another safety measure is continuous pressure flushing of the guiding catheter in the ECA to prevent blood clots. Additionally, we carefully rinse the microcatheter after application of particles before coil embolization of SPA and IMA to avoid dislocation of particles. In general, you have to keep in mind that stained micorparticles may be visible through the skin if injected into superficial arteries [34].

Table 1: Patient assessment before and after intervention.

Indication	Refractory posterior epistaxis after 48 h conservative treatment, confirming indication by otorhinolaryngologist and radiologist
Laboratory assessment	Creatinine, thyroid-stimulating hormone, platelet count, hemoglobin, INR
Sedation/anesthesia	Mild sedation with midazolam or general anesthesia when necessary (e.g., restless patient)
Assessment in the operating suite	The patient placed lying down, infusion (500 ml sodium chloride), head sedated with no radiopaque materials in beam path (e.g., remove dental prosthesis)
	One operator, one operator assistant, and an additional suite technician and anesthesiologist when necessary
Assessment after procedure	AngioSeal/ExoSeal occlusion of vessel access (common femoral artery), manual compression for 10–15 minutes, compression bandage overnight, ultrasound control of groin the next day

Table 2: Standard protocol of procedure (see also Figure 2).

Step 1	Femoral artery access, 5 F introducer sheath
Step 2	Administration of 5000 I.E. heparin to avoid blood clots
Step 3	Catheterize common carotid artery (CCA) with 5 F guide catheter (100 cm) and hydrophilic guide wire
Step 4	Angiogram of the carotid bifurcation (40° RAO or LAO, resp.)
Step 5	Catheterize external carotid artery (ECA) with guide wire and guide wire—tip of catheter approx. 2 cm above the bifurcation
Step 6	Angiogram of ECA to find hazardous anastomoses or other unusual causes of epistaxis, e.g., AVM, tumor, pseudoaneurysm of sinonasal arteries
Step 7	Pressure flushing of guiding catheter in ECA with heparinised normal saline and introduce microcatheter and microwire
Step 8	Identify internal maxillary artery (IMA) and sphenopalatine artery (SPA) and catheterize
Step 9	Angiogram of IMA/SPA ("dangerous anastomoses" and MMA (Figure 2)
Step 10	When there are no hazardous anastomoses, embolize SPA/pterygopalatine segment of IMA with calibrated microparticles in dilution with contrast medium (500 μm) until flow begins to slow. Important: avoid reflux, especially avoid embolization of MMA (headaches and hazardous anastomoses; Figure 2) When there are ECA-ICA anastomoses, directly go to step 12
Step 11	Rinse the microcatheter properly to avoid dislocation of microparticles
Step 12	Embolize SPA and distal IMA with microcoils
Step 13	Control angiogram
Step 14	Quick removal of all catheters from the carotid arteries
Step 15	Removal of introducer sheath, AngioSeal, or ExoSeal occlusion of vessel, compression bandage until the next day
Step 16	Nasal packing is left intact overnight and removed for inspection for bleeding the next day

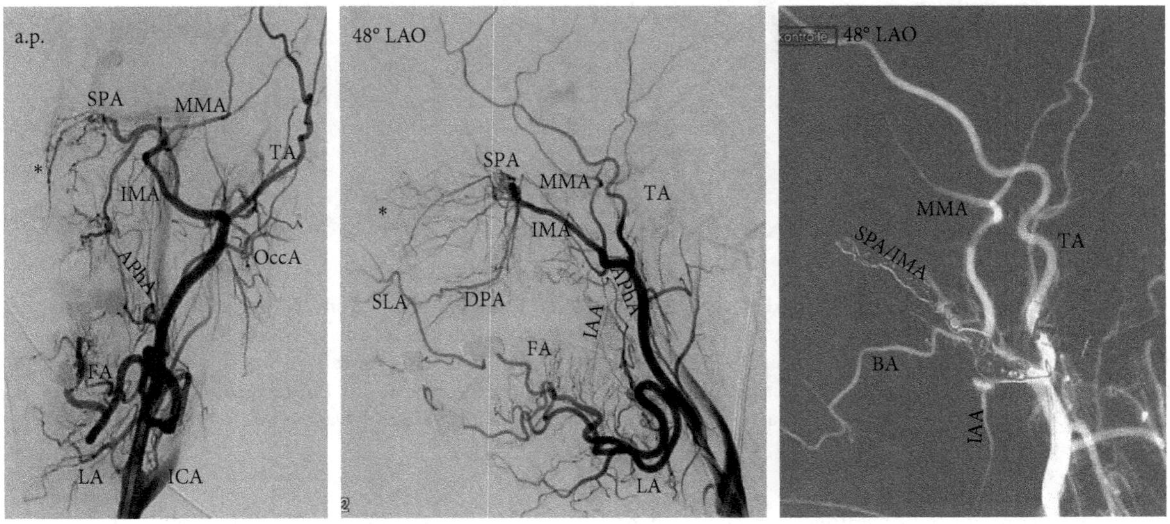

(a) (b) (c)

Figure 2: Embolization of the left internal maxillary artery/sphenopalatine artery (IMA/SPA) in a 49-year-old female patient with hereditary hemorrhagic telangiectasia. A.p. (a) and 48° LAO (b, c) Angiogram of left external carotid artery (ECA) shows arterial supply of nasal cavity via IMA. (a, b) Main supply of Kiesselbach's plexus (asterisk) is provided via SPA, but there also collaterals to the superior labial artery (SLA, a branch of the facial artery FA). (c) Angiogram after embolization with micospheres and coils: there is no contrast flow in the SPA. Particle embolization of the SPA/distal IMA needs to be done very carefully to avoid accidental nontarget embolization of the middle meningeal artery (MMA) with possible hazardous anastomoses to ICA branches. Also shown is the labial artery (LA), temporal artery (TA), buccal artery (BA), occipital artery (OccA), descending palatine artery (DPA), and inferior alveolar artery (IAA).

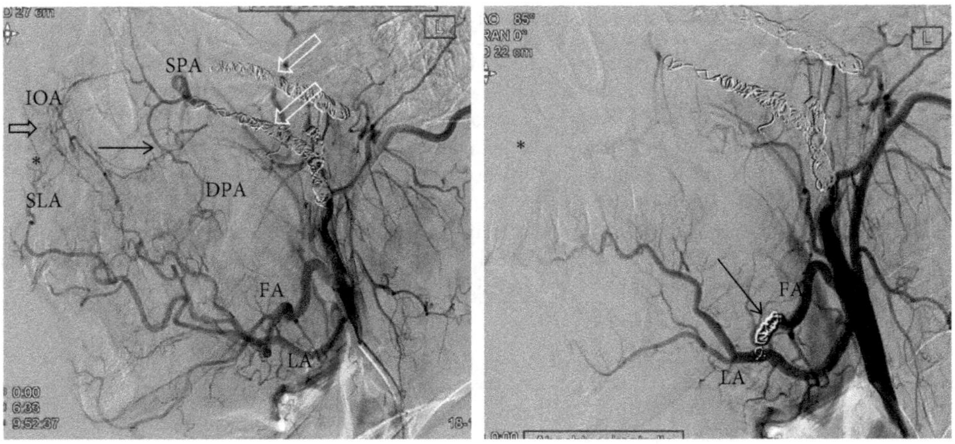

(a) (b)

Figure 3: Embolization of left facial artery (FA) in a 25-year-old male patient with epistaxis and hereditary hemorrhagic telangiectasia having had a double-sided embolization 5 years ago. (a) Angiogram of the external carotid artery (ECA) shows coils in both SPA/IMA (right and left; white open arrows) after a successful double-sided embolization in 2014. Examination shows an extended collateral network via the facial artery (FA) in 2019. The collateral network consists of cross-connections of the superior labial artery (SLA)/infraorbital artery (IOA, open black arrow) and branches of FA/descending palatine artery (DPA, black arrow). (b) Coil embolization of FA was performed (black arrow). Control angiogram after embolization shows no significant contrast flow in the collateral network and Kiesselbach's plexus. Also shown is the labial artery (LA).

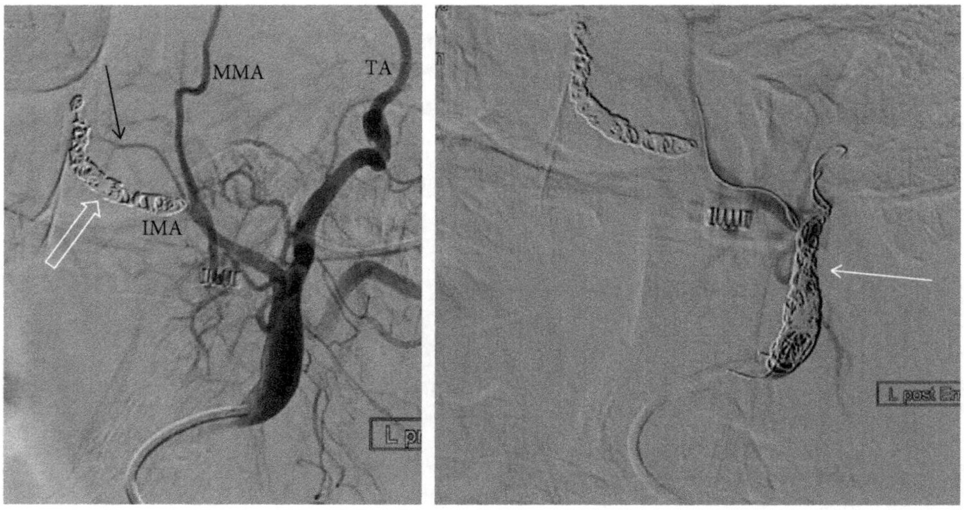

(a) (b)

Figure 4: Re-embolization of left external carotid artery (ECA) due to an accessory artery from IMA in a 72-year-old male patient with epistaxis (risk factor: anticoagulation). (a) Angiogram of ECA shows coils in the internal maxillary artery (IMA) and sphenopalatine artery (SPA, open white arrow) after embolization 53 days earlier. However, there is an accessory artery rising from of the proximal IMA (black arrow), then running to the dorsal part of the nasal cavity, potentially being responsible for the rebleeding. (b) Decision was made to embolize the ECA to stop the blood supply to this artery. No particles were used. Embolization was performed with coils (white arrow). Also shown are middle meningeal artery (MMA) and temporal artery (TA).

Therefore, we make sure to use nonstained particles for head and neck embolizations. The size of microspheres for embolization is carefully chosen. While smaller particles are able to penetrate more distally into capillary beds, they can also cause injury to the vasa nervorum resulting in cranial nerve palsies or enter the intracranial circulation through ECA/ICA anastomoses. When using microspheres, it is recommended to oversize these particles for head and neck embolization compared with polyvinyl alcohol (PVA) particles [20]. We use 500 μm calibrated microparticles for embolization. The application should be performed in highest magnification and dose of continuous fluoroscopy to detect a reflux instantly to prevent nontarget embolization. Particle embolization is halted when flow starts to slow. If there was any doubt about (1) ICA/ECA-anastomoses, (2) the need for a second embolization during the first week, or (3) the need to embolize other arteries than IMA/SPA, no particles were used at all to avoid CVA or facial necrosis. The embolization with coils only had a slightly higher failure rate than particle plus coil-embolization (one of 6 patients

Table 3: Etiologies of epistaxis.

Etiology	No. of patients
Idiopathic epistaxis (no risk factor could be detected)	45
Anticoagulant therapy	26
Hypertension	23
Anticoagulant therapy and hypertension	8
Low platelet count	1
Alcohol withdrawal	1
Surgical complication/preliminary surgery	7
Malignant tumor	8
Trauma	1
Hereditary hemorrhagic telangiectasia	3

Table 4: Outcome of patients in a follow-up period of at least 6 months.

In 111 patients, embolization controlled active hemorrhage and no surgery was necessary	90.2%
(i) In 101 patients, a one-sided embolization was sufficient to stop the bleeding	
(ii) 2 patients had a rebleeding **at the third and fourth days** after intervention and needed embolization of contralateral side; embolization of the contralateral site was performed without particles to avoid facial necrosis, since there was only a short interval to the first embolization	
(iii) 4 patients had a rebleeding **at the 7th till 14th day** after intervention and needed embolization of the contralateral side	
(iv) 2 patients had a rebleeding **after 31 and 32 days** after intervention and needed embolization of contralateral side	
(v) 1 patient had a rebleeding **after 5 months** after intervention and needed embolization of the contralateral side	
(vi) 1 patient with hereditary hemorrhagic telangiectasia had a successful double-sided embolization in 2014 (rebleeding after 36 days) and a rebleeding in 2019; in 2019, an embolization of the facial artery was performed without particles (Figure 3)	
12 patients needed additional surgery	9.7%
(i) 4 patients had **surgery at the following** day after one-sided embolization due to recurrence of bleeding	
(ii) 1 patient had a rebleeding **7 days** after one-sided embolization and received surgery	
(iii) 3 patients had a rebleeding after **7, 22, and 28 days**, respectively, after successful endovascular treatment, and contralateral embolization failed to stop the rebleeding, surgery was performed	
(iv) 1 patient had a rebleeding **one week** after successful embolization; embolization failed due to lack of possibility to catheterize contralateral IMA (technical failure); the patient received surgery	
(v) 2 patients with hereditary hemorrhagic telangiectasia had a rebleeding **49 and 97 days**, respectively, after a successful embolization; contralateral embolization was not successful in stopping the bleeding; surgery was performed	
(vi) 1 patient had a successful embolization of left IMA/SPA and **53 days** later had a rebleeding on the left side; an embolization of the left external carotid artery (ECA) was performed due to an atypical accessory artery (Figure 4); **7 days** later, a rebleeding occurred and embolization of the right IMA/SPA was performed; due to recurrence of bleeding, surgery was performed	

needed further surgery; success rate: 83.3%). Some reports criticize the use of coils in general, because the possibility of repetition of distal embolization could be lost [23]. We use particle and coil embolization of SPA/IMA as we have the impression that, by doing so, we reduce also the residual flow and pressure via the IMA in prevention of a relapse. Furthermore, revascularization after embolization often occurs either via the contralateral side or via the facial artery, thus these arteries can be easily embolized during a second procedure. Should a revascularization occur via the ethmoidal arteries, a surgical therapy would be required.

Rebleeding is a known problem for the treatment of epistaxis. Primary double-sided or triple-artery embolizations are described in the literature postulating that the rate of early recurrences decreases with the number of arteries embolized [19]. However, this group had a certain rate of nose necrosis and several cases of facial edema. A case analysis from 2018 even found out that bilateral particle embolization including facial artery was the treatment method associated with a significant risk of complications [35]. With the exception of patients with hereditary hemorrhagic telangiectasia, one-sided embolization was very efficient in most cases. All 3 patients with hereditary hemorrhagic telangiectasia needed at least a double-sided embolization, and two of them had further surgery after primary bleeding control. In general, these patients are difficult to treat.

The only observed major complications were access site complications with a slightly increased rate of arterial occlusions (1.4% vs. 0.1–0.9% [36]). The reason for this could be the introduction of vascular closure devices in 2008 with no extensive experience during the first month of use. A few cases of headache after embolization could be well handled with analgesics.

The limitation of our case series is of course the small case number of 141 procedures. Although this is to our knowledge one of the largest primary case series in literature, it does not allow postulating general rules at statistical significance. Our protocol has been proved to be safe and effective with a primary efficiency of 95% with no neurological complications. So, we would like to present our protocol or aspects of our protocol as a suggestion for the reader or as basis of a further discussion.

4. Conclusions

Despite reports in the literature describing a higher rate of cerebrovascular complications compared to surgery, we think that when implementing the abovementioned security precautions, embolization of sphenopalatine artery with microcoils and microparticles is a safe, fast, and effective method to stop posterior epistaxis without requiring general anesthesia. Today, there is still no uniform standard in embolization of epistaxis and a complex data situation with different techniques and materials described. We feel the strong need for a systematic comparison of different embolization techniques and recommend further investigations to compare outcome/complication rate of different protocols to develop a uniform standard.

References

[1] M. Small, J. Murray, and A. G. D. Maran, "A study of patients with epistaxis requiring admission to hospital," *Health Bulletin (Edinburgh)*, vol. 40, pp. 20–29, 1982.

[2] R. A. Viducich, M. P. Blanda, and L. W. Gerson, "Posterior epistaxis: clinical features andacute complications," *Annals of Emergency Medicine*, vol. 25, pp. 592–969, 1995.

[3] W. Brinjikji, D. F. Kallmes, and H. J. Cloft, "Trends in epistaxis embolization in the United States: a study of the nationwide inpatient sample 2003–2010," *Journal of Vascular and Interventional Radiology*, vol. 24, no. 7, pp. 969–973, 2013.

[4] P. A. Pollice and M. G. Yoder, "Epistaxis: a retrospective review of hospitalized patients," *Otolaryngology—Head and Neck Surgery*, vol. 117, pp. 49–5311, 1997.

[5] D. A. Klotz, M. R. Winkle, J. Richmon et al., "Surgical management of posterior epistaxis: a changing paradigm," *The Laryngoscope*, vol. 112, no. 9, pp. 1577–8212, 2002.

[6] B. Schaitkin, M. Strauss, and J. R. Houck, "Epistaxis: medical versus surgical therapy—a comparison of efficacy, complications, and economic considerations," *Laryngoscope*, vol. 97, pp. 1392–1396, 1987.

[7] R. Beck, M. Sorge, A. Schneider, and A. Dietz, "Current approaches to epistaxis treatment in primary and secondary care," *Deutsches Arzteblatt International*, vol. 115, no. 1-2, pp. 12–22, 2018.

[8] E. D. Monte, M. J. Belmont, and M. K. Wax, "Management paradigms for posterior epistaxis: a comparison of costs and complications," *Otolaryngology-Head and Neck Surgery*, vol. 121, no. 1, pp. 103–106, 1999.

[9] C. Swords, A. Patel, M. E. Smith, R. J. Williams, I. Kuhn, and C. Hopkins, "Surgical and interventional radiological management of adult epistaxis: systematic review," *The Journal of Laryngology & Otology*, vol. 131, no. 12, pp. 1108–1130, 2017.

[10] A. Asanau, A. P. Timoshenko, P. Vercherin, C. Martin, and J.-M. Prades, "Sphenopalatine and anterior ethmoidal artery ligation for severe epistaxis," *Annals of Otology, Rhinology & Laryngology*, vol. 118, no. 9, pp. 639–644, 2009.

[11] V. Srinivasan, I. W. Sherman, and G. O'Sullivan, "Surgical management of intractable epistaxis: audit of results," *The Journal of Laryngology & Otology*, vol. 114, pp. 697–700, 2000.

[12] N. Umapathy, A. Quadri, and D. W. Skinner, "Persistent epistaxis: what is the best practice?" *Rhinology*, vol. 43, pp. 305–308, 2005.

[13] S. A. R. Nouraei, T. Maani, D. Hajioff, H. A. Saleh, and I. S. Mackay, "Outcome of endoscopic sphenopalatine artery occlusion for intractable epistaxis: a 10-year experience," *The Laryngoscope*, vol. 117, no. 8, pp. 1452–1456, 2007.

[14] J. Sokoloff, I. Wickbom, D. McDonald, F. Brahme, T. G. Goergen, and L. E. Goldberger, "Therapeutic percutaneous embolization in intractable epistaxis," *Radiology*, vol. 111, no. 2, pp. 285–287, 1974.

[15] P. Lasjaunias, K. Marsot-Dupuch, and D. Doyon, "The radio-anatomical basis of arterial embolisation for epistaxis," *Journal of Neuroradiology*, vol. 6, no. 1, pp. 45–53, 1979.

[16] P. Huyett, B. T. Jankowitz, E. W. Wang, and C. H. Snyderman, "Endovascular embolization in the treatment of epistaxis," *Otolaryngology-Head and Neck Surgery*, vol. 160, no. 5, pp. 822–828, 2019.

[17] I. C. Duncan, P. A. Fourie, C. E. le Grange, and H. A van der Walt, "Endovascular treatment of intractable epistaxis—results of a 4-year local audit," *South African Medical Journal*, vol. 94, no. 5, pp. 373–378, 2004.

[18] K. Nishimoto, R. Minoda, R. Yoshida et al., "A case of periodontal necrosis following embolization of maxillary artery for epistaxis," *Case Rep Otolaryngol*, vol. 2016, Article ID 6467974, 6 pages, 2016.

[19] R. Gottumukkala, Y. Kadkhodayan, C. J. Moran, D. W. T. Cross, and C. P. Derdeyn, "Impact of vessel choice on outcomes of polyvinyl alcohol embolization for intractable idiopathic epistaxis," *Journal of Vascular and Interventional Radiology*, vol. 24, no. 2, pp. 234–239, 2013.

[20] N. N. Khoury, P.-O. Champagne, M. Kotowski, J. Raymond, D. Roy, and A. Weill, "Unexpected complications with head and neck hydrogel microsphere particle embolization: a case series and a technical note," *Interventional Neuroradiology*, vol. 23, no. 1, pp. 107–111, 2017.

[21] G. J. Dubel, S. H. Ahn, and G. M. Soares, "Transcatheter embolization in the management of epistaxis," *Seminars in Interventional Radiology*, vol. 30, no. 3, pp. 249–262, 2013.

[22] Q. A. Shah, "Bilateral tri-arterial embolization for the treatment of epistaxis," *Journal of Vascular and Interventional Neurology*, vol. 1, no. 4, pp. 102–105, 2008.

[23] A. Krajina and V. Chrobok, "Radiological diagnosis and management of epistaxis," *CardioVascular and Interventional Radiology*, vol. 37, no. 1, pp. 26–36, 2014.

[24] A. Reyre, J. Michel, L. Santini et al., "Epistaxis: the role of arterial embolization," *Diagnostic and Interventional Imaging*, vol. 96, no. 7-8, pp. 757–773, 2015.

[25] D. K. Filippiadis, C. Binkert, O. Pellerin, R. T. Hoffmann, A. Krajina, and P. L. Pereira, "Cirse quality assurance document and standards for classification of complications: the cirse classification system," *CardioVascular and Interventional Radiology*, vol. 40, no. 8, pp. 1141–1146, 2017.

[26] M. J. Sylvester, S. Y. Chung, L. A. Guinand, A. Govindan, S. Baredes, and J. A. Eloy, "Arterial ligation versus embolization in epistaxis management: counterintuitive national trends," *The Laryngoscope*, vol. 127, no. 5, pp. 1017–1020, 2017.

[27] A. J. Prior, P. Q. Montgomery, and V. Srinivasan, "Eye protection in ear, nose and throat surgery," *The Journal of Laryngology & Otology*, vol. 107, no. 7, pp. 618-619, 1993.

[28] R. Riemann, "Tipps & Tricks—Epistaxis Management unter Berücksichtigung der Kontamination," *Laryngo-Rhino-Otologie*, vol. 95, no. 1, pp. 11–14, 2016.

[29] R. Antonovic, J. Rosch, and C. Dotter, "The value of systemic arterial heparinization in transfemoral angiography: a prospective study," *American Journal of Roentgenology*, vol. 127, no. 2, pp. 223–225, 1976.

[30] A. F. AbuRahma, P. A. Robinson, J. P. Boland et al., "Complications of arteriography in a recent series of 707 cases: factors affecting outcome," *Annals of Vascular Surgery*, vol. 7, no. 2, pp. 122–129, 1993.

[31] J. E. Heiserman, B. L. Dean, J. A. Hodak et al., "Neurologic complications of cerebral angiography," *American Society of Neuroradiology*, vol. 15, pp. 1408–1411, 1994.

[32] J. E. Dion, P. C. Gates, A. J. Fox, H. J. Barnett, and R. J. Blom, "Clinical events following neuroangiography: a prospective study," *Stroke*, vol. 18, no. 6, pp. 997–1004, 1987.

[33] P. W. A. Willems, R. I. Farb, and R. Agid, "Endovascular treatment of epistaxis," *American Journal of Neuroradiology*, vol. 30, no. 9, pp. 1637–1645, 2009.

[34] http://www.bostonscientific.com/en-US/products/embolization/Embozene-Microspheres/Embozene-Microspheres-Indications-Safety-and-Warnings.html.

[35] G. de Bonnecaze, Y. Gallois, F. Bonneville, S. Vergez, B. Chaput, and E. Serrano, "Transnasal endoscopic sphenopalatine artery ligation compared with embolization for intractable epistaxis: a long-term analysis," *American Journal of Rhinology & Allergy*, vol. 32, no. 3, pp. 188–193, 2018.

[36] R. Reich, E. R. Rabelo-Silva, S. M. D. Santos et al., "Vascular access complications in patients undergoing percutaneous procedures in hemodynamics: a scoping review," *Revista Gaúcha de Enfermagem/EENFUFRGS*, vol. 38, no. 4, Article ID e68716, 2018.

27

COVID-19 Viral Pneumonia Complicated with Acute Pulmonary Embolism: A Descriptive Study

Hoda Salah Darwish ,[1,2] Mohamed Yasser Habash,[3] and Waleed Yasser Habash[4]

[1]*Radiology Department, Faculty of Medicine, Suez Canal University, Ismailia, Egypt*
[2]*Dallah Hospital, Riyadh, Saudi Arabia*
[3]*Faculty of Medicine, Kasr Alainy Cairo University, Cairo, Egypt*
[4]*Faculty of Medicine, New Giza University, Giza, Egypt*

Correspondence should be addressed to Hoda Salah Darwish; darwish.hoda@yahoo.com

Academic Editor: Daniele La Forgia

Objective. To evaluate acute pulmonary embolism in patients with 2019 novel coronavirus (COVID-19) pneumonia using pulmonary CT angiography. *Subjects and Methods.* From 95 symptomatic patients confirmed with COVID-19 by RT-PCR from 1 May to 14 July 2020 in Dallah Hospital, Riyadh, Saudi Arabia, CT angiography was done for 25 patients suspected to have pulmonary embolism and have no contraindication for contrast study. 11 cases of them showed CT evidence of acute pulmonary embolism (PE). Retrospectively, CT angiography was analyzed and detailed findings were recorded. This study was approved by the Institutional Review Board of our hospital, and the patient consent was waived. *Results.* The mean age of the included patients was 49 ± 11 years; the youngest was 22 years, and the oldest was 64 years. Common symptoms in the 25 cases that underwent CT angiography were fever that was noted in 21/25 cases (84%), shortness of breath in 18/25 cases (72%), cough in 16/25 cases (64%), and severe myalgia/body fatigue in 13/25 cases (52%). The less common symptoms were sore throat in 11/25 cases (44%) and headache in 10/25 cases (40%). Regarding CT findings, 4/25 cases (16%) had unilateral lung disease and 21/25 cases (84%) had bilateral disease, with slight predilection for the right lower lobe (10/25 cases, 40%). Pure ground-glass opacity (GGO) was seen in 13/25 cases (52%), and GGO with consolidation was seen in 12/25 cases (48%). Common accompanying CT signs included crazy paving stone sign in 15/25 cases (60%) and air bronchogram in 12/25 cases (48%). From the 25 patients that showed respiratory deterioration and elevated serum D-dimer level, 11 cases confirmed to have acute pulmonary embolism, while 14 cases showed negative result for pulmonary embolism. 6/11 were male and 5/11 were female. Pulmonary embolism was diagnosed at a mean of 21 days from symptom onset. Unilateral acute pulmonary embolism was seen in 3/11 cases, while 8/11 cases showed bilateral distribution. Among 11 cases with acute pulmonary embolism, no emboli at the central level could be seen, but 3 cases showed pulmonary embolism at the lobar level, 3 cases at the segmental level, and 5 cases at lobar, segmental, and subsegmental levels. *Conclusion.* In patients with confirmed COVID-19, we should maintain a high suspicion for its thromboembolic complications such as acute pulmonary embolism that was mainly diagnosed at the end of 3rd week from symptom onset. We suggest that whenever a CT evaluation of the parenchymal involvement of COVID-19 pneumonia is performed, a simultaneous evaluation of the pulmonary arteries is also essential in order to identify early signs of associated pulmonary embolism.

1. Introduction

An outbreak of pneumonia of unknown etiology occurred in Wuhan, China, in December 2019, and 2019 novel coronavirus disease (COVID-19) was responsible [1]. The WHO declared it as a pandemic on March 11, 2020, in the following weeks; the disease has swept rapidly across most of the countries of the world, causing a global health emergency [2].

It is thought that viral spreading beyond the respiratory system to other organ systems in the 2nd week of the disease course (correlating with clinical worsening) leads to increased immune-mediated injury and hypercoagulability [3]. Some authors reported that acute pulmonary embolism is a cause of clinical deterioration in viral pneumonia [4, 5].

Han et al. reported disturbed coagulation function in patients infected with SARS-CoV-2 as compared to healthy controls, including elevated D-dimer, fibrin/fibrinogen degradation products, and fibrinogen levels [6]. Also, there is a positive correlation between elevated D-dimer levels on admission and in-hospital COVID-19 mortality [7, 8].

To date, most radiologic literature has focused on the distinctive chest CT abnormalities caused by COVID-19, including peripheral basal-predominant areas of ground-glass opacities and/or consolidation, often in a bilateral distribution [9].

However, emerging research has demonstrated that the inflammation and hypoxemia caused by COVID-19 may result in deranged coagulation parameters and increased risk of thromboembolic complications, which are associated with significant morbidity and mortality [10, 11]. They suggested that as patients with COVID-19 are admitted for treatment and isolation, it is important to follow prophylactic measures to prevent venous thromboembolism. In this condition, respiratory deterioration with other clinical evidence of venous thrombosis should raise suspicion for pulmonary embolism [12].

In our retrospective study, we focus on the development of acute pulmonary embolism as a related complication in patients with COVID-19 viral pneumonia.

2. Subjects and Methods

This study was approved by the Institutional Review Board of our hospital. The requirement for informed patient consent was waived by the ethics committee.

Out of 95 positive cases of COVID-19 in Dallah Hospital, Riyadh, Saudi Arabia, CT angiography was done for 25 patients suspected to have pulmonary embolism and have no contraindication for contrast study. 11 of them who showed CT evidence of acute pulmonary embolism were admitted to the ICU.

All CT scans were performed using a CT scanner (Light Speed™ 7.X CT scanner, GE Medical Systems, USA). Gantry position rotation period was 0.4 s, with an X-ray tube voltage of 140 kV and a current of 230–350 mA. Craniocaudal image acquisition of the entire thorax was carried out with a collimation of 1.25 mm (pitch of six) and a reconstruction increment of 0.8 mm. Mean scan time was 2.30 s. All patients underwent CTPA after administration of 100 ml standard contrast media (Xenetix 350 mg/ml, Guerbet, France) with an injection rate of 4.5–5 ml/s via a 16-gauge catheter inserted into the antecubital vein. Contrast bolus was followed by a 10 ml saline flush using Enhanced Xtream Injector (Nemoto Dual Shot Alpha (CiA425 Class IV/GE)), and delay was estimated using a semiautomatic bolus tracking system (SmartPrep, GE Medical Systems, USA) with a threshold of 80 HU for all examinations. ROI for bolus tracking was measured in the right atrium.

All reformations were performed by a senior CT technologist. From the axial CT data sets, multiplanar volume reconstruction (MPVR) and maximum intensity projection images were reformatted.

All images were sent to the workstation (Sectra, Sweden) and, retrospectively, CT angiography was analyzed and detailed findings were recorded.

We defined PE as a partial or complete intraluminal filling defect surrounded by the contrast medium and occupying the entire arterial vessel section [13]. The central, lobar, segmental, and subsegmental vessels of each lung were assessed for evidence of PE. We considered the main pulmonary artery, left and right pulmonary arteries, and interlobar arteries as the central vessel [14].

Presence or absence of emboli in the pulmonary artery or its branches was identified by using the nomenclature outlined by Remy-Jardin and Remy [13], which is based on the standard descriptions given by Boyden [15]; a 4-point scale was formulated to score different anatomical levels of pulmonary arteries of each lobe: (1) central (main, right and left, and interlobar), (2) lobar, (3) segmental, and (4) subsegmental levels.

2.1. Statistical Analysis. Statistical analyses were performed with SPSS for Windows software package (version 17.0, SPSS Inc.). Data were expressed as mean ± standard deviation (SD).

3. Results

Out of 95 cases confirmed to have COVID-19 viral pneumonia, 25 patients showed respiratory deterioration.

The mean age of the included patients was 49 ± 11 years; the youngest was 22 years, and the oldest was 64 years.

Common symptoms in the 25 cases that underwent CT angiography were fever that was noted in 21/25 cases (84%), shortness of breath in 18/25 cases (72%), cough in 16/25 cases (64%), and severe myalgia/body fatigue in 13/25 cases (52%). The less common symptoms were sore throat in 11/25 cases (44%) and headache in 10/25 cases (40%).

Regarding CT findings, 4/25 cases (16%) had unilateral lung disease and 21/25 cases (84%) had bilateral disease, with slight predilection for the right lower lobe in 10/25 cases (40%) and the middle lobe in 8/25 cases (32%). Pure ground-glass opacity (GGO) was seen in 13/25 cases (52%), and GGO with consolidation was seen in 12/25 cases (48%). Common accompanying CT signs included crazy paving stone sign in 15/25 cases (60%) and air bronchogram in 12/25 cases (48%).

In our study, acute pulmonary embolism was diagnosed at a mean of 21 days from symptom onset (range: from 19 to 24 days).

Unilateral acute pulmonary embolism was seen in 3/11 cases, while 8/11 cases showed bilateral distribution of acute pulmonary embolism.

Among the included 11 cases with acute pulmonary embolism, no emboli could be detected at the central level (main, right, left, and interlobar pulmonary arteries), but 3 cases showed acute pulmonary embolism at the lobar level, 3 cases at the segmental level (Figure 1), and 5 cases at lobar, segmental, and subsegmental levels (Figures 2 and 3).

The respiratory rate in the 11 cases with acute pulmonary embolism was 16/min–18/min, and oxygen saturation was 95%–93% on room air. Blood sampling of patients showed leucopenia, lymphopenia, and thrombopenia. Laboratory

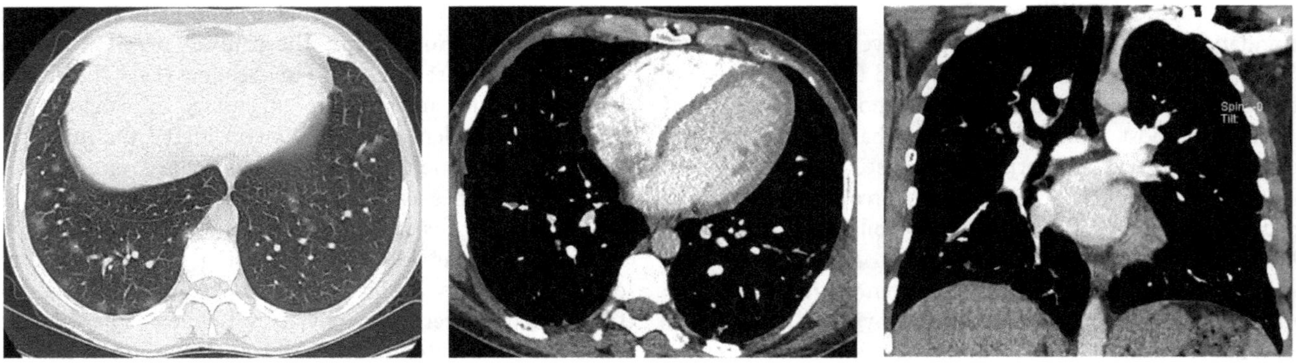

(a) (b) (c)

Figure 1: Images in a 38-year-old male with COVID-19 pneumonia complaining of fever and cough. (a) Axial unenhanced chest CT scan (lung window) obtained on day 5 after the onset of symptoms shows bilateral multiple patchy areas of ground-glass opacities more peripherally. (b) Axial CT pulmonary angiography scan. (c) Coronal reformatted images (mediastinum window) on day 19 after the onset of symptoms demonstrate filling defects (white arrow) within the segmental pulmonary artery branch supplying the lateral basal segment of the right lower lobe.

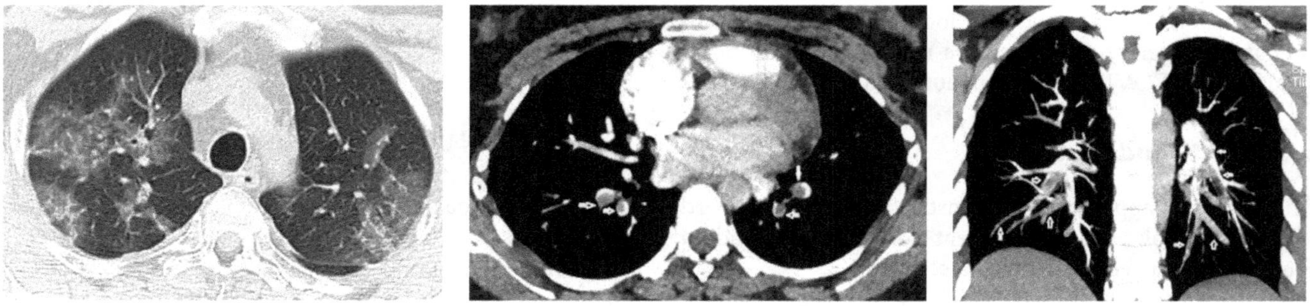

(a) (b) (c)

Figure 2: Images in a 22-year-old female with COVID-19 pneumonia complaining of fever, cough, and headache. (a) Axial unenhanced chest CT scan (lung window) obtained on day 6 after the onset of symptoms shows bilateral areas of central and peripheral ground-glass opacities and mixed density pattern. (b) Axial CT pulmonary angiography scan (mediastinum window). (c) Coronal thick maximum intensity projection slab of CT pulmonary angiography on day 24 after the onset of symptoms demonstrates filling defects (white arrows) in the left lower lobar as well as in both the right and left segmental/subsegmental pulmonary artery branches of the lower lobes.

tests showed prolongation of the prothrombin time (range: 14.2–16.3) with elevated D-dimer level (1.56 mg/ml–8.8 mg/ml).

The 11 COVID-19 cases positive for pulmonary embolism were admitted to the ICU and followed by the cardiologist and intensivists. Echocardiography was not done for any of our cases.

4. Discussion

Several recent studies have explored the link between COVID-19 and hypercoagulability, suggesting that the most common laboratory test result abnormalities include elevated D-dimer levels and mild thrombocytopenia [16]. In our study, all our positive cases for acute pulmonary embolism showed high D-dimer level.

The most typical finding in patients with COVID-19 and coagulopathy is an increased D-dimer concentration, a relatively modest decrease in the platelet count, and a prolongation of the prothrombin time; the combination of thrombocytopenia, prolonged prothrombin time, and increased D-dimer level is suggestive of DIC [17], which was evident in our cases.

In our study, acute pulmonary embolism was seen in 11/95 cases (11.6%), which is less than other studies that showed more frequent pulmonary embolism in patients with COVID-19 and reported almost a quarter of the COVID-19 pneumonia patients [18]; this may be because of a small number of our study cases and also because of early diagnosis of positive cases and good treatment plans in our hospital. This may also be because CT angiography was done only in deteriorating patients (25/95 cases), with high D-dimer levels and high possibility for acute pulmonary embolism, and not in all COVID-19 pneumonia patients.

Some authors reported that lung injury and impaired gas exchange lead to increased production of proinflammatory cytokines, and contributing viral infection may result in vascular endothelium direct damage [19].

Another study demonstrated severe endothelial injury associated with intracellular virus and disrupted cell membranes, as well as extensive thrombosis, microangiopathy, alveolar capillary microthrombi, and more new vessel growth,

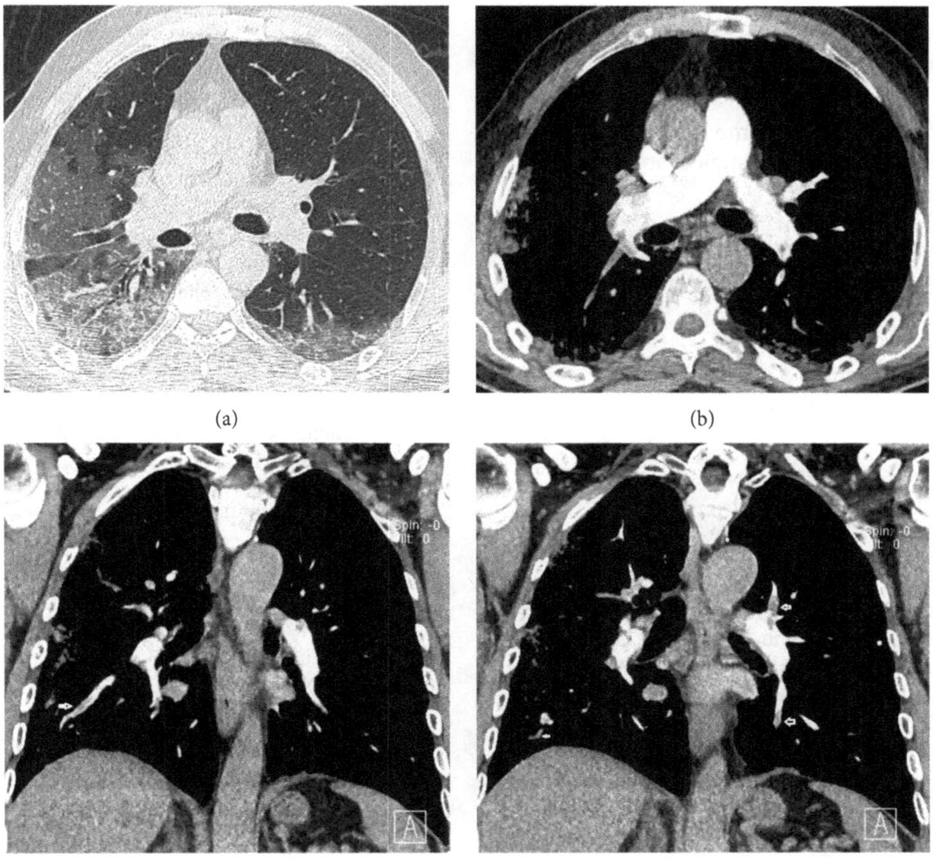

FIGURE 3: Images in a 64-year-old man with COVID-19 pneumonia complaining of body ache, fever, and cough. (a) Axial unenhanced chest CT scan (lung window) obtained on day 9 after the onset of symptoms shows bilateral areas of peripheral ground-glass opacities more at the right side with interlobular septal thickening (crazy paving sign), vascular sign, and air bronchogram sign being seen. (b) Axial CT pulmonary angiography scan. (c, d) Coronal reformatted images (mediastinum window) on day 24 after the onset of symptoms demonstrate multiple bilateral filling defects (white arrows) involving lobar, segmental, and subsegmental branches of the pulmonary artery.

compared with those lungs obtained at autopsy from patients who died from influenza [20].

Our study suggests that COVID-19 patients with severe clinical features such as respiratory deterioration and elevated serum D-dimer level may have associated acute pulmonary embolism and need contrast-enhanced CT angiography study for diagnosis.

Our results revealed that pulmonary embolism was noted at lobar, segmental, and subsegmental pulmonary artery levels with a clear central pulmonary artery (main, right, and left branches).

Imaging features of acute pulmonary embolism in our study in patients with COVID-19 are nonspecific and similar in appearance to those seen in other pathologic conditions, which were also reported by other authors [21].

4.1. Limitations of the Study. Our finding is preliminary in nature in our initial experience with COVID-19 cases. CT angiography was not systematically used for all COVID-19 patients, but only for deteriorating patients with high D-dimer levels, so we cannot assess the incidence of PE in COVID-19 patients. No lower limb venous Doppler ultrasound study was done for our patients to evaluate the presence of deep venous thromboembolism. In addition to a small number of our subjects, further study with more numbers is needed.

5. Conclusion

In patients with confirmed COVID-19, we should maintain a high suspicion for its thromboembolic complications such as acute pulmonary embolism that was mainly diagnosed at the end of 3rd week from symptom onset.

Whenever a CT evaluation of the parenchymal involvement of COVID-19 pneumonia is performed, a simultaneous evaluation of the pulmonary arteries is also essential in order to identify early signs of associated pulmonary embolism.

In any case, early anticoagulant therapy initiated in the early stages of infection will make the CT pictures much less striking compared to the first case studied in the literature and, therefore, the CT could maintain a role in the follow-up of pumonary embolsim in case of disappearnce of symptoms.

Abbreviations

COVID-19: 2019 novel coronavirus
NCP: Novel coronavirus pneumonia
CTA: Computed tomography angiography
GGO: Ground-glass opacity
WHO: World Health Organization
PE: Pulmonary embolism
RT-PCR: Real-time reverse transcription polymerase chain reaction
SOB: Shortness of breath
ICU: Intensive care unit
DIC: Disseminated intravascular coagulopathy.

References

[1] N. Zhu, D. Zhang, W. Wang et al., "A novel coronavirus from patients with pneumonia in China, 2019," *New England Journal of Medicine*, vol. 382, no. 8, pp. 727–733, 2020.
[2] WHO, "Novel corona virus (2019-nCoV) situation reports," 2020, https://www.who.int/emergencies/diseases/novel-coronavirus-2019/situation-reports.
[3] W. Cao and T. Li, "COVID-19: towards understanding of pathogenesis," *Cell Research*, vol. 30, no. 5, pp. 367–369, 2020.
[4] O. M. P. Jolobe, "Similarities between community-acquired pneumonia and pulmonary embolism," *The American Journal of Medicine*, vol. 132, no. 12, p. e863, 2019.
[5] T. Ishiguro, K. Matsuo, S. Fujii, and N. Takayanagi, "Acute thrombotic vascular events complicating influenza-associated pneumonia," *Respiratory Medicine Case Reports*, vol. 28, Article ID 100884, 2019.
[6] H. Han, L. Yang, R. Liu et al., "Prominent changes in blood coagulation of patients with SARS-CoV-2 infection," *Clinical Chemistry and Laboratory Medicine (CCLM)*, vol. 58, no. 7, p. 1116, 2020.
[7] F. Zhou, T. Yu, R. Du et al., "Clinical course and risk factors for mortality of adult in patients with COVID-19 in Wuhan, China: a retrospective cohort study," *Lancet*, vol. 395, pp. 1054–1062, 2020.
[8] N. Tang, D. Li, X. Wang, and Z. Sun, "Abnormal coagulation parameters are associated with poor prognosis in patients with novel coronavirus pneumonia," *Journal of Thrombosis and Haemostasis*, vol. 18, no. 4, p. 844, 2020.
[9] J. P. Kanne, B. P. Little, J. H. Chung, B. M. Elicker, and L. H. Ketai, "Essentials for radiologists on COVID-19: an update-radiology scientific expert panel," *Radiology*, vol. 296, no. 2, 2020.
[10] F. A. Klok, M. J. H. A. Kruip, N. J. M. van der Meer et al., "Incidence of thrombotic complications in critically ill ICU patients with COVID-19," *Thrombosis Research*, vol. 191, pp. 145–147, 2020.
[11] J. M. Connors and J. H. Levy, "COVID-19 and its implications for thrombosis and anticoagulation," *Blood*, vol. 135, no. 23, pp. 2033–2040, 2020.
[12] Y. Xie, X. Wang, P. Yang, and S. Zhang, "COVID-19 complicated by acute pulmonary embolism," *Radiology: Cardiothoracic Imaging*, vol. 2, no. 2, Article ID e200067, 2020.
[13] M. Remy-Jardin and J. Remy, "Spiral CT angiography of the pulmonary circulation," *Radiology*, vol. 212, no. 3, pp. 615–636, 1999.
[14] E. E. Chiang, P. M. Boiselle, V. Raptopoulos, K. F. Reynolds, M. P. Rosen, and M. Simon, "Detection of pulmonary embolism: comparison of paddlewheel and coronal CT reformations-initial experience," *Radiology*, vol. 228, no. 2, pp. 577–582, 2003.
[15] E. A. Boyden, *Segmental Anatomy of the Lungs*, McGraw-Hill, New York, NY, USA, 1955.
[16] B. Bikdeli, M. V. Madhavan, D. Jimenez et al., "COVID-19 and thrombotic or thromboembolic disease: implications for prevention, antithrombotic therapy, and follow-up," *Journal of the American College of Cardiology*, vol. 75, no. 23, pp. 2950–2973, 2020.
[17] M. Levi and M. Scully, "How I treat disseminated intravascular coagulation," *Blood*, vol. 131, no. 8, pp. 845–854, 2018.
[18] F. Bompard, H. Monnier, I. Saab et al., "Pulmonary embolism in patients with COVID-19 pneumonia," *European Respiratory Journal*, vol. 56, no. 1, Article ID 2001365, 2020.
[19] J. Thachil, "The versatile heparin in COVID-19," *Journal of Thrombosis and Haemostasis*, vol. 18, no. 5, pp. 1020–1022, 2020.
[20] M. Ackermann, S. E. Verleden, M. Kuehnel et al., "Pulmonary vascular endothelialitis, thrombosis, and angiogenesis in COVID-19," *New England Journal of Medicine*, vol. 383, no. 2, p. 120, 2020.
[21] M. C. Olson, M. G. Lubner, C. O. Menias et al., "RadioGraphics update: venous thrombosis and hypercoagulability in the abdomen and pelvis-findings in COVID-19," *RadioGraphics*, vol. 40, no. 5, pp. E24–E28, 2020.

28

Unresectable Hepatic Metastasis of Uveal Melanoma: Hepatic Chemosaturation with High-Dose Melphalan—Long-Term Overall Survival Negatively Correlates with Tumor Burden

R. Brüning,[1] M. Tiede,[1] M. Schneider,[1] P. Wohlmuth,[2] H. Weilert,[3] K. Oldhafer,[4,5] and A. Stang[3,4]

[1]*Radiology and Neuroradiology, Asklepios Hospital Barmbek, Ruebenkamp 220, 22307 Hamburg, Germany*
[2]*Biostatistics, ProResearch, Asklepios Hospital St. Georg, Lohmuehlenstrasse 5, 20099 Hamburg, Germany*
[3]*Oncology, Asklepios Hospital Barmbek, Ruebenkamp 220, 22307 Hamburg, Germany*
[4]*Faculty of Medicine, Semmelweis University Campus Hamburg, Lohmuehlenstrasse 5, 20099 Hamburg, Germany*
[5]*Surgery, Asklepios Hospital Barmbek, Ruebenkamp 220, 22307 Hamburg, Germany*

Correspondence should be addressed to R. Brüning; r.bruening@asklepios.com

Academic Editor: Paul Sijens

Introduction. Percutaneous hepatic perfusion with melphalan (PHP-M) for hepatic metastasis of uveal melanoma (LMUM) achieves high local response rates, but the individual clinical benefit is poorly defined. We aimed to determine cofactors of response and clinical outcomes including the probability of long-term (5-years) overall survival (OS) in PHP-M-treated patients with LMUM. *Patients and Methods.* We retrospectively reviewed clinicopathological, radiological, and outcome data of 19 patients with unresectable LMUM treated with 43 PHP-M (median 2 PHP-M) between 2014 and 2019. Tumor response and adverse events were evaluated using RECIST 1.1 and the Clavien–Dindo classification. Kaplan–Meier methods and Cox regression hazard proportional models were used. *Results.* Of 19 patients, 10 (53%) achieved a partial response (PR) and 9 (47%) had stable disease (SD). There was no progressive disease (PD) and no adverse events exceeding Clavien–Dindo grade IV. Median OS was 16.7 months after the first PHP-M treatment and 26.4 months after initial diagnosis. Low hepatic tumor volume (median of 10 mL vs. 150 mL) was an independent predictor of favorable OS (hazard ratio (95% confidence interval): 0.190 (0.041, 0.893); $p < 0.05$), and female patients were at a lower risk compared with males (0.146 (0.017, 1.240)). Estimates of the overall survival were 0.213 (0.0449, 1) from first imaging (95% confidence interval) to 5 years and 0.793 (0.609, 1) and 0.604 (0.380, 0.960) for 1 and 2 years after chemosaturation, respectively. *Discussion.* PHP-M for nonresectable LMUV provides a safe and locally efficient liver-directed procedure that offers patients a chance for long-term OS, especially for patients with a low hepatic tumor burden.

1. Introduction

Metastatic uveal melanoma (UM) carries a poor prognosis with 1-year survival rates reported as low as 10–25% [1, 2]. Up to 50% of uveal melanomas develop hepatic metastasis [3] with reported median survival ranging from 4 to 15 months [4], suggesting a role for liver-directed local therapy in patients without extrahepatic disease.

No effective adjuvant systemic therapy has been demonstrated to reduce the risk of metastasis, as stated by Triozzi and Singh [5]. A meta-analysis of 29 phase II trials in metastatic uveal melanoma until 2015 aimed to define progression-free survival (PFS) and OS. Poor outcomes such as a median PFS of 3.3 months (6-month PFS 27%) and median OS of 10.2 months (1-year OS 43%) were described across all treatment groups based on more than 900 patients [6].

Immune checkpoint inhibitors, such as ipilimumab, nivolumab, and pembrolizumab, achieve long-term OS with 5-year OS rates of 34–52% in metastatic cutaneous melanoma [7–9] but yield poor outcome results in metastatic uveal melanoma (UM) with a median OS of 10–14 months

[10–13]. At present, there is no standard therapy for metastatic UM, and the limited activity of systemic therapy compared with cutaneous melanoma poses a treatment challenge.

Percutaneous isolated hepatic perfusion with melphalan (PHP-M) has been licensed in the European Union (EU) with a CE mark. Although evidence to date is limited, liver-targeted therapies such as PHP-M chemosaturation hold promising results for patients in this setting. However, the OS reported so far was within a large range from 245 days to 27 months [14, 15], and data from randomized trials regarding long-term outcomes are not available.

To enable better stratification of patient selection for this procedure in the future, we sought to evaluate cofactors of prognosis in this setting using a retrospective search from our database. We also aimed to determine cofactors of response and clinical outcomes including the probability of long-term (5-years) OS in PHP-M-treated patients with LMUM.

2. Material and Methods

Patients: from 2014 to 2019, patients were treated by percutaneous PHP-M as a last-line therapy in our center. All treatments were recommended by the multidisciplinary tumor board for clinical indication, and all cases were treated according to the Declaration of Helsinki of 1964. Informed consent was obtained. Patients' baseline and outcome data are given in Table 1.

For this evaluation, data were collected and evaluated in a retrospective fashion based on the medical records and the PACS database; these data are available on request.

Only patients with an Eastern Cooperative Oncology Group (ECOG) performance status of 0–1 and with adequate hematologic, renal, and hepatic function data (e.g. hemoglobin > 8 g/dL; platelets > 150 thsd/μL, bilirubin ≤ 3 × upper limit of normal (ULN)) were included.

Distant extrahepatic metastasis exceeding 10 mm in lymph nodes or in relevant other locations, recent history of transient ischemic attacks, heart failure (left ventricular ejection fraction <40%), contraindications to general anesthesia, or significant chronic obstructive or restrictive pulmonary disorders were considered as contraindications for PHP-M.

The patients had to have at least one follow-up including an MRI- or CT-based restaging; patients lost to follow-up were not included in this evaluation ($n = 1$).

Seven patients received previous systemic treatment (most often pembrolizumab), four patients received trans-arterial chemoembolization (TACE) or transarterial chemoperfusion (not chemosaturation), and three patients received previous surgical of ablative therapy, and these therapies were terminated for either side effects or progressive disease. Six patients had no specified previous therapy.

2.1. Procedure. For the procedure itself, a dedicated filter system (CHEMOSAT® Second Generation; Delcath Systems Inc., New York, NY, USA) was used as previously described [16]. For arterial infusion, a 6 French catheter was inserted through the femoral artery into the common hepatic artery, and a 2.7 French microcatheter (ProGreat®, Terumo, Japan) was used for selective chemoperfusion of the liver. This transarterial chemoperfusion was performed with a dosage of 3.0 mg/kg ideal body weight up to a maximum dose of 220 mg of melphalan (Alkeran®). For venous access, a 18 French double-balloon catheter, inserted through the contralateral femoral vein, facilitated isolation of the hepatic inferior cava segment, the upper balloon by being inflated in the right atrium and being pulled back to cover the diaphragm portion of the inferior vena cava and the lower balloon being inflated in the hepatic portion of the vena cava below entries to the hepatic vein. A separate access in the right internal jugular vein was used for blood return. During the infusion phase, 500 cc of melphalan solution was administered at a rate of 0.4 mL/sec, with intermediate angiograms to ensure correct flow. As suggested by the manufacturer, the subsequent washout was performed with the filtration circuit running for 30 min after cessation of the arterial infusion. In order to maintain an activated clotting time (ACT) above 500 s, which was mandatory for safe extracorporeal hemofiltration, heparin was administered as needed.

These procedures were performed under general anesthesia. All patients were then supervised for the first night under intensive care, in order to monitor blood pressure, coagulation, access sites, and laboratory findings. On the day after the procedure, in our institution, G-CSF (Neulasta®) was given routinely.

2.2. Treatment Outcome. The treatment outcome was measured retrospectively according to the response evaluation criteria in solid tumors (RECIST 1.1) [17], based on the sum of diameter. The sum of diameter was tested as an independent predictor of OS. Therefore, either computed tomography (CT) or magnetic resonance imaging (MRI) was routinely performed at least every 3 months after PHP-M.

Overall survival was calculated from initial diagnosis and from the first PHP-M until the last available follow-up or death. Progression-free survival (PFS) was calculated and is given either from first imaging or from the first PHP. For tumor volume analysis, the patient cohort was stratified to approximately 10 mL tumor volume versus approximately 150 mL.

We monitored for adverse events and they were classified according to the Clavien–Dindo classification [18].

Tumor volume was determined using Advantage Workstation 4.1.2 (GE Healthcare). For volumetric evaluation, the venous phase was chosen, and the lesions were outlined manually. Volumetry was performed on CTs directly prior to chemosaturation. Portal branches and bile ducts were excluded by thresholding the outlined volume.

Tumor stability was defined as stable disease (SD according to RECIST 1.1) in comparison to partial response (PD according to RECIST 1.1).

Table 1: Patients baseline data ($n = 19$).

Patient gender		
Male	11	
Female	8	
Patient age	Mean	SD
	58 years	12 years
RECIST 1.1 after first PHP		
Complete remission (CR)	0	
Partial remission (PR)	10	
Stable disease (SD)	9	
Progressive disease (PD)	0	
	Mean	SD
Time from first (positive) imaging liver to first PHP (days)	324	432
Time between first and second PHP (days)	119	145

2.3. Statistics. Continuous data were summarized as means ± standard deviations or as medians [25th and 75th percentiles] as appropriate. Categorical data were presented as N (%).

Overall survival was estimated with the Kaplan–Meier method. Univariable Cox proportional hazards models were used to associate the covariables to overall survival. Effects on mortality were presented with hazard ratios and 95% confidence intervals.

Univariable logistic regression models were used to relate age, gender, and tumor size to tumor stability (which is considered as an undesired event compared to partial remission). The logistic regression models were presented with parameter estimates, standard errors, odds ratios and 95% confidence intervals.

p values of likelihood ratio tests were presented. All p values were two-sided and a p value <0.05 was considered significant. All calculations were performed with the statistical analysis software R (R Core Team, 2018).

3. Results

In 19 patients, there were 43 procedures of chemosaturation with a median of 2 chemosaturation per patient. The interval between first and second PHP was on average of 119 days (SD of 145 days).

3.1. Overall Survival. Median OS following initial diagnosis was 26.4 months and following first PHP-M treatment was 16.7 month, as determined by the Kaplan–Meier method (Figure 1(a)). Progression-free survival (PFS) was 751.8 days since first imaging (SD 515.5 days) and 427.8 days since first PHP (SD 295.2 days) (Figure 1(b)).

A lower tumor volume decreases the risk of mortality: increased OS was found associated with lower tumor volume (hazard ratio (95% confidence interval) for the tumor volume as stratified in 10 mL versus 150 mL: 0.190 (0.041, 0.893)). However, there was only a weak correlation between age and survival (HR (95% CI) for 65 versus 50 years: 0.627 (0.187, 2.100); Figure 2). The influence of gender was also estimated: in our patient cohort, the risk to females was only 15% of the risk to male patients (HR: 0.146 [0.017, 1.240]) (Figure 3). A correlation of OS to "time from initial diagnosis" showed a hazard ratio of 1.071 (lower/upper HR: 0.759/1.512), and the p value was not significant (0.695).

Elevation of serum LDH (in steps of 200 units) resulted in a hazard ration of 1.934 (lower/upper HR: 0.873/4.282); however, this trend was not significant ($p = 0.104$). An increase in the sum of tumor diameter had a hazard ration of 2.503 (lower/upper HR: 0.732 8.556) in our cohort; but did not reach statistical significance (p 0.143).

Estimates of OS were 0.213 (0.0449, 1) from first imaging (95% confidence interval) to 5 years and 0.793 (0.609, 1) and 0.604 (0.380, 0.960) for 1 and 2 years after chemosaturation, respectively.

3.2. Restaging by RECIST. Ten of 19 patients achieved a partial response (PR; 53%), and 9/19 had stable disease (SD; 47%) following the initial treatment. There was no progressive disease (PD) and no complete response (CR).

For the statistical analysis, SD and tumor stability (compared to partial remission) were referred to as an undesired event. Tumor stability (and not partial response) was inversely correlated to lower age (odds ratio (95% confidence interval) of age = 50 years versus age = 65 years: 0.179 (0.031, 1.040)) (Figure 3). However, there was only weak evidence that female gender (OR (95% CI): 0.500 (0.078, 3.210)) or a lower tumor volume were associated with a marginally lower risk of SD (OR (95% CI): 0.623 (0.226, 1.710)).

3.3. Adverse Events. Adverse events according to the Clavien–Dindo classification until discharge: In our cohort of the 43 procedures, there were no or minor complications—grade ≤1 in 39 procedures, one case with grade II, in 2 cases grade IIIa (coronary ischemia), and in one case grade IIIb (transfemoral bleeding with following surgery); no grade IV-V occurred. Details are given in Table 2.

There were changes in the hematological state, most profoundly in platelet count (from 251.7/nL (SD 65.8) before the first PHP-M procedure to an average of 104.2/nL (SD 45.4) following the procedure). Bilirubin following the procedure was stable at an average of 0.9 (SD 0.6), and erythrocytes following the procedure were stable at 4.1/pL (SD 0.5).

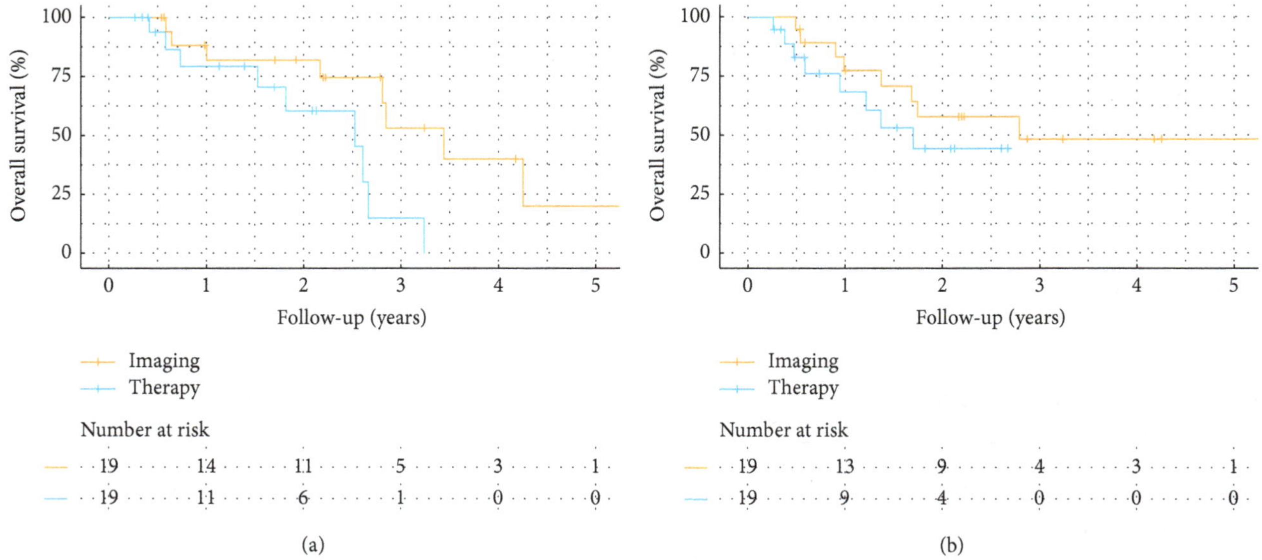

FIGURE 1: Kaplan–Meier plots. (a) Overall survival estimates (OS) (and patients at risk) from initial diagnosis/imaging and from initial chemosaturation therapy. (b) Estimates of progression-free survival (PFS) (and patients at risk) from initial diagnosis/imaging and from initial chemosaturation therapy.

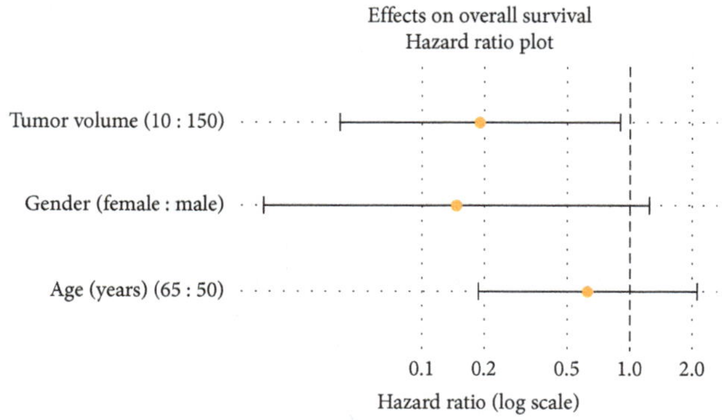

FIGURE 2: Plot of hazard ratios (95% confidence intervals) for overall survival.

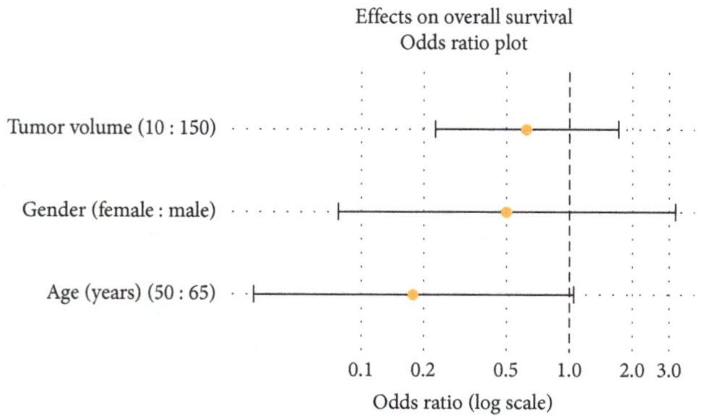

FIGURE 3: Plot of the odds ratios (95% confidence intervals) regarding tumor stability (tumor stability refers to stable disease RECIST 1.1, and compared to partial remission, it is referred to as an undesired event).

4. Discussion

Uveal melanoma (UM) once metastatic carries a poor prognosis. Unfortunately, even modern agents such as immune checkpoint inhibitors—ipilimumab, nivolumab and pembrolizumab—yield poor outcome results in metastatic uveal melanoma (UM) with a median OS of 10–14 months [10–12]. At present, there is no standard therapy for metastatic UM, and the limited activity of systemic therapy compared with cutaneous melanoma poses a treatment challenge.

Of the metastatic UM, more than every second uveal melanoma develops hepatic metastasis [3], suggesting a role for liver-directed local therapy in patients without extrahepatic disease. As a consequence of this known predilection of uveal melanoma for hepatic metastasis, liver-directed therapies represent an important research focus in the treatment of metastatic disease [19, 20].

In our study treating unresectable liver metastasis with PHP-M and in part refractory to systemic therapy, median OS was 26.4 months following initial diagnosis and 16.7 months from first PHP-M treatment. Thus, we were able to show that PHP offers as second-line option the chance of the long-term OS outcome.

Our data on OS were compared positively with published reports. Karydis et al. reported an overall survival of 15.3 months following treatment in a larger retrospective bicenter evaluation with over 50 patients [21]. Data from a multicenter trial report a median OS of 9.6 months with a range from 1.6 to 41.0 months [19]. However, this work was a retrospective analysis of data acquired from multiple centers throughout Germany, resulting in a substantially higher heterogeneity of data [19]. An initial phase III trial of

TABLE 2: Complications after PHP chemosaturation during hospital stay according to the Clavien–Dindo classification [18].

Clavien–Dindo classification after 1 PHP	Clavien–Dindo classification after 2 PHP	Clavien–Dindo classification after 3 PHP	Clavien–Dindo classification after 4 PHP
0	0		
0	0	0	
0	0	0	
0			
IIIa	0		
0	0	0	IIIB
0	0	0	0
0	0	0	
0	0	0	
0	0		
1			
1	1		
0			
0	0		
0	0	II	
1	1		
IIIa	0	1	
0			
0			

PHP with melphalan compared with best alternative care in 93 patients with ocular (88%) or cutaneous (12%) melanoma demonstrated an overall response rate with PHP-M therapy; OS was similar between the two arms; however, this was confounded by allowing crossover [22]. Further analysis on this patient cohort exhibited that while the hPFS was significantly better for the PHP-M group ($p < 0.0001$), the median OS was not significantly different (PHP-Mel 10.6 months vs. BAC 10.0 months) [23].

In our cohort, the main factor found to be beneficial for prolonged OS was lower tumor volume. This observation needs to be verified; however, no such tumor volume-associated analysis has, to the best our knowledge, been published. Also, the influence of gender was estimated: in our patient cohort, females had only 15% of the risk of male patients; this is in accordance with a recently published multivariate analysis on an international patient population that showed male patients (and those with elevated LDH and elevated ALP) were all associated with a shorter PFS [6]. In our patient cohort, there was only weak evidence that age was associated with survival. However, we did observe a trend that elevated serum LDH had an elevated hazard ration, but this did not reach statistical significance. Estimates of 5-year OS (95% confidence interval) from first imaging were 0.213 (0.0449, 1). This again may prove a strong argument toward the use of PHP-M.

In this retrospective single-institutional study, we observed a disease control in all of the metastatic melanoma patients after the first PHP-M, either by SD or by PR as classified by RECIST 1.1. There was no case of progressive disease following the PHP-M treatment by chemosaturation in our cohort.

A factor found to be beneficial for a PR (in comparison to SD) was lower age (odds ratio (95% confidence interval) of age = 50 years versus age = 65 years: 0.179 (0.031, 1.040)); however, there was only weak evidence that female gender or a lower tumor volume was associated with a lower risk of SD instead of a PR.

The PHP-M procedure itself can be considered as standardized and safe, as no AEs of grades 4-5 occurred during the procedure or in the hospitalization period; thereafter, the observed adverse events up to grade IIIB were within the range of previously published data [19].

We did monitor hematological changes with a most pronounced drop in platelets; these changes were within the range of previous reports and occurred after the PHP-M procedure, frequently improving after 5–7 days. These known effects were most likely due to side effects of dilution and the use of the extracorporeal filter system, as previously described [14, 21]. A study of de Leede et al. reports an overall filter efficiency of 86% (range 71.1–95.5%) and bone marrow depression up to 80.0% of procedures [24].

However, as other authors have recommended, we suggest that patients with a tumor volume higher than 50% of the total liver volume and with abnormal liver functions (ECOG) and especially with inadequate hematological and renal functions (our exclusion limit was hemoglobin > 8 g/dL; platelets > 150 thsd/μL, bilirubin $\leq 3 \times$ upper limit) should be excluded from PHP-M [19, 23].

A wide range of other transarterial therapies are presently available for the treatment of hepatic malignancy, including bland arterial embolization, chemoembolization using a variety of chemotherapeutic agents (e.g. cisplatin) [25] or radioembolization using yttrium-90-labeled microspheres (Y90). One study to date is available reporting a direct comparison between PHP-M and SIRT (=Y90 radioembolization). This study also showed a doubled overall survival time using PHP-M chemosaturation compared with SIRT and TACE (median OS from time of treatment for PHP at 608 days versus Y90 (295 d) and CE (265 d)) [26]. However, as this was a retrospective evaluation in a single center, more work is necessary to confirm these encouraging data. For future directions, a phase III trial comparing IHP with the best alternative care in uveal melanoma is underway. The combination of 90Y-labeled microspheres with sorafenib is being studied in a phase I trial (NCT01893099), and the combination with ipilimumab is being assessed in a phase 0 study (NCT01730157).

Limitations of the reported observations comprise mainly its single-center database, its retrospective nature, and the cutoff in follow-up. Uveal melanoma is a relatively rare disease overall, and larger patient numbers are likely to be achieved only by the use of pooled data analysis from multiple centers. This retrospective approach in turn may be limited due to the inconsistency of treatment regimens and postprocedural patient care. As a result, a single center was used to minimize these confounding effects at the cost of a more limited sample size.

In conclusion, PHP-M for nonresectable liver metastasis of uveal melanoma provides a safe and locally efficient liver-directed procedure that offers patients a chance for long-term survival. PHP offers as second-line option the chance of long-term OS outcome, especially for patients with a low hepatic tumor burden.

Acknowledgments

The authors acknowledge the input of M. Zeile, J. Tesdorff, and H. Hentschel in patient handling. The authors appreciate the most valuable co-operation with Dr. Peter Mohr. The authors also acknowledge the precious assistance by Mrs. Anke Anstadt and Gabriela Ramlow. The authors declare that there was no external funding.

References

[1] E. S. Gragoudas, K. M. Egan, J. M. Seddon et al., "Survival of patents with metastases from uveal melanoma," *Ophthalmology*, vol. 98, no. 3, pp. 383–390, 1991.

[2] Group COMS, "Development of metastatic disease after enrollment in the COMS trials for treatment of choroidal melanoma: collaborative ocular melanoma study group report no. 26," *JAMA Ophthalmology*, vol. 123, no. 12, pp. 1639–1643, 2005.

[3] R. D. Carvajal, G. K. Schwartz, T. Tezel, B. Marr, J. H. Francis, and P. D. Nathan, "Metastatic disease from uveal melanoma: treatment options and future prospects," *British Journal of Ophthalmology*, vol. 101, no. 1, p. 38, 2017.

[4] Group COMS, "The COMS randomized trial of iodine 125 brachytherapy for choroidal melanoma: V. Twelve-year mortality rates and prognostic factors: COMS report no. 28," *JAMA Ophthalmology*, vol. 124, no. 12, pp. 1684–1693, 2006.

[5] P. L. Triozzi and A. D. Singh, "Adjuvant therapy of uveal melanoma: current status," *Ocular Oncology and Pathology*, vol. 1, no. 1, pp. 54–62, 2015.

[6] L. Khoja, E. G. Atenafu, A. M. Joshua, and Group TIRCsI-OM, "Meta-analysis of phase II trials in metastatic uveal melanoma (MUM) to determine progression-free (PFS) and overall survival (OS) benchmarks for future phase II trials: an irci-ocular melanoma initiative," *Journal of Clinical Oncology*, vol. 34, no. 15, p. 9567, 2016.

[7] O. Hamid, C. Robert, A. Daud et al., "Five-year survival outcomes for patients with advanced melanoma treated with pembrolizumab in KEYNOTE-001," *Annals of Oncology*, vol. 30, no. 4, pp. 582–588, 2019.

[8] J. Larkin, V. Chiarion-Sileni, R. Gonzalez et al., "Combined nivolumab and ipilimumab or monotherapy in untreated melanoma," *New England Journal of Medicine*, vol. 373, no. 1, pp. 23–34, 2015.

[9] C. Robert, A. Ribas, J. Schachter et al., "Pembrolizumab versus ipilimumab in advanced melanoma (KEYNOTE-006): post-hoc 5-year results from an open-label, multicentre, randomised, controlled, phase 3 study," *The Lancet Oncology*, vol. 20, no. 9, pp. 1239–1251, 2019.

[10] C. Mignard, A. Deschamps Huvier, A. Gillibert et al., "Efficacy of immunotherapy in patients with metastatic mucosal or uveal melanoma," *Journal of Oncology*, vol. 2018, Article ID 1908065, 9 pages, 2018.

[11] A. P. Algazi, K. K. Tsai, A. N. Shoushtari et al., "Clinical outcomes in metastatic uveal melanoma treated with PD-1 and PD-L1 antibodies," *Cancer*, vol. 122, no. 21, pp. 3344–3353, 2016.

[12] M. V. Heppt, L. Heinzerling, K. C. Kähler et al., "Prognostic factors and outcomes in metastatic uveal melanoma treated with programmed cell death-1 or combined PD-1/cytotoxic T-lymphocyte antigen-4 inhibition," *European Journal of Cancer*, vol. 82, pp. 56–65, 2017.

[13] C. Robert, J. Schachter, G. V. Long et al., "Pembrolizumab versus ipilimumab in advanced melanoma," *New England Journal of Medicine*, vol. 372, no. 26, pp. 2521–2532, 2015.

[14] H. A. Lillemoe and H. Alexander, "Current status of percutaneous hepatic perfusion as regional treatment for patients with unresectable hepatic metastases: a review," *Am Oncology and Hematology*, vol. 2014, pp. 15–23, 2014.

[15] C. Artzner, O. Mossakowski, G. Hefferman et al., "Chemosaturation with percutaneous hepatic perfusion of melphalan for liver-dominant metastatic uveal melanoma: a single center experience," *Cancer Imaging*, vol. 19, no. 1, p. 31, 2019.

[16] S. Marquardt, M. M. Kirstein, R. Brüning et al., "Percutaneous hepatic perfusion (chemosaturation) with melphalan in patients with intrahepatic cholangiocarcinoma: European multicentre study on safety, short-term effects and survival," *European Radiology*, vol. 29, no. 4, pp. 1882–1892, 2019.

[17] E. A. Eisenhauer, P. Therasse, J. Bogaerts et al., "New response evaluation criteria in solid tumours: revised RECIST guideline (version 1.1)," *European Journal of Cancer*, vol. 45, no. 2, pp. 228–247, 2009.

[18] D. Dindo, N. Demartines, and P.-A. Clavien, "Classification of surgical complications: a new proposal with evaluation in a cohort of 6336 patients and results of a survey," *Annals of Surgery*, vol. 240, no. 2, pp. 205–213, 2004.

[19] T. J. Vogl, S. A. Koch, G. Lotz et al., "Percutaneous isolated hepatic perfusion as a treatment for isolated hepatic metastases of uveal melanoma: patient outcome and safety in a multi-centre study," *Cardiovascular and Interventional Radiology*, vol. 40, no. 6, pp. 864–872, 2017.

[20] Group TCOMS, "Assessment of metastatic disease status at death in 435 patients with large choroidal melanoma in the collaborative ocular melanoma study (COMS): COMS report no. 15," *Archives of Ophthalmology*, vol. 119, no. 5, pp. 670–676, 2001.

[21] I. Karydis, A. Gangi, M. J. Wheater et al., "Percutaneous hepatic perfusion with melphalan in uveal melanoma: a safe and effective treatment modality in an orphan disease," *Journal of Surgical Oncology*, vol. 117, no. 6, pp. 1170–1178, 2018.

[22] J. F. Pingpank, M. S. Hughes, H. R. Alexander et al., "A phase III random assignment trial comparing percutaneous hepatic perfusion with melphalan (PHP-mel) to standard of care for patients with hepatic metastases from metastatic ocular or cutaneous melanoma," *Journal of Clinical Oncology*, vol. 28, no. 18, 2010.

[23] M. S. Hughes, J. Zager, M. Faries et al., "Results of a randomized controlled multicenter phase III trial of percutaneous hepatic perfusion compared with best available care for patients with melanoma liver metastases," *Annals of Surgical Oncology*, vol. 23, no. 4, pp. 1309–1319, 2016.

[24] E. M. de Leede, M. C. Burgmans, T. S. Meijer et al., "Prospective clinical and pharmacological evaluation of the Delcath system's second-generation (GEN2) hemofiltration system in patients undergoing percutaneous hepatic perfusion with melphalan," *Cardiovascular and Interventional Radiology*, vol. 40, no. 8, pp. 1196–1205, 2017.

[25] Y. Shibayama, K. Namikawa, M. Sone et al., "Efficacy and toxicity of transarterial chemoembolization therapy using cisplatin and gelatin sponge in patients with liver metastases from uveal melanoma in an Asian population," *International Journal of Clinical Oncology*, vol. 22, no. 3, pp. 577–584, 2017.

[26] A. M. Abbott, M. P. Doepker, Y. Kim et al., "Hepatic progression-free and overall survival after regional therapy to the liver for metastatic melanoma," *American Journal of Clinical Oncology*, vol. 41, no. 8, pp. 747–753, 2018.

Solid Indeterminate Pulmonary Nodules Less Than or Equal to 250 mm^3: Application of the Updated Fleischner Society Guidelines in Clinical Practice

Andrea Borghesi,[1] Silvia Michelini,[2] Giorgio Nocivelli,[1] Mario Silva,[3] Alessandra Scrimieri,[1] Stefania Pezzotti,[2] Roberto Maroldi,[1] and Davide Farina[1]

[1] *Department of Radiology, University and Spedali Civili of Brescia, Piazzale Spedali Civili 1, 25123 Brescia, Italy*
[2] *Department of Radiology, Fondazione Poliambulanza Istituto Ospedaliero, Via Leonida Bissolati, 57, 25124 Brescia, Italy*
[3] *Section of Radiology, Department of Medicine and Surgery, University of Parma, Pad. Barbieri, Via Gramsci 14, 43126 Parma, Italy*

Correspondence should be addressed to Andrea Borghesi; andrea.borghesi@unibs.it

Academic Editor: Paul Sijens

Background. The latest version of the Fleischner Society guidelines for management of incidental pulmonary nodules was published in 2017. The main purpose of these guidelines is to reduce the number of unnecessary computed tomography (CT) examinations during the follow-up of small indeterminate nodules. *Objective.* The present study aimed to evaluate the performance of these guidelines for management of solid indeterminate pulmonary nodules (SIPNs) ≤ 250 mm^3. *Materials and Methods.* During a 7-year period, we retrospectively reviewed the chest CT scans of 672 consecutive patients with SIPNs. The study sample was selected according to the following inclusion criteria: solitary SIPN; diameter ≥ 3 mm; volume ≤ 250 mm^3; two or more CT scans performed with the same scanner and same acquisition/reconstruction protocol; thin-section 1-mm images in DICOM format; histologic diagnosis or follow-up ≥ 2 years; and no oncological history. Applying these criteria, a total of 27 patients with single SIPNs ≤ 250 mm^3 were enrolled. For each SIPN, the volume and doubling time were calculated using semiautomatic software throughout the follow-up period. For each SIPN, we applied the Fleischner Society guidelines, and the recommended management was compared to what was actually done. *Results.* A significant volumetric increase was detected in 5/27 (18.5%) SIPNs; all growing nodules were observed in high-risk patients. In these SIPNs, a histologic diagnosis of malignancy was obtained. Applying the Fleischner Society recommendations, all five malignant nodules would have been identified. None of the SIPNs < 100 mm^3 in low-risk patients showed significant growth during the follow-up period. The application of the new guidelines would have led to a significant reduction in follow-up CT examinations (Hodges-Lehmann median difference, -2 CT scans; p = 0.0001). *Conclusion.* The application of the updated Fleischner Society guidelines has been shown to be effective in the management of SIPNs ≤ 250 mm^3 with a significant reduction in radiation dose.

1. Introduction

A pulmonary nodule is defined as a focal opacity measuring less than 3 cm in diameter [1]. Pulmonary nodules are a frequent incidental finding on routine chest computed tomography (CT) [1, 2], but their prevalence in the general population is not known precisely. Pulmonary nodules smaller than 8 mm in diameter are considered small nodules [3], while nodules ranging between 3 and 5 mm in diameter are classified as very small nodules. These very small nodules, so called "ditzels" (i.e., *little things that could mean a lot*) [4, 5], represent approximately 50% of all pulmonary nodules detected on CT [6]. Micronodule is a term that should be reserved only for nodules smaller than 3 mm [7]. In patients without malignancy, these micronodules should be considered benign until proven otherwise.

The improvement in spatial resolution and broad availability of multidetector-row CT (MDCT) has significantly increased the detection rate of pulmonary nodules, particularly those smaller than 8 mm. Many small pulmonary nodules are benign (i.e., hamartomas or granulomas) [1, 2]. However, the majority of these nodules remain indeterminate. In fact, a confident diagnosis of benignity can be formulated only for fully calcified and fat-containing nodules.

The malignancy rate of small pulmonary nodules is very low but not zero. In their high-risk cohort, Swensen et al. [8] identified a malignancy rate of 1% among 3072 nodules smaller than 8 mm. Therefore, the most challenging category of nodules is represented by indeterminate pulmonary nodules (i.e., noncalcified and non-fat-containing) with a diameter ranging from 3 to 8 mm.

The goal of the radiological evaluation of small pulmonary nodules is to differentiate benign from malignant lesions as noninvasively and as accurately as possible. In clinical practice, small indeterminate nodules usually require monitoring with serial chest CT scans for a minimum of 2 years [9]. For these nodules, fluorine-18 FDG PET is inaccurate for discriminating between benign and malignant lesions. Therefore, the only indicator of malignancy is the growth rate.

The first version of the Fleischner Society guidelines for management of small pulmonary nodules was published in 2005. In this statement, only solitary solid nodules were considered, and the recommendations were based on nodule diameter and patient risk factors for lung cancer [9]. In the latest version of the Fleischner Society guidelines for management of incidental pulmonary nodules, which was published at the beginning of 2017 [10], the recommendations include both solid and subsolid nodules and, in addition to nodule diameter, also consider other nodule features, such as volume, multiplicity, morphology, and location.

The main purpose of these updated guidelines is to reduce the number of unnecessary CT examinations during the follow-up of small indeterminate nodules while providing radiologists and clinicians with greater power in the decision-making process.

The main purpose of the present study was to evaluate the performance of the updated Fleischner Society guidelines in a group of solitary solid indeterminate pulmonary nodules (SIPNs) ≤ 250 mm^3 that were incidentally detected on routine chest CT scans.

2. Materials and Methods

2.1. Patient and Nodule Selection. During a 7-year period, from January 2005 to January 2012, a retrospective search was performed in the department radiology information system/picture archiving and communication system (RIS/PACS) to retrieve all MDCT reports containing findings indicative of SIPNs ≤ 8 mm in diameter.

The search identified a total of 672 patients with one or more SIPNs ≤ 8 mm in diameter. The images contained in these MDCT reports were reviewed by an experienced radiologist (A.B. who had 14 years of experience in thoracic imaging), and the study sample was selected according to the following inclusion criteria: (a) solitary SIPN (i.e., noncalcified and non-fat-containing); (b) nodule diameter (i.e., the average between the longest axis and its perpendicular short axis on the image with the largest cross-sectional area of the lesion) ≥ 3 mm; (c) nodule volume ≤ 250 mm^3; (d) two or more MDCT examinations performed with the same scanner and the same acquisition/reconstruction protocol; (e) thin-section 1-mm lung window images in DICOM format; (f) histologic diagnosis or follow-up more than two years. Patients who were younger than 35 years, those who were immunocompromised, and those who had an oncologic history or previous granulomatous disease were excluded.

TABLE 1: Characteristics of the study patients (n = 27).

Characteristics	
Age (years)	65 ± 10.6
Sex	
Male	15 (55.6)
Female	12 (44.4)
Risk status	
Low risk	16 (59.3)
High risk	11 (40.7)

Data are presented as numbers (%) or means ± standard deviations.

Applying these criteria, a total of 27 patients with single SIPNs ≤ 250 mm^3 were enrolled in the study. The selected patients were classified as having a low or high risk of lung cancer based on their smoking history and exposure to other carcinogens. Patients with a minimal or absent history of smoking and no occupational exposure to carcinogens (such as asbestos, silica, coal mine dust, beryllium, hard-metal dust, or uranium) were classified as low risk for lung cancer. On the other hand, patients with a smoking history and/or occupational exposure to carcinogens were classified as high risk for lung cancer. The characteristics of the study patients are listed in Table 1.

2.2. Image Acquisition. All chest CT examinations were performed with the same MDCT scanner (Somatom Sensation 16; Siemens, Germany) and the same acquisition/reconstruction protocol. The MDCT scanner used the following parameters: collimation, 16 × 0.75 mm; beam pitch, 1.0; rotation time, 0.5 s; tube voltage, 120 kVp; and tube current, 180 mAs. The acquisition, extending from the lung apex to the lung base, was performed at end inspiration. The volume was reconstructed as 1-mm thick sections, applying a sharp reconstruction algorithm and preset windowing suited for lung parenchyma assessment. No contrast material was used.

2.3. Image Analysis. For each SIPN, the axial diameter (i.e., the long and short axes on the image with the largest cross-sectional area) and the volume at baseline and at the last follow-up CT scan were calculated using three-dimensional semiautomatic software (SAT module, classic version, Terarecon Inc., United States). The volumetric variation in each SIPN between baseline and the last CT scan was automatically calculated by matching the volumes. The volume doubling time (VDT) was generated only when a positive variation was detected by the software. A volumetric increase of more than

Table 2: 2017 Fleischner Society management protocol for single solid indeterminate pulmonary nodules ≤ 250 mm^3.

Nodule volume	Patient risk status	
	Low risk	High risk
< 100 mm^3	No routine follow-up	Optional CT at 12 months∗
100-250 mm^3	Initial CT at 6-12 month, then consider CT at 18-24 months	Initial CT at 6-12 month, then CT at 18-24 months

∗ High-risk patients with nodules < 100 mm^3 with a suspicious morphology and/or an upper lobe location should repeat CT at 12 months.

Table 3: Characteristics of the 27 SIPNs ≤ 250 mm^3 on baseline MDCT in the low- and high-risk groups.

Characteristic	Patient risk status		Chi-square test
	Low risk	High risk	*p* value
Volume			
< 100 mm^3	8 (29.6)	8 (29.6)	0.247
100-250 mm^3	8 (29.6)	3 (11.1)	
Margins			
Smooth	13 (48.1)	8 (29.6)	0.383∗
Lobulated	3 (11.1)	2 (7.4)	
Spiculated		1 (3.7)	
Lobe location			
Middle/Lower	9 (33.3)	5 (18.5)	0.588
Upper	7 (25.9)	6 (22.2)	

Data are presented as numbers (%).
∗Chi-squared test for trend.

25% [11] with a VDT < 600 days was considered clinically significant.

Prior to the computerized analysis, visual assessment of the nodule margins and lobe location on the baseline CT scan was performed.

For each SIPN, we applied the updated Fleischner Society guidelines (*in their less conservative version*) (Table 2), and the recommended management was compared to what was actually done.

The computerized analysis and visual assessment of the nodule margins and lobe location were performed by the same experienced thoracic radiologist (A.B.).

The present study was retrospective, and patient management was not altered; thus, no specific consent was required. However, informed consent for the use of personal data was obtained from all patients.

2.4. Statistical Analysis. The data are presented as numbers (%) or the mean ± standard deviation for normally distributed data or as the median and interquartile range (IQR) for not normally distributed data. A chi-square test was used to analyze differences in the distribution of the nodule characteristics (size, margins, and location) between the low- and high-risk groups. A chi-square test was also used to investigate significant relationships between nodule outcome and certain independent variables (such as sex, patient risk status, nodule size, nodule margins, and nodule location). The Wilcoxon matched-pairs test was used to analyze the difference between the number of CT scans actually performed and the number of CT scans required according to the new Fleischner Society guidelines.

Statistical analysis was performed using dedicated software (MedCalc Software Version 18.2.1). p values <0.05 were considered statistically significant.

3. Results

Segmentation and computerized analysis were successfully performed in all 27 SIPNs.

At the baseline MDCT, 16/27 (59.3%) SIPNs had a volume < 100 mm^3 (8 SIPNs in low-risk patients and 8 SIPNs in high-risk patients), and 11/27 (40.7%) SIPNs had a volume ranging between 100 and 250 mm^3 (8 SIPNs in low-risk patients and 3 SIPNs in high-risk patients). No statistically significant differences were observed in the distribution of the nodule characteristics (size, margins, and location) between the low- and high-risk groups (Table 3).

A significant increase in volume (more than 25% with a VDT < 600 days) between baseline and the last CT scan was observed in 5/27 (18.5%) SIPNs (2 SIPNs < 100 mm^3 and 3 SIPNs measuring between 100 and 250 mm^3). In this group exhibiting growth, the volume increased from 71% to 292% (mean, 173 ± 101%) with VDT ranging from 93 to 447 days (mean, 257 ± 164 days); the time interval between baseline and the last CT scan ranged from 165 to 411 days (mean, 287 ± 108 days). These growing nodules were observed in high-risk patients and were surgically removed with a histological diagnosis of non-small cell lung cancer. The characteristics and histological features of the malignant nodules are listed in Table 4.

Applying the new Fleischner Society guidelines, all 5 malignant nodules would have been identified: in 2/5 (40%)

TABLE 4: Characteristics and histological features of the malignant nodules.

Nodule	Volume∗ (mm^3)	Margins∗	Lobe location	Time interval 1st-last CT (days)	Volume increment (%)	VDT (days)	Histology	Stage$
1	135	Spiculated	Upper	316	71	407	ADC	IA2
2	55	Smooth	Upper	184	292	93	ADC	IA1
3	80	Lobulated	Upper	411	254	226	SCC	IA2
4	107	Lobulated	Lower	360	75	447	SCC	IA1
5	102	Smooth	Upper	165	175	113	SCC	IA1

∗At the baseline MDCT. $According to the 8th edition of the TNM staging.
VDT, volume doubling time; ADC, adenocarcinoma; SCC, squamous cell carcinoma.

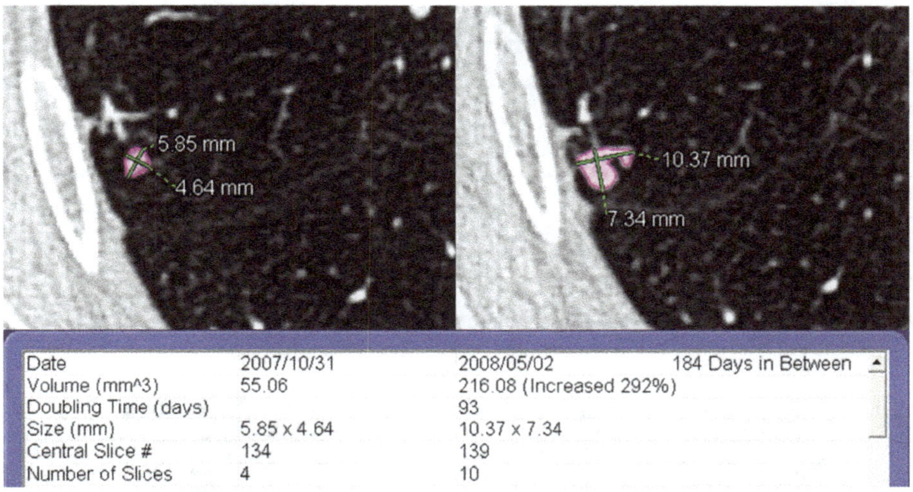

FIGURE 1: Solid pulmonary nodule smaller than 100 mm^3 with smooth margins located in the right upper lobe in a 71-year-old high-risk male patient. Baseline (left) and follow-up CT scans (right). The interval between the two CT examinations was 184 days. The software calculated significant growth between the baseline and follow-up CT scans with a relative volume variation of 292% (from 55 mm^3 to 216 mm^3) and a volume doubling time of 93 days. The nodule was surgically removed and proven to be a pulmonary adenocarcinoma. In this case, the new Fleischner Society guidelines would have recommended a follow-up CT examination at 12 months.

nodules, the radiological diagnosis would have been formulated with similar timing (within 45 days); in 2/5 (40%) nodules, there would have been an earlier diagnosis (136 and 180 days, respectively); and in the remaining nodule (20%), there would have been a diagnostic delay of 181 days (see Figure 1).

None of the SIPNs < 100 mm^3 identified in low-risk patients showed significant growth during the follow-up period (see Figure 2).

The application of the new Fleischner Society guidelines in our sample would have led to a significant reduction in the number of follow-up CT examinations (Hodges-Lehmann median difference, -2 CT scans; 95% confidence interval, -2.5 to -1.5; p = 0.0001).

A statistically significant relationship was observed between nodule outcome, patient risk status, and nodule margins (Table 5). On the other hand, no statistically significant relationships were observed among nodule outcome, sex, nodule size, and nodule location (Table 5). However, considering only the high-risk group, we found a significant relationship between nodule outcome and nodule size (p = 0.034), as all three nodules with volumes ranging from 100 mm^3 to 250 mm^3 were malignant (Table 4). Moreover, we observed that 4/5 (80%) malignant nodules were located in the upper lobe (Table 4).

4. Discussion

Pulmonary nodules are classified as solid or subsolid nodules based on their consistency on thin-section CT. Subsolid nodules are further classified as part-solid or pure ground-glass nodules according to the presence or absence of a solid component within the lesion [12, 13].

Among all pulmonary nodules incidentally detected on MDCT, solid nodules are the most frequent, followed by pure ground-glass nodules and part-solid nodules [5, 14]. The malignancy rate of solid nodules is very low, particularly in nodules smaller than 8 mm [8]. Therefore, the characterization of these small solid nodules remains a diagnostic challenge for radiologists.

The size and morphology (especially nodule margins) are considered the main parameters to estimate lung cancer risk [5, 15]. However, small solid nodules frequently remain indeterminate, and a follow-up CT examination is usually recommended to exclude growth.

Table 5: Association between nodule outcome and independent variables (sex, risk status, volume, margins, and lobe location).

Independent variables	Nodule Outcome		Chi-square test
	Stable ≥ 2 years	Malignant	*p* value
Sex			
Male	13 (48.1)	2 (7.4)	0.447
Female	9 (33.3)	3 (11.1)	
Risk status			
Low risk	16 (59.3)	-	0.003
High risk	6 (22.2)	5 (18.5)	
Volume			
< 100 mm^3	14 (51.9)	2 (7.4)	0.340
100-250 mm^3	8 (29.6)	3 (11.1)	
Margins			
Smooth	19 (70.4)	2 (7.4)	0.009*
Lobulated	3 (11.1)	2 (7.4)	
Spiculated	-	1 (3.7)	
Lobe location			
Middle/Lower	13 (48.1)	1 (3.7)	0.121
Upper	9 (33.3)	4 (14.8)	

Data are presented as numbers (%).
*Chi-squared test for trend.

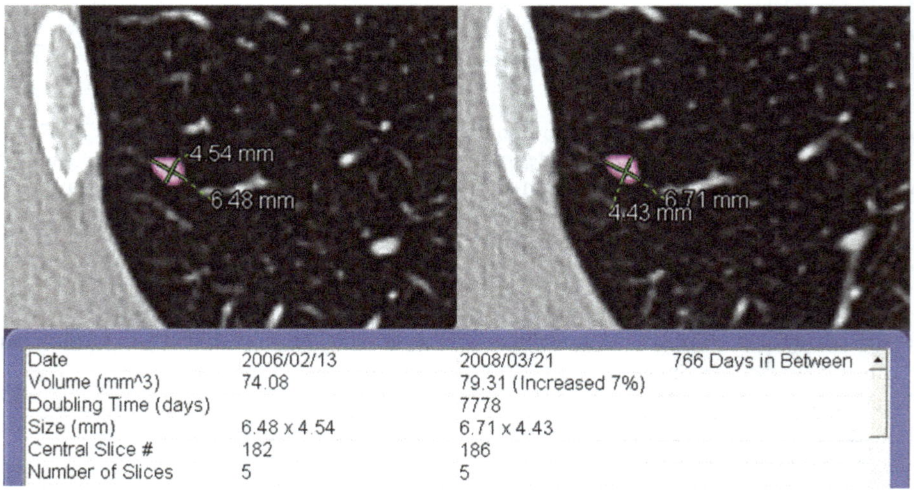

Figure 2: Solid pulmonary nodule smaller than 100 mm^3 with smooth margins located in the right lower lobe in a 36-year-old low-risk male patient. Baseline (left) and last follow-up CT scans (right). The interval between the two CT examinations was 766 days. The software did not show significant growth of the nodule (relative volume variation of 7% with a volume doubling time of 21 years). The unequivocal nodule stability after more than 2 years indicates the benign nature of the lesion. In this case, the new Fleischner Society guidelines would not have recommended a follow-up CT scan.

In the NELSON trial, the 2-year risk of lung cancer in nodules smaller than 100 mm^3 was 0.6% and did not differ significantly from the 2-year lung cancer risk for participants without baseline lung nodules [16, 17]. On the basis of this low risk of malignancy, the updated Fleischner Society guidelines suggest no routine CT follow-up for solid nodules with a volume < 100 mm^3 (or smaller than 6 mm) [10, 18]. This recommendation has been proposed for all patients, regardless of their clinical risk status. The threshold size of 100 mm^3 was established to exclude from CT follow-up all solid nodules with a cancer risk less than 1% [10, 18]. However, the presence of a suspicious morphology (such as spiculation), an upper lobe location or both in nodules < 100 mm^3, increases the cancer risk up to 5%. Thus, high-risk patients with solid nodules < 100 mm^3 with a suspicious morphology and/or an upper lobe location should undergo a CT scan after one year [10, 18].

With regard to solitary SIPNs ranging from 100 mm^3 to 250 mm^3, the new guidelines recommend an initial CT follow-up at 6-12 months [10, 18]. For patients at low risk, a single follow-up is usually sufficient to demonstrate the stability of the nodule [10, 18]. However, when a suspicious morphology is present or volumetric stability is uncertain, an additional CT follow-up at 18-24 months should be considered [10, 18]. Conversely, for patients at high risk, a second follow-up at 18-24 months is strongly recommended because, in this size range, the cancer risk grows up to 2% [10, 15–19].

To the best of our knowledge, the present study is the first to evaluate the performance of the updated Fleischner Society guidelines in a group of solitary SIPNs ≤ 250 mm^3 incidentally detected in routine clinical settings. Our study found that the retrospective application of the new Fleischner Society guidelines has proven to be effective in the management of SIPNs ≤ 250 mm^3, as all malignant nodules would have been identified, and none of the SIPNs < 100 mm3 in low-risk patients showed significant growth during the follow-up period. Moreover, we observed that the new guidelines would have led to a significant reduction in the number of CT examinations performed, resulting in a significant reduction in the radiation dose delivered to the patients.

The only critical aspect in the application of the new guidelines was observed in a malignant nodule with a baseline volume of 55 mm^3 that would have been identified with a delay of 6 months (see case 2 in Table 4 and Figure 1). However, considering the baseline volume and the VDT of this nodule (Figure 1), we believe that the diagnostic delay of 6 months would not have been clinically significant because the expected size of the nodule at 12 months (approximately 12 mm) would have led to only a minimal variation in T category (from T1a to T1b).

In a literature search of the PubMed database, we found only one other study published in 2018 in which the performance of the new Fleischner Society guidelines was assessed in a clinical setting [20]. In that study, Scholtz et al. [20] retrospectively evaluated the performance of the new Fleischner Society guidelines for the management of pulmonary nodules incidentally detected during emergent coronary CT angiography. Similar to our study, they found that the application of the new guidelines would have significantly reduced the number of recommended follow-up CT examinations [20]. The main aspect that differentiates the present study from that performed by Scholtz et al. is the sample size (which was smaller in our study); however, in their study, both solid and subsolid (single and multiple) nodules of any size were included. In contrast, only solitary SIPNs with a diameter ≥ 3 mm and volume ≤ 250 mm^3 were selected in our study. Another aspect that differentiates the two studies is that, in our sample, the CT images and nodule characteristics (type, size, morphology, and location) of all cases were reviewed by an experienced thoracic radiologist, and volumetric analysis using three-dimensional semiautomatic software was performed. In contrast, in Scholtz's study [20], the two-dimensional nodule data were extracted from CT reports, and only in incomplete cases the CT images were reviewed by a board-certified radiologist.

According to the literature [9, 10, 15–19, 21], we found that the patient risk status, nodule margins, and nodule size (for the high-risk group only) were significantly related to the nodule outcome. In contrast to many studies [5, 6, 8–10, 15, 16, 18, 19], no significant relationships were found between the nodule outcome and nodule location; however, we found that 80% of malignant nodules were located in the upper lobes (Table 4).

This study has some limitations. First, it was retrospectively performed. Second, only a small number of SIPNs were included; however, the inclusion criteria were very strict. Third, the image analysis was performed by one observer; however, his experience may have improved the accuracy of the analysis.

5. Conclusion

This retrospective study noted that, in the selected sample, the application of the updated Fleischner Society guidelines was effective for managing solitary SIPNs ≤ 250 mm^3, with a significant reduction in the number of follow-up CT examinations performed, resulting in a significant reduction in the overall radiation dose per patient. We also found that the patient risk status, nodule margins, and nodule size (for the high-risk group only) were significantly related to the nodule outcome.

Disclosure

The present manuscript is a revised, corrected, and expanded version of a conference poster presented at the European Congress of Radiology (ECR) 2018, Vienna, Austria, February 28-March 4 2018.

References

[1] M. T. Truong, J. P. Ko, S. E. Rossi et al., "Update in the evaluation of the solitary pulmonary nodule," *RadioGraphics*, vol. 34, no. 6, pp. 1658–1679, 2014.

[2] V. R. Papapietro, G. Milanese, A. Borghesi, N. Sverzellati, and M. Silva, "Look around your target: a new approach to early diagnosis of lung cancer," *Annals of Translational Medicine*, vol. 6, no. S1, pp. S77–S77, 2018.

[3] M. Sánchez, M. Benegas, and I. Vollmer, "Management of incidental lung nodules <8 mm in diameter," *Journal of Thoracic Disease*, vol. 10, no. S22, pp. S2611–S2627, 2018.

[4] R. F. Munden and K. R. Hess, ""Ditzels" on chest CT: Survey of members of the society of thoracic radiology," *American Journal of Roentgenology*, vol. 176, no. 6, pp. 1363–1369, 2001.

[5] S. C. van't Westeinde, H. J. de Koning, D. Xu, H. C. Hoogsteden, and R. J. van Klaveren, "How to deal with incidentally detected pulmonary nodules less than 10mm in size on CT in a healthy person," *Lung Cancer*, vol. 60, no. 2, pp. 151–159, 2008.

[6] C. I. Henschke, D. F. Yankelevitz, D. P. Naidich et al., "CT screening for lung cancer: suspiciousness of nodules according to size on baseline scans," *Radiology*, vol. 231, no. 1, pp. 164–168, 2004.

[7] D. M. Hansell, A. A. Bankier, H. MacMahon, T. C. McLoud, N. L. Müller, and J. Remy, "Fleischner Society: glossary of terms for

thoracic imaging," *Radiology*, vol. 246, no. 3, pp. 697–722, 2008.

[8] S. J. Swensen, J. R. Jett, and T. E. Hartman, "CT screening for lung cancer: five-year prospective experience," *Radiology*, vol. 235, no. 1, pp. 259–265, 2005.

[9] H. MacMahon, J. H. M. Austin, G. Gamsu et al., "Guidelines for management of small pulmonary nodules detected on CT scans: a statement from the Fleischner Society," *Radiology*, vol. 237, no. 2, pp. 395–400, 2005.

[10] H. MacMahon, D. P. Naidich, J. M. Goo et al., "Guidelines for management of incidental pulmonary nodules detected on CT images: from the Fleischner Society 2017," *Radiology*, vol. 284, no. 1, pp. 228–243, 2017.

[11] D. Wormanns, G. Kohl, E. Klotz et al., "Volumetric measurements of pulmonary nodules at multi-row detector CT: in vivo reproducibility," *European Radiology*, vol. 14, no. 1, pp. 86–92, 2004.

[12] A. Borghesi, D. Farina, S. Michelini et al., "Pulmonary adenocarcinomas presenting as ground-glass opacities on multidetector CT: Three-dimensional computer-assisted analysis of growth pattern and doubling time," *Diagnostic and Interventional Radiology*, vol. 22, no. 6, pp. 525–533, 2016.

[13] A. Borghesi, S. Michelini, F. Bertagna, A. Scrimieri, S. Pezzotti, and R. Maroldi, "Hilly or mountainous surface: a new CT feature to predict the behavior of pure ground glass nodules?" *European Journal of Radiology Open*, vol. 5, pp. 177–182, 2018.

[14] C. I. Henschke, D. F. Yankelevitz, R. Mirtcheva, G. McGuinness, D. McCauley, and O. S. Miettinen, "CT screening for lung cancer: frequency and significance of part-solid and nonsolid nodules," *American Journal of Roentgenology*, vol. 178, no. 5, pp. 1053–1057, 2002.

[15] A. McWilliams, M. C. Tammemagi, J. R. Mayo et al., "Probability of cancer in pulmonary nodules detected on first screening CT," *The New England Journal of Medicine*, vol. 369, no. 10, pp. 910–919, 2013.

[16] N. Horeweg, J. van Rosmalen, M. A. Heuvelmans et al., "Lung cancer probability in patients with CT-detected pulmonary nodules: A prespecified analysis of data from the NELSON trial of low-dose CT screening," *The Lancet Oncology*, vol. 15, no. 12, pp. 1332–1341, 2014.

[17] J. E. Walter, M. A. Heuvelmans, and M. Oudkerk, "Small pulmonary nodules in baseline and incidence screening rounds of low-dose CT lung cancer screening," *Translational Lung Cancer Research*, vol. 6, no. 1, pp. 42–51, 2017.

[18] J. Bueno, L. Landeras, and J. H. Chung, "Updated fleischner society guidelines for managing incidental pulmonary nodules: common questions and challenging scenarios," *RadioGraphics*, vol. 38, no. 5, pp. 1337–1350, 2018.

[19] A. R. Larici, A. Farchione, P. Franchi et al., "Lung nodules: size still matters," *European Respiratory Review*, vol. 26, no. 146, p. 170025, 2017.

[20] J. Scholtz, M. T. Lu, S. Hedgire et al., "Incidental pulmonary nodules in emergent coronary CT angiography for suspected acute coronary syndrome: Impact of revised 2017 Fleischner Society Guidelines," *Journal of Cardiovascular Computed Tomography*, vol. 12, no. 1, pp. 28–33, 2018.

[21] C. Rampinelli, S. F. Calloni, M. Minotti, and M. Bellomi, "Spectrum of early lung cancer presentation in low-dose screening CT: a pictorial review," *Insights into Imaging*, vol. 7, no. 3, pp. 449–459, 2016.

Permissions

All chapters in this book were first published by Hindawi Publishing Corporation; hereby published with permission under the Creative Commons Attribution License or equivalent. Every chapter published in this book has been scrutinized by our experts. Their significance has been extensively debated. The topics covered herein carry significant findings which will fuel the growth of the discipline. They may even be implemented as practical applications or may be referred to as a beginning point for another development.

The contributors of this book come from diverse backgrounds, making this book a truly international effort. This book will bring forth new frontiers with its revolutionizing research information and detailed analysis of the nascent developments around the world.

We would like to thank all the contributing authors for lending their expertise to make the book truly unique. They have played a crucial role in the development of this book. Without their invaluable contributions this book wouldn't have been possible. They have made vital efforts to compile up to date information on the varied aspects of this subject to make this book a valuable addition to the collection of many professionals and students.

This book was conceptualized with the vision of imparting up-to-date information and advanced data in this field. To ensure the same, a matchless editorial board was set up. Every individual on the board went through rigorous rounds of assessment to prove their worth. After which they invested a large part of their time researching and compiling the most relevant data for our readers.

The editorial board has been involved in producing this book since its inception. They have spent rigorous hours researching and exploring the diverse topics which have resulted in the successful publishing of this book. They have passed on their knowledge of decades through this book. To expedite this challenging task, the publisher supported the team at every step. A small team of assistant editors was also appointed to further simplify the editing procedure and attain best results for the readers.

Apart from the editorial board, the designing team has also invested a significant amount of their time in understanding the subject and creating the most relevant covers. They scrutinized every image to scout for the most suitable representation of the subject and create an appropriate cover for the book.

The publishing team has been an ardent support to the editorial, designing and production team. Their endless efforts to recruit the best for this project, has resulted in the accomplishment of this book. They are a veteran in the field of academics and their pool of knowledge is as vast as their experience in printing. Their expertise and guidance has proved useful at every step. Their uncompromising quality standards have made this book an exceptional effort. Their encouragement from time to time has been an inspiration for everyone.

The publisher and the editorial board hope that this book will prove to be a valuable piece of knowledge for researchers, students, practitioners and scholars across the globe.

List of Contributors

Soulafa Almazrooa, Nada O. Binmadi, Hanadi M. Khalifa, Fatima M. Jadu, Ahmed M. Jan and Dalia E. Meisha
Faculty of Dentistry, King Abdulaziz University, Jeddah, Saudi Arabia

Hesham N. Alrowayeh and Talal A. Alshatti
Kuwait University, Faculty of Allied Health Sciences, Physical Therapy Department, Kuwait City, Kuwait

Musaed Z. Alnaser
Kuwait University, Faculty of Allied Health Sciences, Occupational Therapy Department, Kuwait City, Kuwait

Raed S. Saeed
Kuwait University, Faculty of Allied Health Sciences, Radiological Science Department, Kuwait City, Kuwait

Guiswe Gnowe
Department of Biomedical Sciences, Faculty of Sciences, University of Ngaoundere, Cameroon
Higher Institute of Sciences, Health Technics and Management of Garoua, Cameroon

Fouda H. P. Ekobena
University Institute of Technology, University of Ngaoundere, Cameroon

Amvene J. Mbo
Faculty of Medicine and Biomedical Sciences of Garoua, Cameroon

Guena M. Neossi
Department of Biomedical Sciences, Faculty of Sciences, University of Ngaoundere, Cameroon
Department of Radiology and Medical Imaging, Regional Hospital of Ngaoundere, Cameroon

Bashiru Babatunde Jimah
Department of Medical Imaging, College of Health Sciences, University of Cape Coast, Cape Coast, Ghana
Department of Medical Imaging, School of Medical Sciences, University of Cape Coast, Cape Coast, Ghana

Lingam Amara Swapna, Nada Tarek AlMegbil and Alhanouf Othman Almutlaq
Department of Surgical and Diagnostic Sciences, College of Dentistry, Dar Al Uloom University, Riyadh 13314, Saudi Arabia

Pradeep Koppolu
Department of Preventive Dental Sciences, College of Dentistry, Dar Al Uloom University, Riyadh 13314, Saudi Arabia

Penala Soumya
Department of Dentistry, Mahavir Institute of Medical Sciences, Vikarabad, Telangana, India

Krishnajaneya Reddy Pathakota
Department of Peroiodontics, Sri Sai College of Dental Surgery, Vikarabad, India

Vani Chappidi
Department of Oral Medicine and Radiology, Sri Sai College of Dental Surgery, Vikarabad, Telangana, India

Ron C. Gaba and Ali Kord
Department of Radiology, University of Illinois at Chicago, Chicago, IL, USA
Division of Interventional Radiology, University of Illinois at Chicago, Chicago, IL, USA

Behnam Rabiee, Sara Rostami and Karen L. Xie
Department of Radiology, University of Illinois at Chicago, Chicago, IL, USA

Siwen Wang
Biomedical Visualization Graduate Program, University of Illinois at Chicago, Chicago, IL, USA

Anthony Baffour Appiah
Ghana Field Epidemiology and Laboratory Training Programme, University of Ghana, Accra, Ghana

Benjamin Dabo Sarkodie
Department of Radiology, University of Ghana, School of Medicine Sciences, Accra, Ghana

Dorothea Anim
Department of Radiology, Korle Bu Teaching Hospital, Accra, Ghana

Wanyin Lim
Dr Jones and Partners Medical Imaging, Adelaide, South Australia, Australia
Department of Radiology, Royal Adelaide Hospital, Adelaide, South Australia, Australia
Dr Jones and Partners, 226 Greenhill Road, Eastwood 5065, Australia

Christen D. Barras
Dr Jones and Partners Medical Imaging, Adelaide, South Australia, Australia
Department of Radiology, Royal Adelaide Hospital, Adelaide, South Australia, Australia
South Australian Health and Medical Research Institute and the University of Adelaide, Adelaide, South Australia, Australia

Steven Zadow
Dr Jones and Partners Medical Imaging, Adelaide, South Australia, Australia
Flinders Medical Centre, Bedford Park, South Australia, Australia

Ephrem Awulachew, Kuma Diriba, Asrat Anja, Eyob Getu and Firehiwot Belayneh
Dilla University, College of Health Science and Medicine, Dila, Ethiopia

Koichi Shibata
Graduate School of Healthcare Science, Suzuka University of Medical Science, 1001-1, Kishioka-cho, Suzuka, Mie 510-0293, Japan

Hironobu Tomita
Graduate School of Healthcare Science, Suzuka University of Medical Science, 1001-1, Kishioka-cho, Suzuka, Mie 510-0293, Japan
Department of Radiology, Saiseikai Kawaguchi General Hospital, 5-11-5, Nishikawaguchi, Kawaguchi, Saitama 332-0021, Japan

Cleverson Alex Leitão, Gabriel Lucca de Oliveira Salvador, Priscilla Tazoniero, Danny Warszawiak, Cristian Saievicz and Dante Luiz Escuissato
Department of Radiology, Universidade Federal do Paraná, Curitiba, Paraná, Brazil

Rosangela Requi Jakubiak
Universidade Tecnológica Federal do Paraná, Curitiba, Paraná, Brazil

Ghufran Aref Saeed, Asad Shah, Abeer Ahmed Al Helali and Safaa Almazrouei
Department of Radiology, Sheikh Khalifa Medical City, Abu Dhabi, UAE

Waqar Gaba, Emadullah Raidullah, Ameirah Bader Al Ali, Mohammed Elghazali, Deena Yousef Ahmed and Shaikha Ghanam Al Kaabi
Department of Internal Medicine, Sheikh Khalifa Medical City, Abu Dhabi, UAE

Chantelle Ip and Michael Croft
Royal Adelaide Hospital, Port Road, Adelaide 5000, Australia

Edward H. Wang
Flinders Medical Centre, Flinders Dr, Bedford Park 5042, Australia

Fabienne Jordana
Oral and Maxillofacial Radiology, Dentistry Department, University Health Centre, University of Nantes, Orvault, France

Antoinette Pelé and Pierre-Alexandre Berry
Oral and Maxillofacial Radiology, Dentistry Department, University Health Centre, University of Nantes, Orvault, France
Private Practice, 34 Rue Jules Verne, 44700 Orvault, France

Charles Evanno
Private Practice, 34 Rue Jules Verne, 44700 Orvault, France
Oral Implantology, Dentistry Department, University Health Centre, University of Nantes, Nantes, France

Sándor Csizmadia
Affidea Hungary Ltd. Budapest, 44-46 Bókay János Street, Budapest H-1083, Hungary

Gergely H. Fodor
Department of Medical Physics and Informatics, University of Szeged, Faculty of General Medicine, 9 Korányi Alley, Szeged H-6725, Hungary

András Palkó and Erika Vörös
Department of Radiology, University of Szeged, Faculty of General Medicine, 6 Semmelweis Street, Szeged H-6725, Hungary

Ahmed B. Salem Salamh
Institute of Science, Material Science and Engineering, Kastamonu University, Kuzey Kent Kastamonu, Kastamonu, Turkey

Abdulrauf A. Salamah
Tripoli Central Hospital, Tripoli, Libya

Halil Ibrahim Akyüz
Computer and Teaching Technologies Education, Kastamonu University, Kuzey Kent Kastamonu, Kastamonu, Turkey

Labib Ghulmiyyah, Anwar Nassar, Dib Sassine, Sally Khoury, Joseph Nassif and Hadi Ramadan
Department of Obstetrics and Gynecology, American University of Beirut Medical Center, Lebanon

Elie Najem and Ghina Berjawi
Department of Diagnostic Radiology, American University of Beirut Medical Center, Lebanon

Saul N. Friedman
Division of Nuclear Medicine, Mallinckrodt Institute of Radiology, Washington University School of Medicine, Saint Louis, MO 63110, USA

Miriam Grushka
974 Eglington Avenue West, Toronto, Ontario M6C 2C5, Canada

Hussam K. Beituni, Madhu Rehman and Lawrence Friedman
Department of Medical Imaging, North York General, 4001 Leslie Street, Toronto, Ontario M2K 1E1, Canada

Hart B. Bressler
Department of Family and Community Medicine, University of Toronto, Mount Sinai Hospital, 600 University Ave, Toronto, Ontario M5G 1X5, Canada

Emmanuel Kobina Mesi Edzie, Philip Narteh Gorleku, Abdul Raman Asemah, Henry Kusodzi and Richard Ato Edzie
Department of Medical Imaging, School of Medical Sciences, College of Health and Allied Sciences, University of Cape Coast, P.M.B. University of Cape Coast, Cape Coast, Ghana

Klenam Dzefi-Tettey
Department of Radiology, Korle Bu Teaching Hospital, Korle Bu, Accra, Ghana

James William Ampofo and Albert Dayor Piersson
Department of Imaging Technology and Sonography, School of Allied Health Sciences, College of Health and Allied Sciences, University of Cape Coast, P.M.B. University of Cape Coast, Cape Coast, Ghana

Yusuke Inoue and Keiji Matsunaga
Department of Diagnostic Radiology, Kitasato University School of Medicine, Sagamihara, Kanagawa, Japan

Hirofumi Hata, Yusuke Ohzeki, Tetsuya Hashimoto and Ai Nakajima
Department of Radiology, Kitasato University Hospital, Sagamihara, Kanagawa, Japan

Hiroki Haradome
Department of Diagnostic Radiology, Kitasato University Hospital, Sagamihara, Kanagawa, Japan

Lori C. Jordan
Department of Radiology, Vanderbilt University Medical Center, Nashville, TN, USA
Department of Pediatrics, Division of Pediatric Neurology, Vanderbilt University Medical Center, Nashville, TN, USA
Department of Neurology, Vanderbilt University Medical Center, Nashville, TN, USA

Olivia Justice, Spencer Waddle, Sumit Pruthi and L. Taylor Davis
Department of Radiology, Vanderbilt University Medical Center, Nashville, TN, USA

Chelsea A. Lee and Niral J. Patel
Department of Radiology, Vanderbilt University Medical Center, Nashville, TN, USA
Department of Pediatrics, Division of Pediatric Neurology, Vanderbilt University Medical Center, Nashville, TN, USA

Adetola A. Kassim
Department of Pediatrics, Vanderbilt-Meharry Center for Excellence, Sickle Cell Disease, Vanderbilt University Medical Center, Nashville, TN, USA
Department of Internal Medicine, Division of Hematology/Oncology, Vanderbilt University Medical Center, Nashville, TN, USA

Manus J. Donahue
Department of Radiology, Vanderbilt University Medical Center, Nashville, TN, USA
Department of Neurology, Vanderbilt University Medical Center, Nashville, TN, USA
Department of Psychiatry, Vanderbilt University Medical Center, Nashville, TN, USA

Callen Kwamboka Onyambu and Alfred Otieno Odhiambo
Department of Diagnostic Imaging and Radiation Medicine, University of Nairobi, Nairobi, Kenya

Mufaddal Nuruddin Wajihi
Nairobi West Hospital, Nairobi, Kenya

Kathryn E. Keenan, Slávka Rýger and Stephen E. Russek
National Institute of Standards and Technology, Physical Measurement Laboratory, 325 Broadway, Boulder, CO 80305, USA

Ben P. Berman and Joseph Dagher
The MITRE Corporation, 7515 Colshire Dr, McLean, VA 22102, USA

Wen-Tung Wang and Dzung L. Pham
Henry M. Jackson Foundation, 10 Center Drive, Bethesda, MD 20892, USA

John A. Butman
Clinical Center, National Institutes of Health, 10 Center Drive, Bethesda, MD 20814, USA

Ahmed Kamel Abdel Aal
Department of Diagnostic and Interventional Imaging, University of Texas Health Science Center at Houston, Houston, TX 77030, USA

Khalid Mahmoud, Noha Alaaeldin Aboueldahab, Anas Souid and Andrew Gunn
Department of Radiology, University of Alabama at Birmingham, Birmingham, AL 35233, USA

Amr Soliman Moustafa
Department of Radiology, University of Arkansas for Medical Sciences, Little Rock, AR 72205, USA
Department of Radiology, Zagazig University, Zagazig, Egypt

Yufeng Li and Zhixin Wang
Department of Medicine, Division of Preventive Medicine, University of Alabama at Birmingham, Birmingham, AL 35233, USA

Ammar Almehmi
Department of Medicine, Division of Nephrology, University of Alabama at Birmingham, Birmingham, AL 35233, USA

Mareike Franke
Diagnostic and Interventional Radiology, Dr. Hancken Clinic, 21680 Stade, Germany
Department of Radiology, Wesling Hospital Minden, University Hospital of the Ruhr University Bochum, 32429 Minden, Germany

Christian Saager, Sven Barthel and Kersten Mueckner
Diagnostic and Interventional Radiology, Dr. Hancken Clinic, 21680 Stade, Germany

Jasper Franke
53 N Studios, 21682 Stade, Germany

Randolf Riemann
Otorhinolaryngology, Head and Neck Surgery, Elbe Hospitals, 21680 Stade, Germany

Hoda Salah Darwish
Radiology Department, Faculty of Medicine, Suez Canal University, Ismailia, Egypt
Dallah Hospital, Riyadh, Saudi Arabia

Mohamed Yasser Habash
Faculty of Medicine, Kasr Alainy Cairo University, Cairo, Egypt

Waleed Yasser Habash
Faculty of Medicine, New Giza University, Giza, Egypt

R. Brüning, M. Tiede and M. Schneider
Radiology and Neuroradiology, Asklepios Hospital Barmbek, Ruebenkamp 220, 22307 Hamburg, Germany

P. Wohlmuth
Biostatistics, ProResearch, Asklepios Hospital St. Georg, Lohmuehlenstrasse 5, 20099 Hamburg

H. Weilert
Oncology, Asklepios Hospital Barmbek, Ruebenkamp 220, 22307 Hamburg, Germany

K. Oldhafer
Faculty of Medicine, Semmelweis University Campus Hamburg, Lohmuehlenstrasse 5, 20099 Hamburg, Germany
Surgery, Asklepios Hospital Barmbek, Ruebenkamp 220, 22307 Hamburg, Germany

A. Stang
Oncology, Asklepios Hospital Barmbek, Ruebenkamp 220, 22307 Hamburg, Germany
Faculty of Medicine, Semmelweis University Campus Hamburg, Lohmuehlenstrasse 5, 20099 Hamburg, Germany

Andrea Borghesi, Giorgio Nocivelli, Alessandra Scrimieri, Roberto Maroldi and Davide Farina
Department of Radiology, University and Spedali Civili of Brescia, Piazzale Spedali Civili 1, 25123 Brescia, Italy

Silvia Michelini and Stefania Pezzotti
Department of Radiology, Fondazione Poliambulanza Istituto Ospedaliero, Via Leonida Bissolati, 57, 25124 Brescia, Italy

Mario Silva
Section of Radiology, Department of Medicine and Surgery, University of Parma, Pad. Barbieri, Via Gramsci 14, 43126 Parma, Italy

Index

www.ingramcontent.com/pod-product-compliance
Lightning Source LLC
LaVergne TN
LVHW082156200926
848484LV00008B/2170